Transcranial Brain Stimulation for Treatment of Psychiatric Disorders

Advances in Biological Psychiatry

Vol. 23

Transcranial Brain Stimulation for Treatment of Psychiatric Disorders

Volume Editors

M.A. Marcolin, São Paulo
F. Padberg, Munich

34 figures, 4 in color, and 19 tables, 2007

KARGER

Basel · Freiburg · Paris · London · New York ·
Bangalore · Bangkok · Singapore · Tokyo · Sydney

Marco Antonio Marcolin, MD, MPH, PhD
Institute of Psychiatry
University of São Paulo
05403-010 São Paulo (Brazil)

Priv. Doz. Dr. med. Frank Padberg
Department of Psychiatry and
Psychotherapy
Ludwig-Maximilian University Munich
DE-80336 Munich (Germany)

Library of Congress Cataloging-in-Publication Data

Transcranial brain stimulation for treatment of psychiatric disorders /
volume editors, M.A. Marcolin, F. Padberg.
p. ; cm. – (Advances in biological psychiatry, ISSN 0378-7354 ; v.
23)
Includes bibliographical references and indexes.
ISBN-13: 978-3-8055-8186-8 (hard cover : alk. paper)
1. Transcranial brain stimulation. 2. Mental illness–Treatment. I.
Marcolin, M. A. (Marco Antonio) II. Padberg, F. (Frank) III. Series.
[DNLM: 1. Transcranial Magnetic Stimulation–methods. 2.
Brain–physiology. 3. Deep Brain Stimulation–methods. 4.
Electroconvulsive Therapy–methods. 5. Mental Disorders–therapy. W1 AD44
v.23 2007 / WL 141 T772 2007]
RC386.6.M32T58 2007
616.89′1–dc22

2007002876

Bibliographic Indices. This publication is listed in bibliographic services, including Current Contents® and Index Medicus.

www.karger.com
Printed in Switzerland on acid-free paper by Reinhardt Druck, Basel
ISSN 0378–7354
ISBN 978–3–8055–8186–8

Contents

Preface

Modern neuropsychopharmacology has led to important insights into the pathophysiology of mental disorders and the development of effective drugs since the 1950s. More recently, findings derived from functional neuroimaging studies have emphasized the neuroanatomical perspective in mental disorders. This is directly linked to the idea of focally stimulating distinct brain regions in order to exert therapeutic effects.

Many different brain stimulation approaches have been considered during the last decades and some of them have been developed into effective therapeutic interventions. Electroconvulsive therapy (ECT), for example, is a well-established treatment for depression and catatonia, and deep brain stimulation (DBS) is widely applied in patients suffering from severe Parkinson's disease. Many of these methods converge in terms of underlying mechanisms of action based on fundamental principles of brain function. Sometimes they even show common neurobiological effects, demonstrated by functional neuroimaging, neurophysiology methods and molecular neuroscience techniques. One example are the effects of antidepressant interventions on regional cerebral activity demonstrated by functional neuroimaging: antidepressant drugs and ECT as well as DBS of the subgenual cingulate cortex, which has most recently been investigated [Mayberg et al., 2005], act in a similar manner on dysfunctional regional brain activity in depression, i.e. modulating limbic and paralimbic brain activity in rest towards a state normally observed in healthy volunteers and associated with mental health. However, it is often difficult or impossible to identify the key mechanisms of action and to distinguish them from epiphenomena purely associated with the recovery from disease, but not related to a specific action of an intervention.

The different brain stimulation methods can principally be distinguished by specific characteristics. (1) They act on neuronal circuits through various neuroanatomic 'windows'. In some interventions these 'windows' can be defined in terms of neuroanatomic structures as in vagal nerve stimulation (VNS), DBS or repetitive transcranial magnetic stimulation (rTMS), and in some interventions the action on the brain is not focal at all as in ECT, magnetic seizure therapy (MST) and transcranial direct current stimulation (tDCS). (2) The methods range in terms of their invasiveness from practically noninvasive approaches (rTMS, tDCS), to ECT and MST, which provoke an epileptic seizure, require general anesthesia and may somehow be regarded as 'more invasive' than rTMS and tDCS, to clearly invasive techniques (VNS and DBS) where stimulation electrodes and a neurostimulator are implanted. (3) Finally, they differ in terms of the duration of the intervention, i.e. ECT, rTMS, MST and tDCS represent acute treatments normally applied over several weeks and rarely extended towards maintenance treatment, whereas VNS and DBS work through a permanent stimulator and are per se long-term treatment strategies, particularly suitable for chronic or frequently relapsing disorders.

Our book focuses on transcranially applied, non- or low-invasive interventions not requiring surgery, i.e. ECT, rTMS, MST and tDCS. Recent progress in this field has prompted us to edit this book in order to provide an overview on this spectrum of fascinating techniques – not only for scientists, but also for clinicians who are interested in these methods and who may even consider applying one or the other approach for the treatment of their patients. However, it is important to emphasize that the different methods are at different stages of development in specific disorders. To reflect this range, the book contains a state-of-the-art chapter on ECT, which still represents a kind of gold standard in this field. It reviews more recent methods, particularly rTMS, which is just about to become clinically applicable as treatment for several mental disorders and introduces the most recent achievements: MST, tDCS and two novel variants of rTMS, i.e. theta burst stimulation and deep rTMS. The latter chapters do not present ready-to-use approaches, but are thought to stimulate a wider interest in methodology and trigger a substantial discussion about options for method development which is clearly needed in this field.

We are extremely grateful to our colleagues who have spent their valuable time writing for this book, despite the large number of publication duties a scientist faces in our times. All authors have contributed to the benefit of our readers. Moreover, we thank the staff of S. Karger AG, Basel for their excellent, accurate and speedy work during the editorial process. Finally, we particularly acknowledge the initiative and the input of the series editors (K.P. Ebmeier, W.P. Kaschka, D. Ebert and W.F. Gattaz) who made this book possible.

Marco Antonio Marcolin
Frank Padberg
São Paulo and Munich

Reference

Mayberg HS, Lozano AM, Voon V, McNeely HE, Seminowicz D, Hamani C, Schwalb JM, Kennedy SH: Deep brain stimulation for treatment-resistant depression. Neuron 2005;45:651–660.

Marcolin MA, Padberg F (eds): Transcranial Brain Stimulation for Treatment of Psychiatric Disorders.
Adv Biol Psychiatr. Basel, Karger, 2007, vol 23, pp 1–17

Electroconvulsive Therapy: Update and New Research

Daniela Eser, Cornelius Schüle, Rainer Rupprecht, Thomas C. Baghai

Department of Psychiatry and Psychotherapy, Ludwig-Maximilian University Munich, Munich, Germany

Abstract

Electroconvulsive therapy (ECT) is a nonpharmacologic biological treatment, which has been proven to be a highly effective treatment option. Several studies indicated the clinical efficacy and clinical effectiveness of ECT predominantly for major depression, but also for other psychiatric disorders. Particularly in major depression, ECT still has to be considered as the most effective treatment option, especially in treatment-resistant depression. In patient populations not fulfilling the criteria of therapy resistance, response rates of 80–90%, which are superior to pharmacotherapy response rates, have been reported. Although the crucial neurobiological mechanisms underlying the clinical effectiveness of ECT are still under investigation, recent research enhanced the knowledge about possible mechanisms and indicated that ECT does not only affect neurotransmission but may also induce structural changes in neuronal networks. In addition, modified stimulation techniques and the progress in modern anesthesia have obviously enhanced the safety and tolerability of ECT during the last decades. Former absolute contraindications became relative during the last years; therefore, ECT today can be offered as a safe treatment also to patients with higher somatic risks. ECT still offers a highly effective therapeutic option that should not be kept back especially from patients who did not respond to other treatments such as combined pharmacotherapy and psychotherapy.

Since the first publication of a placebo-controlled double-blind study in the early 1960s indicating the efficacy of electroconvulsive therapy (ECT) in the treatment of depression [1], a variety of reports, which have been summarized in a recent review [2], described the excellent therapeutic efficacy of ECT. Particularly in major depression, ECT still has to be considered as the most effective biological treatment option, especially in patients after medication treatment failures. Therefore, pharmacoresistant depressive disorders are still one of the main indications for the treatment with ECT. In patients suffering from depression and treated with ECT, a markedly better improvement has been shown compared to pharmacological treatment strategies such as tricyclic antidepressants (TCAs) [3], monoamine oxidase inhibitors [3] and selective serotonin reuptake inhibitors [4]. In addition, compared to pharmacotherapeutic approaches, the amelioration of depressive symptoms can be achieved more rapidly with ECT [5, 6]. Response rates of up to 80–90%, which have been reported in depressed patients treated with ECT [5, 7], are not yet achieved with pharmacotherapy. Furthermore, in those cases in which depressive symptoms are not ameliorated with pharmacotherapy, response rates of about 50–60% can nevertheless be achieved by ECT [8]. Although pharmacoresistant major depression is still the most frequent indication for ECT, other psychiatric conditions like delirious mania, malignant catatonia, or malignant neuroleptic syndrome have to be considered as urgent first-line indications for the treatment with ECT. Furthermore, ECT has been shown as an effective treatment strategy in schizophrenia in combination with antipsychotic pharmacotherapy [9] and in several other psychiatric disorders like bipolar disorder [10, 11], obsessive-compulsive disorder [12] or personality disorders comorbid with depression [13, 14] in cases of resistance to pharmacotherapy. In a recent study of the National Institute of Health and Clinical Excellence on the economic analysis of ECT [15] the economic modelling results suggested that ECT has no clear economic benefit compared to psychopharmacotherapy and has to be considered as a second-line treatment strategy in depression due to enhanced relapse rates following ECT [15]. However, this conclusion has recently been criticized due to the limited number of included trials and due to a bias in the included trials in favor of medication [16].

The current standard of ECT with the induction of a series of generalized epileptic seizures using brief-pulse stimulation techniques under anesthesia and muscle relaxation has to be considered as one of the best tolerated and as safe biological treatment strategies with low risk for severe complications, even lower risk compared to antidepressant treatment with TCAs [17, 18].

Mechanisms of Action of Electroconvulsive Therapy

Although many decades of research and clinical experience have improved the technique and practice of ECT, the underlying crucial mechanisms which contribute to the superior therapeutic effects of ECT in distinct psychiatric disorders are still under investigation. Most research investigating the neurobiological effects of ECT focused on the antidepressive potential of ECT and revealed that ECT particularly affects neurotransmitter systems which may be involved in the pathophysiology of depression, e.g. the serotonergic, dopaminergic, GABAergic or glutaminergic system (for a current review, see Wahlund and von Rosen [19]). In accordance with the so-called catecholamine and serotonin deficiency hypothesis in depression, several studies indicated that ECT attenuates serotonergic and noradrenergic neurotransmission. However, animal studies revealed conflicting results as an enhanced sensitivity of presynaptic hippocampal 5-HT1A receptors [20] but also a decreased sensitivity of hippocampal 5-HT1A receptors [21] has been described after treatment with electroconvulsive shocks (ECS) in rats. However, in patients suffering from major depression ECT has been shown to increase tryptophan plasma levels [22, 23], suggesting that an increased availability of the serotonin precursor may contribute to the therapeutic effects of ECT [23].

In addition, a compensatory increase in γ-aminobutyric acid (GABA) neurotransmission has been suggested as a possible mechanism of ECT. In line with the anticonvulsive effects of ECT and the GABA deficit hypothesis of depression [24], a proton magnetic resonance spectroscopy study showed that occipital cortex GABA concentrations [25] are increased in depressed patients treated with ECT. Furthermore, an iomazenil SPECT study in depressed patients treated with ECT showed a significant increase in iomazenil binding to the $GABA_A$-receptor-associated benzodiazepine binding site in most cortical areas [26], suggesting an enhanced GABAergic neurotransmission as a possible mechanism of ECT [26]. Recently, ECT has been shown to enhance activity of inhibitory circuits in the human motor cortex, which was assessed by transcranial magnetic stimulation, further indicating that ECT has marked effects on GABAergic neurotransmission [27].

Furthermore, current studies indicated that also effects on glutamate, the most important excitatory neurotransmitter, may play a role for the therapeutic effects of ECT. In patients suffering from major depression, ECT increased glutamate plasma levels [23] and normalized reduced glutamate/glutamine levels in the left cingulum in those patients who responded to ECT [28].

In addition to the effects on neurotransmitter systems, the therapeutic effects of ECT have also been attributed to its influence on hormonal levels, particularly the putative effects of ECT on the hypothalamic-pituitary-adrenal (HPA) system. A dysregulation of the HPA axis comprising elevated levels of corticotropin-releasing hormone, adrenocorticotropic hormone (ACTH) and cortisol during depressive episodes which normalize after clinical remission is one of the most consistent and stable biological finding in depressive disorders [29]. Acute elevations of ACTH and cortisol plasma levels have been observed immediately after ECT [30, 31] and might be interpreted as a physiological stress response. However, during the course of ECT, ACTH and cortisol plasma levels have been found to decrease, suggesting that a downregulation of the HPA axis [32] might comprise a therapeutic effect of ECT in major depression.

In addition, in the last decades, considerable evidence has emerged that certain so-called neuroactive steroids, which alter neuronal excitability via nongenomic mechanisms, might be involved in the pathophysiology of depression and that the attenuation of such neuroactive steroids might contribute to the therapeutic effects of antidepressant drugs [33]. Although no alterations of positive GABAergic 3α-reduced neuroactive steroids have been detected in depressed patients after treatment with ECT [34], elevated plasma levels of dehydroepiandrosterone sulfate (DHEAS), which is a potent negative modulator of the $GABA_A$ receptor, have been found in psychotic depressed patients and were associated with nonresponse to ECT in these patients [35]. Therefore, it has been suggested that DHEAS plasma levels might serve as a predictive marker of nonresponsiveness to ECT [35]. Furthermore, in a genetic rat model of depression, DHEAS pretreatment abolished the antidepressive effects of ECS [36], suggesting that a pharmacologically induced decrease in DHEAS levels might serve as a putative intervention to restore the treatment response in depressed patients resistant to ECT [36].

Recently, growing evidence has emerged for a major role of downstream signal transduction pathways, e.g. the cyclo-AMP-responsive element binding protein (CREB) cascade, and their effects on neurotrophic factors like the brain-derived neurotrophic factor (BDNF) in the pathogenesis and treatment of depressive disorders [37]. In this context, in vivo and animal studies suggested that the antidepressive effects of ECS may be attributed to its putative effects on neurogenesis and neuroplasticity. Single ECS have been shown to rise BDNF mRNA [38–40] and tyrosine kinase B mRNA, which is an effector of BDNF [40]. Furthermore, comparable to the observations after pharmacological antidepressant treatment [41], BDNF mRNA and tyrosine kinase B mRNA are continuously increased after a course of ECS [42]. Moreover, several studies indicated that ECS increase synaptic connectivity. Chronic ECS induce mossy fiber sprouting in the hippocampus [43, 44] and in other brain regions such as the amygdala and frontal areas [45]. In addition, ECS are followed by an increase in neuron formation in the hippocampus [43, 46, 47], an effect that was already observed after a single ECS [47] but which was even more pronounced after a series of ECS [46, 47], suggesting a dose-dependent mechanism of ECT on neurogenesis [47]. In addition, increased levels of CREB and an enhanced transcription mediated by CREB have been detected in the hippocampus after ECS in experimental animals [41]. In humans, current proton magnetic resonance spectroscopy studies supported the hypothesis that ECT does not induce neuronal damage or cell death, because ECT does not induce a decrease in the N-acetylaspartate signal, a sign of cell atrophy [28, 48].

Further SPECT studies in depressed patients indicated a reduced cerebral blood flow in frontal areas briefly after ECT [49]. In contrast to these acute effects, cerebral blood flow has been shown to increase and therefore to normalize in depressed patients after a course of ECT [26, 50]. In the frontal and parietal cortex and in the anterior and posterior cingulate gyrus of depressed patients, a decreased regional cerebral glucose metabolism has been observed after ECT [51, 52]. Responders compared to nonresponders had a reduced cerebral glucose metabolism in frontal regions [53], suggesting that the decrease in glucose metabolism might contribute to the therapeutic effects of ECT [51].

Stimulus Wave Form, Stimulus Intensity and Electrode Placement

Although the underlying crucial mechanisms contributing to the clinical efficacy of ECT are still under investigation, there is increasing evidence that stimulus wave form, electrode placement and stimulus intensity have a major influence on the efficacy and safety of ECT.

With regard to stimulus wave forms, a recent meta-analysis [2] indicated no significant differences between brief-pulse and sine wave stimulation in the amelioration of depressive symptoms. However, due to enhanced rates of cognitive impairment following sine wave ECT [54], this method of stimulation has been replaced by brief-pulse stimulation techniques, which have to be considered as the stimulation method of choice nowadays.

In general, bilateral ECT is considered to be more effective than unilateral (UL) ECT, which requires higher stimulus dosage to achieve the same efficacy. Therefore, stimulus intensity depends on electrode placement.

Several studies and a recent meta-analysis [2] concerning the effectiveness of UL ECT in depressed patients indicated that higher electrical dosage is associated with increased effectiveness and more rapid response than low-dosage ECT [6, 8, 55] (for a review, see UK ECT Review Group [2] and Abrams [18]). Compared to response rates of 35% in patients treated with low-dosage, right UL ECT (1.5× above the titrated seizure threshold), high-dosage ECT (6× above the titrated seizure threshold) was associated with a response rate of 65% [8]. Interestingly, response rates did not differ in patients treated with high-dosage right UL or bilateral ECT, although former publications using lower UL stimulation energy reported a superior efficacy of bilateral ECT [2, 6, 56]. Furthermore, UL high-dosage ECT has been shown to induce less severe cognitive side effects compared to bilateral ECT [8] and high-dosage right UL ECT (403 mC) has been shown to be followed by a significantly more rapid response compared to titrated low-dosage right UL ECT (2.25× initial seizure threshold) in depressed patients [55]. Therefore, it has been suggested that high-dosage UL ECT is superior compared to moderately titrated suprathreshold treatment strategies [18].

However, in a recent meta-analysis, bilateral ECT has still been found to be more effective than UL ECT [2]. In contrast to UL ECT, consistent response rates of 70–90% have been reported in depressed patients treated with bilateral ECT with stimulus doses limited to 1–2.5 times above the convulsive threshold [6, 8, 57], suggesting that the relation between clinical efficacy and stimulus intensity is less pronounced in bilateral ECT. Nevertheless, electrode placement has been suggested as a crucial factor for cognitive side effects induced by bilateral ECT. Bifrontal electrode placement has been shown to be as efficacious as bitemporal placement but might induce less cognitive impairment [57, 58].

In contrast to the results in major depression, the influence of electrode placement or stimulus intensity on the efficacy of ECT is less obvious in schizophrenic patients. A recent Cochrane review on ECT for schizophrenia [9] found no evidence for a difference in efficacy between UL and bilateral ECT and only limited data indicated a faster improvement but no differences in the extent of improvement in high-dosage UL ECT [9].

Clinical Indications of Electroconvulsive Therapy

ECT as a First-Line Treatment Strategy

Acute psychiatric conditions that may require ECT as a first-line treatment are severe excitement, e.g. in delirious mania and malignant catatonia. Intensive ECT, usually administered daily, has been shown to relieve the high rates of mortality associated with these psychiatric conditions [59, 60]. In addition, also in case of a malignant neuroleptic syndrome or severe medication toxicity ECT serves as a first-line treatment strategy [18, 61].

Although the most frequent indication for ECT in major depression is non-response to psychopharmacological treatment strategies, the occurrence of depressive stupor and inanition as in melancholic or psychotic depression may constitute a first-line indication for ECT. ECT has been shown to be one of the safest therapeutic options with the fastest relief of symptoms in case of refusal of food and drinking and of severe psychomotor retardation [62]. Also in severe psychotic depression or in patients at high risk of suicide, ECT should be considered earlier than other therapeutic options [17]. Particularly in psychotic depressed patients remission rates of approximately 90% with relief experienced already 10–14 days after the beginning of treatment have been observed after ECT [63, 64]. Furthermore, the risks of suicide have been shown to relieve quickly by ECT, although attention to continuation treatments is essential to sustain the benefit [65].

ECT has to be considered further as a first-line treatment for depression, mania and psychotic symptoms in patients suffering from severe systemic illnesses at risk of worsening the somatic status due to psychopharmacological treatment [66–68] and in women during early pregnancy and during the breast-feeding postpartum period when the administration of psychotropic medications is precluded.

ECT as a Second-Line Treatment

Most commonly, ECT is applied in patients after psychopharmacological treatment failures or in those cases where medication toxicity interrupted the course of therapy [18, 61]. In psychopharmacological treatment-resistant depressed patients, ECT has been shown to enhance response rates significantly [4, 69, 70], particularly in patients suffering from psychotic depression, even if antipsychotic pharmacotherapy has been applied adequately before ECT [4, 17].

Intolerable side effects of antidepressant medications, somatic comorbidities emerging during the pharmacological treatment [17, 71] or worsening of depressive symptoms including severe suicidality during an antidepressant pharmacotherapy constitute further second-line treatment indications for ECT [17]. Clinical indications for ECT are summarized in table 1.

Continuation ECT

After successful acute treatment with ECT, continuation ECT (C-ECT) might also offer a further possibility in maintenance therapy. Although absence of controlled studies limits the scientific evidence for the use of C-ECT, clinical observations indicated that ECT may serve as an efficacious prophylactic tool [65, 72] in the treatment of depression. C-ECT should be considered if the prior history of an individual patient shows an enhanced risk for recurrence of depression during continued pharmacotherapy including both antidepressants and mood stabilizers [73–75]. After acute treatment, which usually consists of 2 or 3 ECT treatments per week, the treatment intervals should be prolonged usually to 1 treatment per week for 4–8 weeks. Afterwards the frequency of 1 treatment every 2 weeks and 1 treatment every 4 weeks should be maintained for at least 6 months. An alternative frequently used strategy (the so-called *cafeteria style*) is based on the individual decision, whether a C-ECT treatment is administered when the first signs of recurrence of depressive symptoms are reported [18, 76].

Table 1. Indications for ECT (adopted from Baghai et al. [61])

Category of ECT indications	Indication
ECT as a first-line treatment	febrile catatonia [60] malignant neuroleptic syndrome [60] severe depressive episode[1] schizoaffective psychosis[1] schizophrenia[1] [97] in case of life-threatening or intolerable side effects of psychopharmacological treatments
ECT as a second-line treatment	medication treatment failures in depression schizoaffective psychosis schizophrenia mania depression or psychotic symptoms in case of organic diseases
ECT as a last-resort treatment	treatment-resistant OCD treatment-resistant dyskinesias treatment-resistant Gilles de la Tourette syndrome treatment-resistant epilepsy Parkinson's disease (treatment resistant)

[1]With suicidality which cannot be handled even on protected wards, psychotic symptoms or depressive stupor, with positive symptoms or acute danger of self-harm or harm of others.

Efficacy of Electroconvulsive Therapy

The general efficacy and superiority of ECT in comparison to antidepressant pharmacotherapy has been described in several controlled clinical trials and meta-analyses [2]. In a recent meta-analysis of the UK ECT Review Group [2], ECT has been found to be significantly superior in major depression compared to antidepressant pharmacotherapy. In non-treatment-resistant depression response rates between 80–90% [5, 7] and even up to 100% [8] have been observed, although in drug-resistant depression lower response rates of about 50–60% have to be expected [8]. However, a more rapid improvement [5, 6, 63, 18] and a faster treatment response during ECT has been consistently reported in patients suffering from major depression compared to pharmacotherapy [17]. In those patients not responding to ECT, the concomitant prescription of antidepressants may enhance the clinical efficacy of ECT. However, study results regarding the putative benefits of combined ECT and psychopharmacological treatment are still controversial, reporting an amelioration of depression under ECT and TCA treatment [77, 78] but a lack of clinical effectiveness for selective serotonin reuptake inhibitors [77].

ECT is also an effective antidepressant treatment strategy if depressive episodes occur in bipolar disorder [17, 18], although infrequent switches from depression to mania have been described during the course of ECT [17]. However, randomized controlled trials on the switch rates during ECT compared to pharmacological antidepressant treatment strategies are lacking so far. Therefore, no definite conclusion can be drawn at the moment if a switch to mania is indeed a side effect of ECT or whether it has to be interpreted as an artifact [79]. In contrast to antidepressant pharmacotherapy, in cases of a switch ECT treatment does not have to be stopped due to the antimanic properties of ECT. In patients suffering from obsessive-compulsive disorder (OCD) not responsive to pharmacotherapy, response after ECT may be expected if OCD is accompanied by depressive symptoms [17] and a beneficial effect of ECT during OCD continuation therapy has been reported [17].

Comorbid personality disorder is a predictor of poor response to ECT and the recommendation for ECT should be cautious in such patients [18, 80]. Nevertheless, in patients suffering from major depression and personality disorders, a recent meta-analysis indicated that ECT may be of benefit [14]. Therefore, ECT should be taken into account as an additional treatment strategy in such patients if no response can be achieved with pharmacotherapy [17].

In comparison to major depression, in patients suffering from organic depression due to somatic disorders, lower response rates to ECT have been described [81–83]. However, ECT has been proven as a clinically effective treatment strategy in patients suffering from poststroke depression [8, 56, 83].

In patients suffering from schizophrenia, the Cochrane Schizophrenia Group ECT review [9] found that ECT monotherapy is less effective than antipsychotic [9] drug treatment, although the combination of ECT with antipsychotic drugs resulted in greater improvement in mental state compared to antipsychotic pharmacotherapy. Furthermore, compared to antipsychotic monotherapy, the combination with ECT was found to be more effective in the maintenance of response in patients not responding to psychopharmacotherapy [9]. The authors concluded that ECT, combined with antipsychotic drugs, may be considered a therapeutic option in patients with schizophrenia, particularly when rapid global improvement and reduction of symptoms is warranted [9].

Safety of Electroconvulsive Therapy and Clinical Precautions

After many decades of research and clinical experience, clinicians have developed protocols for the safe treatment of patients warranting ECT regardless of age, medical status, or physical state.

In general, ECT is one of the best tolerated antidepressant therapies with low risk for severe complications, even lower than that obtained with TCAs [17, 18]. The mortality rate during ECT varies between 1:50,000 and 1:25,000 treatments [17, 18]. In less than 1 in 10,000 treatments, severe complications have warranted special attention [17]. Therefore, ECT has to be considered as one of the safest medical procedures under anesthesia. Clinical conditions requiring special attention before and during an ECT, which have been described in Abrams [18] and Baghai et al. [61], are summarized in table 2.

No absolute contraindications are acknowledged. Conditions including higher somatic risks are a recent myocardial or cerebral infarction, high intracranial pressure, and every untreated severe medical and life-threatening anesthesiological risk. If treated sufficiently, these conditions become relative contraindications and an individual and interdisciplinary benefit/risk analysis for each patient has to be performed. Conditions enhancing the cardiovascular risks are coronary artery disease, arrhythmias, insufficiently treated hypertonia, or aneurysms. Other medical conditions such as severe lung or liver diseases, disturbances of blood coagulation or an untreated pheochromocytoma can enhance both ECT and anesthesia risk. Neurological diseases such as intracranial tumors or bleeding, vascular malformations, cerebral ischemia or acute infections enhance the treatment risk. In general, each factor enhancing the risk for ECT or anesthesia side effects should be taken into consideration and in case of such specific risks, interdisciplinary counseling may be necessary. Afterwards the higher somatic risk has to be compared to the risk of an insufficiently treated or prolonged psychiatric illness. Patients and relatives or responsible legal guardians have to be informed about risk/benefit ratios to contribute to a shared decision.

Side Effects of Electroconvulsive Therapy

Somatic Side Effects

The most frequent immediate unpleasant effects of ECT are headache, nausea and vomiting (varying with anesthetic). Up to 45% of patients report headache after ECT, which can be treated symptomatically using analgesics such as acetylsalicylic acid or paracetamol and, if severe, by changing the induction medications. Patients suffering from regular migraine attacks are

Table 2. Clinical conditions requiring special attention before and during ECT (adopted from Baghai et al. [61])

Category	Clinical condition
Enhanced intracerebral pressure[1]	at present
Cerebral infarction[1]	not older than 3 months
Myocardial infarction[1]	not older than 3 months
Intracerebral tumor[1]	including intracerebral edema
Any life-threatening anesthesia risk[1]	at present
Cardiovascular disorders	cardiac arrhythmias, instable angina pectoris, myocardial infarction (older than 3 months), myocardial insufficiency, heart valve abnormalities, not sufficiently treated hyper- or hypotonia, aortal aneurysm
Medical disorders	disturbance of blood coagulation, severe liver diseases, severe pulmonary diseases, pheochromocytoma
Neurological disorders	intracerebral neoplasias, intracranial bleeding, intracerebral vascular malformations, cerebral ischemia, cerebral inflammations, hydrocephalus, dementias, diseases of the basal ganglia, craniotomies, severe cerebral traumas
Orthopedic disorders	osteoporosis
Esophageal hernia	increased aspiration risk, intubation recommended
Concomitant pharmacological treatment	if enhancing the ECT risks or reducing ECT efficacy

[1]In former times considered as absolute contraindications; today an individual risk/benefit analysis is necessary.

predisposed to postictal headache after ECT. In this case, triptans, e.g. sumatriptan, can be applied orally or intranasally [84]. Nausea occurs rarely after intravenous anesthesia and can be treated using metoclopramide. Other rare complications of ECT can be cardiovascular events emerging from anesthesia. Furthermore, prolonged seizures beyond the anticipated 30–180 s have been described as a side effect of ECT [17]. An enhanced risk for such prolonged seizures has been reported in patients treated with theophylline [85, 86]. However, the treating anesthesiologist or psychiatrist will end the seizure by the administration of intravenous benzodiazepines (e.g. diazepam), anesthetics or other anticonvulsants. This event is best managed by ictal and postictal EEG monitoring [85], which can also be of use in the treatment of nonconvulsive seizures which rarely occur after ECT [85, 86]. In addition, the rare case of prolonged muscle relaxation either due to an individual predisposition or to a side effect of concomitant lithium therapy [87, 88] might require subsequent measurement of oxygen saturation and assisted respiration to prevent hypoxia. Adequate muscle relaxation prevents aching muscles, which is reported only rarely. In patients suffering from bipolar depression, ECT similar to any other antidepressant agent [84] might induce a switch to hypomania or mania [84]. However, concomitant therapy with lithium or mood stabilizers [89] can reduce the switch risk significantly, although an enhanced risk of side effects and a decreased effectiveness due to the anticonvulsant properties of the mood stabilizers have to be considered [89].

Cognitive Side Effects

In up to one third of patients, transient cognitive side effects have been described after ECT [17]. In general, transient cognitive disturbances are more prominent in bilateral than in UL and in high-dosage than in low-dosage ECT [2]. In such cases, postseizure delirium has to be distinguished from transient memory disturbances such as anterograde or retrograde amnesia and from rarely occurring effects on the autobiographic long-term memory [90]. The duration and the severity of postictal delirium including a prolonged reorientation period may vary with patient age, dosage and type of anesthetic, and the characteristics of the concomitant psychoactive or systemic medications.

In older patients with physical comorbidity, short-term memory disturbances have been reported in up to 28% of ECT-treated patients [91]. In cases of concentration or attention deficits reported after ECT, it might be difficult to differentiate cognitive side effects in an individual patient after treatment from cognitive disturbances caused by the illness itself [92]. In addition, also an amelioration of cognitive impairment has been reported in depressed patients treated with ECT [93]. The rate of cognitive disturbances is generally dependent on dose and application of electrical stimulation, with higher risk of cognitive side effects in bilateral and high-dosage ECT [83, 93]. Nevertheless, using modified ECT techniques such as UL or bifrontal pulse wave stimulation, anesthesia with muscle relaxation and sufficient oxygenation reduced these risks substantially [6, 8, 94].

If, in spite of these precautions, cognitive disturbances occur, a rapid improvement within 1–4 weeks can be observed in most cases [94]. Follow-up investigations showed a complete reversibility of cognitive side effects after an ECT course [61, 94] or even an improvement in comparison to the time interval before ECT treatment [61]. This is in accordance with a variety of case reports and controlled studies confirming that ECT does not cause long-lasting functional [95] or any structural damage of the central nervous system [93, 95, 96].

Conclusion

Besides the extensive development of psychopharmacological treatments and the promising results of studies investigating novel nonpharmacological strategies like repetitive transcranial magnetic stimulation, vagus nerve stimulation and magnetic seizure therapy, so far a significant improvement in response rates and a more rapid amelioration of symptoms has not been achieved with these new treatment strategies. ECT has still to be considered as a highly effective treatment option predominantly for depression, but also for other psychiatric disorders.

References

1 Greenblatt M, Grosser GH, Wechsler HA: Differential response of hospitalized depressed patients in somatic therapy. Am J Psychiatry 1964;120:935–943.
2 UK ECT Review Group: Efficacy and safety of electroconvulsive therapy in depressive disorders: a systematic review and meta-analysis. Lancet 2003;361:799–808.
3 Janicak PG, Davis JM, Gibbons RD, Ericksen S, Chang S, Gallagher P: Efficacy of ECT: a meta-analysis. Am J Psychiatry 1985;142:297–302.
4 Folkerts HW, Michael N, Tolle R, Schonauer K, Mucke S, Schulze-Monking H: Electroconvulsive therapy vs paroxetine in treatment-resistant depression – A randomized study. Acta Psychiatr Scand 1997;96:334–342.
5 Prudic J, Haskett RF, Mulsant B, Malone KM, Pettinati HM, Stephens S, Greenberg R, Rifas SL, Sackeim HA: Resistance to antidepressant medications and short-term clinical response to ECT. Am J Psychiatry 1996;153:985–992.
6 Sackeim HA, Prudic J, Devanand DP, Kiersky JE, Fitzsimons L, Moody BJ, McElhiney MC, Coleman EA, Settembrino JM: Effects of stimulus intensity and electrode placement on the efficacy and cognitive effects of electroconvulsive therapy. N Engl J Med 1993;328:839–846.
7 Prudic J, Sackeim HA, Devanand DP: Medication resistance and clinical response to electroconvulsive therapy. Psychiatry Res 1990;31:287–296.
8 Sackeim HA, Prudic J, Devanand DP, Nobler MS, Lisanby SH, Peyser S, Fitzsimons L, Moody BJ, Clark J: A prospective, randomized, double-blind comparison of bilateral and right unilateral electroconvulsive therapy at different stimulus intensities. Arch Gen Psychiatry 2000;57:425–434.
9 Tharyan P, Adams CE: Electroconvulsive therapy for schizophrenia. Cochrane Database Syst Rev 2005;2:CD000076.
10 Gitlin M: Treatment-resistant bipolar disorder. Mol Psychiatry 2006;11:227–240.
11 Grunze H: Reevaluating therapies for bipolar depression. J Clin Psychiatry 2005;66(suppl 5): 17–25.
12 Dell'Osso B, Altamura AC, Allen A, Hollander E: Brain stimulation techniques in the treatment of obsessive-compulsive disorder: current and future directions. CNS Spectr 2005;10:966–979, 983.
13 DeBattista C, Mueller K: Is electroconvulsive therapy effective for the depressed patient with comorbid borderline personality disorder? J ECT 2001;17:91–98.
14 Newton-Howes G, Tyrer P, Johnson T: Personality disorder and the outcome of depression: meta-analysis of published studies. Br J Psychiatry 2006;188:13–20.
15 Greenhalgh J, Knight C, Hind D, Beverley C, Walters S: Clinical and cost-effectiveness of electroconvulsive therapy for depressive illness, schizophrenia, catatonia and mania: systematic reviews and economic modelling studies. Health Technol Assess 2005;9:1–156, iii–iv.
16 McDonald WM: Is ECT cost-effective? A critique of the National Institute of Health and Clinical Excellence's report on the economic analysis of ECT. J ECT 2006;22:25–29.

17 Weiner RD, Coffey CE, Folk J, Fochtmann LJ, Greenberg RM, Isenberg KE, Kellner CH, Sackeim HA, Moench LM: The Practice of Electroconvulsive Therapy: Recommendations for Treatment, Training and Privileging, ed 2. Washington, American Psychiatric Association, 2001.
18 Abrams R: Electroconvulsive Therapy, ed 4. New York, Oxford University Press, 2002.
19 Wahlund B, von Rosen D: ECT of major depressed patients in relation to biological and clinical variables: a brief overview. Neuropsychopharmacology 2003;28(suppl 1):S21–S26.
20 Newman ME, Gur E, Shapira B, Lerer B: Neurochemical mechanisms of action of ECS: evidence from in vivo studies. J ECT 1998;14:153–171.
21 Gur E, Dremencov E, Garcia F, van De Kar LD, Lerer B, Newman ME: Functional effects of chronic electroconvulsive shock on serotonergic 5-HT(1A) and 5-HT(1B) receptor activity in rat hippocampus and hypothalamus. Brain Res 2002;952:52–60.
22 Hoekstra R, van den Broek WW, Fekkes D, Bruijn JA, Mulder PG, Pepplinkhuizen L: Effect of electroconvulsive therapy on biopterin and large neutral amino acids in severe, medication-resistant depression. Psychiatry Res 2001;103:115–123.
23 Palmio J, Huuhka M, Saransaari P, Oja SS, Peltola J, Leinonen E, Suhonen J, Keranen T: Changes in plasma amino acids after electroconvulsive therapy of depressed patients. Psychiatry Res 2005;137:183–190.
24 Sackeim HA: The anticonvulsant hypothesis of the mechanisms of action of ECT: current status. J ECT 1999;15:5–26.
25 Sanacora G, Mason GF, Rothman DL, Hyder F, Ciarcia JJ, Ostroff RB, Berman RM, Krystal JH: Increased cortical GABA concentrations in depressed patients receiving ECT. Am J Psychiatry 2003;160:577–579.
26 Mervaala E, Kononen M, Fohr J, Husso-Saastamoinen M, Valkonen-Korhonen M, Kuikka JT, Viinamaki H, Tammi AK, Tiihonen J, Partanen J, Lehtonen J: SPECT and neuropsychological performance in severe depression treated with ECT. J Affect Disord 2001;66:47–58.
27 Bajbouj M, Lang UE, Niehaus L, Hellen FE, Heuser I, Neu P: Effects of right unilateral electroconvulsive therapy on motor cortical excitability in depressive patients. J Psychiatr Res 2006;40: 322–327.
28 Pfleiderer B, Michael N, Erfurth A, Ohrmann P, Hohmann U, Wolgast M, Fiebich M, Arolt V, Heindel W: Effective electroconvulsive therapy reverses glutamate/glutamine deficit in the left anterior cingulum of unipolar depressed patients. Psychiatry Res 2003;122:185–192.
29 Holsboer F: The corticosteroid receptor hypothesis of depression. Neuropsychopharmacology 2000;23:477–501.
30 Szuba MP, O'Reardon JP, Evans DL: Physiological effects of electroconvulsive therapy and transcranial magnetic stimulation in major depression. Depress Anxiety 2000;12:170–177.
31 Florkowski CM, Crozier IG, Nightingale S, Evans MJ, Ellis MJ, Joyce P, Donald RA: Plasma cortisol, PRL, ACTH, AVP and corticotrophin releasing hormone responses to direct current cardioversion and electroconvulsive therapy. Clin Endocrinol (Oxf) 1996;44:163–168.
32 Grunhaus L, Zelnik T, Albala AA, Rabin D, Haskett RF, Zis AP, Greden JF: Serial dexamethasone suppression tests in depressed patients treated only with electroconvulsive therapy. J Affect Disord 1987;13:233–240.
33 Rupprecht R: The neuropsychopharmacological potential of neuroactive steroids. J Psychiatr Res 1997;31:297–314.
34 Baghai TC, di Michele F, Schule C, Eser D, Zwanzger P, Pasini A, Romeo E, Rupprecht R: Plasma concentrations of neuroactive steroids before and after electroconvulsive therapy in major depression. Neuropsychopharmacology 2005;30:1181–1186.
35 Maayan R, Yagorowski Y, Grupper D, Weiss M, Shtaif B, Kaoud MA, Weizman A: Basal plasma dehydroepiandrosterone sulfate level: a possible predictor for response to electroconvulsive therapy in depressed psychotic inpatients. Biol Psychiatry 2000;48:693–701.
36 Maayan R, Morad O, Dorfman P, Overstreet DH, Weizman A, Yadid G: The involvement of dehydroepiandrosterone (DHEA) and its sulfate ester (DHEAS) in blocking the therapeutic effect of electroconvulsive shocks in an animal model of depression. Eur Neuropsychopharmacol 2005;15: 253–262.
37 Duman RS, Heninger GR, Nestler EJ: A molecular and cellular theory of depression. Arch Gen Psychiatry 1997;54:597–606.

38 Altar CA: Neurotrophins and depression. Trends Pharmacol Sci 1999;20:59–61.
39 Smith MA, Zhang LX, Lyons WE, Mamounas LA: Anterograde transport of endogenous brain-derived neurotrophic factor in hippocampal mossy fibers. Neuroreport 1997;8:1829–1834.
40 Lindefors N, Brodin E, Metsis M: Spatiotemporal selective effects on brain-derived neurotrophic factor and trkB messenger RNA in rat hippocampus by electroconvulsive shock. Neuroscience 1995;65:661–670.
41 Nibuya M, Nestler EJ, Duman RS: Chronic antidepressant administration increases the expression of cAMP response element binding protein (CREB) in rat hippocampus. J Neurosci 1996;16: 2365–2372.
42 Nibuya M, Morinobu S, Duman RS: Regulation of BDNF and trkB mRNA in rat brain by chronic electroconvulsive seizure and antidepressant drug treatments. J Neurosci 1995;15:7539–7547.
43 Vaidya VA, Siuciak JA, Du F, Duman RS: Hippocampal mossy fiber sprouting induced by chronic electroconvulsive seizures. Neuroscience 1999;89:157–166.
44 Reid IC, Stewart CA: Seizures, memory and synaptic plasticity. Seizure 1997;6:351–359.
45 Reid IC, Stewart CA: How antidepressants work: new perspectives on the pathophysiology of depressive disorder. Br J Psychiatry 2001;178:299–303.
46 Scott BW, Wojtowicz JM, Burnham WM: Neurogenesis in the dentate gyrus of the rat following electroconvulsive shock seizures. Exp Neurol 2000;165:231–236.
47 Madsen TM, Treschow A, Bengzon J, Bolwig TG, Lindvall O, Tingstrom A: Increased neurogenesis in a model of electroconvulsive therapy. Biol Psychiatry 2000;47:1043–1049.
48 Ende G, Braus DF, Walter S, Weber-Fahr W, Henn FA: The hippocampus in patients treated with electroconvulsive therapy: a proton magnetic resonance spectroscopic imaging study. Arch Gen Psychiatry 2000;57:937–943.
49 Scott AI, Dougall N, Ross M, O'Carroll RE, Riddle W, Ebmeier KP, Goodwin GM: Short-term effects of electroconvulsive treatment on the uptake of ^{99m}Tc-exametazime into brain in major depression shown with single photon emission tomography. J Affect Disord 1994;30:27–34.
50 Bonne O, Krausz Y, Shapira B, Bocher M, Karger H, Gorfine M, Chisin R, Lerer B: Increased cerebral blood flow in depressed patients responding to electroconvulsive therapy. J Nucl Med 1996;37:1075–1080.
51 Nobler MS, Oquendo MA, Kegeles LS, Malone KM, Campbell CC, Sackeim HA, Mann JJ: Decreased regional brain metabolism after ECT. Am J Psychiatry 2001;158:305–308.
52 Yatham LN, Clark CC, Zis AP: A preliminary study of the effects of electroconvulsive therapy on regional brain glucose metabolism in patients with major depression. J ECT 2000;16:171–176.
53 Nobler MS, Teneback CC, Nahas Z, Bohning DE, Shastri A, Kozel FA, George MS: Structural and functional neuroimaging of electroconvulsive therapy and transcranial magnetic stimulation. Depress Anxiety 2000;12:144–156.
54 Squire LR, Zouzounis JA: ECT and memory: brief pulse versus sine wave. Am J Psychiatry 1986;143:596–601.
55 McCall WV, Reboussin DM, Weiner RD, Sackeim HA: Titrated moderately suprathreshold vs fixed high-dose right unilateral electroconvulsive therapy: acute antidepressant and cognitive effects. Arch Gen Psychiatry 2000;57:438–444.
56 Sackeim HA, Decina P, Kanzler M, Kerr B, Malitz S: Effects of electrode placement on the efficacy of titrated, low-dose ECT. Am J Psychiatry 1987;144:1449–1455.
57 Bailine SH, Rifkin A, Kayne E, Selzer JA, Vital-Herne J, Blieka M, Pollack S: Comparison of bifrontal and bitemporal ECT for major depression. Am J Psychiatry 2000;157:121–123.
58 Letemendia FJ, Delva NJ, Rodenburg M, Lawson JS, Inglis J, Waldron JJ, Lywood DW: Therapeutic advantage of bifrontal electrode placement in ECT. Psychol Med 1993;23:349–360.
59 Fink M: Electroshock: Restoring the Mind. New York, Oxford University Press, 1999.
60 Fink M, Tayor MA: Catatonia. A Clinician's Guide to Diagnosis and Treatment. Cambridge, Cambridge University Press, 2003.
61 Baghai TC, Eser D, Schüle C, Nothdurfter C, Möller H-J, Rupprecht R: Elektrokonvulsionstherapie bei depressiven Störungen. J Neurol Neurochir Psychiatr 2005;6: 20–28.
62 Gangadhar BN, Kapur RL, Kalyanasundaram S: Comparison of electroconvulsive therapy with imipramine in endogenous depression: a double-blind study. Br J Psychiatry 1982;141: 367–371.

63 Petrides G, Fink M, Husain MM, Knapp RG, Rush AJ, Mueller M, Rummans TA, O'Connor KM, Rasmussen KG Jr, Bernstein HJ, Biggs M, Bailine SH, Kellner CH: ECT remission rates in psychotic versus nonpsychotic depressed patients: a report from CORE. J ECT 2001;17:244–253.
64 Ottoson JO, Fink M: The Ethics in Electroconvulsive Therapy. New York, Brunner-Routledge, 2004.
65 Kellner CH, Fink M, Knapp R, Petrides G, Husain M, Rummans T, Mueller M, Bernstein H, Rasmussen K, O'Connor K, Smith G, Rush AJ, Biggs M, McClintock S, Bailine S, Malur C: Relief of expressed suicidal intent by ECT: a consortium for research in ECT study. Am J Psychiatry 2005;162:977–982.
66 Beliles K, Stoudemire A: Psychopharmacologic treatment of depression in the medically ill. Psychosomatics 1998;39:S2–S19.
67 Franco-Bronson K: The management of treatment-resistant depression in the medically ill. Psychiatr Clin North Am 1996;19:329–350.
68 Rothschild AJ: Management of psychotic, treatment-resistant depression. Psychiatr Clin North Am 1996;19:237–252.
69 Davidson J, McLeod M, Law-Yone B, Linnoila M: A comparison of electroconvulsive therapy and combined phenelzine-amitriptyline in refractory depression. Arch Gen Psychiatry 1978;35: 639–642.
70 Kroessler D: Relative efficacy rates for therapies of delusional depression. Convuls Ther 1985;1: 173–182.
71 Rasmussen KG, Sampson SM, Rummans TA: Electroconvulsive therapy and newer modalities for the treatment of medication-refractory mental illness. Mayo Clin Proc 2002;77:552–556.
72 Sartorius A, Henn FA: Continuation ECT. Psychiatr Prax 2005;32:408–411.
73 Frey R, Schreinzer D, Heiden A, Kasper S: Use of electroconvulsive therapy in psychiatry. Nervenarzt 2001;72:661–676.
74 McCall WV: Electroconvulsive therapy in the era of modern psychopharmacology. Int J Neuropsychopharmacol 2001;4:315–324.
75 Rabheru K, Persad E: A review of continuation and maintenance electroconvulsive therapy. Can J Psychiatry 1997;42:476–484.
76 Fink M, Abrams R, Bailine S, Jaffe R: Ambulatory electroconvulsive therapy: report of a task force of the association for convulsive therapy. Association for Convulsive Therapy. Convuls Ther 1996;12:42–55.
77 Lauritzen L, Odgaard K, Clemmesen L, Lunde M, Ohrstrom J, Black C, Bech P: Relapse prevention by means of paroxetine in ECT-treated patients with major depression: a comparison with imipramine and placebo in medium-term continuation therapy. Acta Psychiatr Scand 1996;94: 241–251.
78 Nelson JP, Benjamin L: Efficacy and safety of combined ECT and tricyclic antidepressant drugs in the treatment of depressed geriatric patients. Convuls Ther 1989;5:321–329.
79 Tayor MA, Fink M: Melancholia: The Diagnosis, Pathophysiology and Treatment of Depressive Illness. Cambridge, Cambridge University Press, 2006.
80 O'Connor MK, Knapp R, Husain M, Rummans TA, Petrides G, Smith G, Mueller M, Snyder K, Bernstein H, Rush AJ, Fink M, Kellner C: The influence of age on the response of major depression to electroconvulsive therapy: a CORE Report. Am J Geriatr Psychiatry 2001;9:382–390.
81 Black DW, Winokur G, Nasrallah A: A multivariate analysis of the experience of 423 depressed inpatients treated with electroconvulsive therapy. Convuls Ther 1993;9:112–120.
82 Coryell W, Pfohl B, Zimmerman M: Outcome following electroconvulsive therapy: a comparison of primary and secondary depression. Convuls Ther 1985;1:10–14.
83 Krystal AD, Coffey CE: Neuropsychiatric considerations in the use of electroconvulsive therapy. J Neuropsychiatry Clin Neurosci 1997;9:283–292.
84 Angst J, Angst K, Baruffol I, Meinherz-Surbeck R: ECT-induced and drug-induced hypomania. Convuls Ther 1992;8:179–185.
85 Grogan R, Wagner DR, Sullivan T, Labar D: Generalized nonconvulsive status epilepticus after electroconvulsive therapy. Convuls Ther 1995;11:51–56.
86 Rao KM, Gangadhar BN, Janakiramaiah N: Nonconvulsive status epilepticus after the ninth electroconvulsive therapy. Convuls Ther 1993;9:128–129.

87 Hill GE, Wong KC, Hodges MR: Lithium carbonate and neuromuscular blocking agents. Anesthesiology 1977;46:122–126.
88 Reimherr FW, Hodges MR, Hill GE, Wong KC: Prolongation of muscle relaxant effects by lithium carbonate. Am J Psychiatry 1977;134:205–206.
89 Zarate CA Jr, Tohen M, Baraibar G: Combined valproate or carbamazepine and electroconvulsive therapy. Ann Clin Psychiatry 1997;9:19–25.
90 Lisanby SH, Maddox JH, Prudic J, Devanand DP, Sackeim HA: The effects of electroconvulsive therapy on memory of autobiographical and public events. Arch Gen Psychiatry 2000;57:581–590.
91 van Waarde JA, Stek ML: Electroconvulsive therapy effective and safe in 55 patients aged 56 years and older with mood disorders and physical comorbidity. Ned Tijdschr Geneeskd 2001;145:1693–1697.
92 Lisanby SH, Luber B, Schlaepfer TE, Sackeim HA: Safety and feasibility of magnetic seizure therapy (MST) in major depression: randomized within-subject comparison with electroconvulsive therapy. Neuropsychopharmacology 2003;28:1852–1865.
93 Devanand DP, Sackeim HA, Prudic J: Electroconvulsive therapy in the treatment-resistant patient. Psychiatr Clin North Am 1991;14:905–923.
94 Ghaziuddin N, Laughrin D, Giordani B: Cognitive side effects of electroconvulsive therapy in adolescents. J Child Adolesc Psychopharmacol 2000;10:269–276.
95 Krause P, Genz A, Knorr W: Prospective study of the late sequelae of electroconvulsive treatment. Psychiatr Neurol Med Psychol (Leipz) 1988;40:532–536.
96 Lisanby SH, Morales O, Payne N, Kwon E, Fitzsimons L, Luber B, Nobler MS, Sackeim HA: New developments in electroconvulsive therapy and magnetic seizure therapy. CNS Spectr 2003;8:529–536.
97 Fink M, Sackeim HA: Convulsive therapy in schizophrenia? Schizophr Bull 1996;22:27–39.

Thomas C. Baghai
Department of Psychiatry and Psychotherapy, Ludwig-Maximilian University Munich
Nussbaumstrasse 7
DE–80336 Munich (Germany)
Tel. +49 89 5160 5731, Fax +49 89 5160 5524
E-Mail Thomas.Baghai@med.uni-muenchen.de

Marcolin MA, Padberg F (eds): Transcranial Brain Stimulation for Treatment of Psychiatric Disorders.
Adv Biol Psychiatr. Basel, Karger, 2007, vol 23, pp 18–34

Repetitive Transcranial Magnetic Stimulation Effects in vitro and in Animal Models

Martin E. Keck

Klinik Schlössli, Oetwil am See/Zurich and Neuroscience Center Zurich,
ETH and University of Zurich, Zurich, Switzerland

Abstract

In recent years, the therapeutic properties of repetitive transcranial magnetic stimulation (rTMS) have been investigated more or less systematically for the treatment of a multitude of psychiatric disorders. Unfortunately, the effects are far from being convincing. Therefore, it is important to acknowledge that the optimal use of rTMS necessitates knowledge concerning the putative neurobiological changes induced by its use. This could finally allow for separating myth from reality. Preclinical studies in suitable animal models and basic studies at the cellular and molecular level are necessary to understand how the induced intracerebral current density is regulated and which regulatory elements might serve as potential treatment targets. rTMS has repeatedly been demonstrated to cause changes in neuronal circuits as reflected by behavioural changes and decreases in the activity of the hypothalamic-pituitary-adrenocortical system. Specific changes in the dynamic release patterns of biogenic amines, amino acids and the neuropeptide vasopressin in response to rTMS (20 Hz) were demonstrated by means of the microdialysis technique. These alterations are reminiscent of those accompanying antidepressant drugs and suggest regional changes in neurotransmitter/neuromodulator release, signalling pathways, and in gene transcription. Most consistently, the data available so far provide evidence that acute rTMS of frontal brain regions can exert a modulatory effect on both the mesolimbic and the mesostriatal dopaminergic systems, brain regions known to be involved in the pathophysiology of deleterious disorders such as major depression, Parkinson's disease and drug addiction. Translational psychiatry should now define which patient and treatment characteristics might lead to satisfactory therapeutic effects with rTMS.

To use repetitive transcranial magnetic stimulation (rTMS) optimally, it is most important to know how it is acting in brain tissue, i.e. knowledge concerning the putative neurobiological changes underlying the observed clinical effects is essential. The limitations of human research necessitate preclinical studies in suitable animal models and basic studies at the cellular and molecular level for a better understanding of how the induced intracerebral current density is regulated and which regulatory elements might serve as potential treatment targets.

By the use of rTMS, charge is moved across the excitable neuronal membranes, creating a transmembrane potential. This in turn causes membrane depolarization and initiates an action potential that propagates along the nerve. Therefore, rTMS can activate the output and input connections of any area of the cortex. Clearly, the effects induced are not limited to the cortical area targeted by rTMS but changes can also occur at distant interconnected sites in the brain. The threshold for producing effects at a distance depends on the intensity of stimulation [1, 2]. As a measure for the strength of TMS applied in preclinical and clinical studies, the biological efficacy of the stimulus in the individual subject is critical [3, 4]. Therefore, the intensity of TMS is typically given as a multiple or percentage of the threshold intensity for evoking a small motor evoked potential in a relaxed hand muscle [5]. It is of note that the strength of association between motor threshold reflecting motor cortex excitability and thresholds for neuronal depolarization in other cortical regions is unknown. However, to date there is no method for determining stimulus strength in other brain areas more relevant for, e.g. mood circuitries [2]. Importantly, motor threshold can also be determined in rodents and should be a prerequisite for conducting basic research in these animals [6–9].

By selectively modulating activity in brain circuitries involved in pathological processes such as depression, mania, and schizophrenia, rTMS could theoretically be able to therapeutically influence such disorders. So far, the largest single area of TMS research in psychiatry has been the exploration of possible therapeutic effects of cortical, usually prefrontal, stimulation on symptoms of major depression [10].

Size Matters: Repetitive Transcranial Magnetic Stimulation in Rodent Studies

To be able to identify new psychiatric treatments, appropriate animal models are indispensable tools. In the case of rTMS, the situation is complicated by the fact that in the vast majority of rodent studies available so far the entire brain is likely to be stimulated due to the usage of commercially obtained stimulation coils [2]. Therefore, it is difficult to relate the effects measured to specific neuronal circuits. To reliably investigate the underlying neurobiological effects in animal models, the adoption of equivalent stimulation conditions is indispensable. Like in clinical studies, another problem arises from the sham stimulation conditions used, which in some cases are likely to elicit biologically active conductive patterns [11].

In the pioneering studies demonstrating that chronic rTMS has an antidepressant-like effect in rats, stimulation patterns used were not tested to be analogous to those used under clinical conditions and the effects observed were most probably due to a stimulation of the entire rat brain [12]. In clinical studies, antidepressant rTMS effects most probably relate to frontal forebrain stimulation [10, 13], and a major point is the appropriateness of extrapolating the effects observed in rodent studies. It is worth noting that magnetic stimulation of rodent brains is not diffuse by necessity [2]. One possibility of working around these problems is to calculate the spatial distribution of current density induced in both the rat and human brain and to adjust the stimulation parameters accordingly.

The coil and stimulation parameters used in the studies conducted at our laboratory [7, 14–23] were selected according to an exact characterization of the conductive phenomena elicited by rTMS in both human and rat brain. This enabled us to accurately adapt the experimental set-up in order to achieve a stimulation pattern which is analogous to the one used in patients during standard clinical treatment. The results of the above procedure show that our experimental set-up allows to obtain a stimulation pattern which exhibits a definite peak in the left frontal region as desired [20, 21]. It is, therefore, justified to interpret subsequently collected data as related to selective stimulation of this brain area.

Antidepressant-Like Effects

To obtain predictions about the clinical condition in human depression, an animal model of depressive-like behaviour with face, construct and predictive validity should be used [24–28]. We, therefore, characterized the effects of rTMS on the regulation of hypothalamic-pituitary-adrenocortical (HPA) system activity, stress coping and anxiety-related behaviour in two Wistar rat lines selectively bred for high (HAB) and low (LAB) anxiety-related behaviour under a regimen adapted from clinical conditions. These two rat breeding lines differ not only in their inborn anxiety, but also in their stress coping strategies and their HPA system susceptibility to external stressors [29–32].

Chronic rTMS treatment in the above-mentioned psychopathological animal model under stimulation conditions adapted from hospital use induced profound changes in acute stress coping strategies [23]. Hargreaves et al. [9] could replicate this finding in commercially obtained rats. The occurrence of changes towards more active coping strategies during exposure to modified versions of the Porsolt's swim test has frequently been shown to predict the antidepressant efficacy of a drug when administered to patients suffering from depression [33]. Therefore, such behavioural effects of rTMS support an antidepressant efficacy of this treatment. This rTMS-induced shift in HAB animals towards active stress coping was markedly higher than has previously been reported in commercially obtained rats, i.e. 'normal' rats [20, 34]. In contrast, rTMS-treated LAB animals, innately displaying rather active stress coping abilities, were unaffected. Our findings that chronic rTMS differentially affected the coping abilities of HAB and LAB rats indicate that these treatment-induced changes are determined by both the rats' innate emotionality and coping strategy. Indeed, it should be emphasized that antidepressant treatment strategies such as psychopharmacological agents exert marked beneficial actions in depressed individuals only, but have no mood-elevating effects in healthy controls.

Interestingly, effects in the forced swim test obtained with frequencies ranging from 1 to 25 Hz were found to be comparable to those seen with the tricyclic antidepressant imipramine [35].

Chronic rTMS (20 Hz) had no effect on anxiety-related behaviour of rats [9, 20, 36]. The observed lack of anxiolytic properties of rTMS is consistent with the finding that benzodiazepine-binding characteristics were found to be unchanged after chronic rTMS treatment [20, 37], suggesting that 20-Hz rTMS might not be beneficial in treating anxiety-related behaviour. In contrast, it was demonstrated that rTMS applied with 25 Hz exerts anxiolytic effects in rats pointing out that such therapeutic effects might depend on the stimulation frequency [38].

Repetitive Transcranial Magnetic Stimulation and Monoamines: Is Dopamine the Key?

Although the monoaminergic synapse finally lost its long-standing relevance for strategies to improve antidepressant therapy, an increase in the disposition of biogenic amines accompanies the therapeutic effects of most antidepressant treatments [39]. Interestingly, a selective stimulation of hippocampal dopamine release, but not serotonin or noradrenaline release, induced by 20-Hz rTMS was monitored [21]. Therefore, the dopaminergic system appeared to be one of the primary candidate neurotransmitter systems which is directly and selectively modulated by rTMS of frontal brain regions. It has been demonstrated that the prefrontal cortex has dense efferent projections to both the ventral tegmental area and the substantia nigra, i.e. the regions of origin of the mesolimbic and mesostriatal dopaminergic pathways [40]. These neuro-anatomical connections may explain how stimulation of frontal brain regions enhances dopamine efflux in axon terminal areas originating from mesencephalic dopaminergic cell groups. Apart from the hippocampus, the ventral (i.e. nucleus accumbens) and dorsal striatum receive dense dopaminergic projections from the ventral tegmental area and substantia nigra, respectively [41, 42], and might therefore be candidate regions for possible rTMS-induced changes in interneuronal communication. Consistent with the hypothesis that stimulation of frontal brain regions by rTMS may increase dopaminergic neurotransmission in areas other than the hippocampus, it has been reported that direct electrical stimulation of the prefrontal cortex enhances dopamine release in the dorsal striatum and nucleus accumbens [43, 44]. In support of this assumption, we found that rTMS applied under the same conditions also increased dopamine release in the striatum and the nucleus accumbens septi [16, 21, 45]. In this respect, the nucleus accumbens septi is of particular interest as it is a major component of the neural circuitry of reward and incentive motivation, which most likely is dysfunctional not only in depression but also in schizophrenia leading to negative symptoms such as anhedonia and loss of interest [41, 46]. Indeed, preliminary clinical evidence suggests that rTMS might be able to improve negative symptoms in patients suffering from schizophrenia [47, 48]. The release of dopamine in the mesolimbic system is supposed to mediate positive reinforcing effects that ultimately shape behaviours for success accompanied by experience of pleasure, whereas disturbances in dopaminergic transmission could result in dysphoric unrewarding states [49, 50]. Not only natural rewards but also many drugs of abuse such as morphine and cocaine have the ability to increase the extracellular dopamine levels in the nucleus accumbens septi after acute administration [51, 52]. In addition, chronic administration of addictive substances produces a number of adaptive changes in the central nervous system that lead to an increase, such as sensitization, or decrease, such as tolerance, of their behavioural effects [53]. In response to a long-lasting overstimulation of dopaminergic neurons, the normal function of the system seems to become dependent on the presence of the exogenous substance. Therefore, drug abstinence might result in understimulation of dopaminergic neurons followed by a relative lack of dopamine in the mesolimbic system thus producing emotional withdrawal symptoms such as dysphoria and anhedonia in both animal models and humans [54–56]. By investigating the influence of 20-Hz rTMS as a tool in re-establishing the dysregulated intra-accumbal dopamine secretion observed during withdrawal in morphine-sensitized rats, we were able to provide first evidence that acute rTMS is able to increase dopamine concentration in the shell region of the nucleus accumbens in morphine-sensitized rats during abstinence [16]. Thus, rTMS has the potential to gain a therapeutic role in the treatment of dysphoric and anhedonic states during drug withdrawal in humans.

Interestingly, evidence from both preclinical and clinical studies supports our finding of an rTMS-induced increase in dopamine release [57–60] and beneficial effects have increasingly been reported in the treatment of patients suffering from Parkinson's disease [2, 61, 62].

Other studies reported effects of rTMS on the brain serotonergic and noradrenergic systems: Levkovitz et al. [63, 64] demonstrated lasting effects of chronic rTMS (25 Hz) on reactivity of the rat's hippocampus to electrode stimulation of its main excitatory afferent pathway, i.e. the perforant path. A long-lasting reduction in noradrenergic and serotonergic functions in the hippocampus of chronically treated rats was reported and animals showed significant changes in motility in an open field as well as an increase in pain sensitivity [64]. Further, 7 days of rTMS (25 Hz) did not affect single population spikes but caused an increase in paired-pulse inhibition. This effect, which was still evident 3 weeks after the last series of daily rTMS, could also be obtained after a 7-day series of treatment with the antidepressants desipramine and mianserin [63]. The efficacy of rTMS in modulating inhibitory circuits of the hippocampus, however, was found to be drastically reduced in aged rats [65]. This finding may contribute to the understanding of the reduced antidepressant efficacy of rTMS in aged patients [66]. Taken together, the data reported by the Levkovitz group suggest that rTMS (25 Hz) affects local inhibitory circuits more than the main excitatory afferent to the hippocampus. The modulation of local inhibition reported may either be a direct action by increasing the efficacy of inhibition pre- or postsynaptically, or an indirect one by reducing the efficacy of GABAergic modulators, e.g. serotonin [65].

Kole et al. [67] monitored a selective increase in 5-HT1A binding sites in the frontal cortex, the cingulate cortex, and the anterior olfactory nucleus in response to a single train of rTMS (20 Hz). As corticosteroids are well known to play an inhibitory role in 5-HT1A mRNA and protein expression [68, 69], this finding is in line with the observation of an attenuated stress-induced HPA system activity in response to rTMS [15, 20, 23, 36, 70]. 5-HT uptake sites, however, showed no changes after rTMS (20 Hz) [67] whereas changes are described after long-term antidepressant drug treatment [30]. While most antidepressant drugs typically upregulate postsynaptic 5-HT2 receptors, Ben-Shachar et al. [71] found postsynaptic 5-HT2A receptors to be downregulated in the frontal cortex and striatum after 10 days of rTMS (15 Hz). By use of in vivo microdialysis of the prefrontal cortex combined with challenges with a 5-HT1A receptor agonist or a 5-HT1B receptor antagonist subsequent to 10 days of rTMS (15 Hz), subsensitivity of presynaptic serotonergic autoreceptor activity was demonstrated, thus revealing parallels to other antidepressant treatments [72]. Three days of rTMS (25 Hz) were shown to be able to reduce stress-induced increase in serotonin release in frontal cortical regions [38]. In common with other antidepressant treatments,

8 days of rTMS (15 Hz) were shown to reduce the sensitivity of hypothalamic 5-HT1A receptors in rats [73].

Taken together, these findings suggest that the serotonergic system might be one of several possible mediators of rTMS treatment efficacy. rTMS-induced changes in intracerebral dopamine release, however, appear to be of higher clinical relevance.

Hypothalamic-Pituitary-Adrenocortical System

Dynamic changes in HPA system regulation are a well-known feature in major depression [74]: normalization of an initial aberrancy might be predictive of a favourable antidepressant drug treatment response whereas persistent HPA abnormality correlates with therapy resistance or relapse [75]. Stress hormone dysregulation was therefore related to causality of depression suggesting that antidepressants may act through normalization of these HPA changes [76, 77]. Accordingly, findings of blunted hormone responses to stress have been obtained in rats after chronic treatment with various antidepressants [78]. Thus, this neuro-endocrine system was hypothesized to be a common denominator for clinically efficacious antidepressant treatments [79]. In line with the above are the findings on rTMS-induced changes in basal and stress-induced corticotropin (ACTH) and corticosterone plasma levels both in commercially obtained rats [15, 20, 36, 70] and – to a higher extent – in a psychopathological animal model [23] suggesting that rTMS of frontal brain regions attenuates the activity of the HPA system.

Within the limits of neuro-endocrine HPA regulation, it seems clear that corticosteroids suppress corticotropin-releasing hormone (CRH; also termed CRF) and arginine vasopressin (AVP) expression [the main corticotropin (ACTH) secretagogues at the level of the anterior pituitary] through activation of hypothalamic glucocorticoid receptors [80]. The mechanism underlying HPA hyperdrive in depression is still under debate, but clinical studies in patients and probands with high genetic risk are consistent with decreased glucocorticoid receptor and mineralocorticoid receptor function, rendering the cortisol-mediated negative feedback on CRH and AVP expression insufficient [81, 82]. Several groups have shown that treatment of rats with various antidepressant drugs increases the binding capacity and gene expression of mineralocorticoid and glucocorticoid receptors in the hippocampus as well as other limbic and cortical brain areas [78, 83, 84]. Thus, the effects of antidepressants on these receptors may be a key phenomenon in the readjustment of HPA regulation in major depression. To date, it is unclear whether or not in the case of rTMS HPA system regulation is changed due to alterations in mineralocorticoid and glucocorticoid receptor function, or if the blunted stress-induced HPA system activity is achieved via different mechanisms leading to a decrease in CRH and AVP gene expression. Most likely, rTMS-induced changes in the neuro-endocrine regulation occur at the hypothalamic level and the findings of a specific activation in terms of immediate-early gene expression in the paraventricular nucleus of the hypothalamus in response to acute rTMS support this notion [85]. Similarly, changes in the dynamic release patterns of AVP and specific amino acids in this hypothalamic region have been reported [21]. The observation of an rTMS-induced blunted HPA activity is also interesting in the light of findings suggesting that the prefrontal cortex may participate in the regulation of the neuro-endocrine response to stressful stimuli and, in particular, can inhibit HPA system response to stress, i.e. CRH and AVP synthesis and release [86]. Accordingly, projections of the prefrontal cortex to the perinuclear area of the hypothalamic paraventricular nucleus have been demonstrated and major depression is known to be frequently accompanied by frontal cortex dysfunction [46]. Therefore, we hypothesize that rTMS-induced stimulation of frontal brain regions may normalize aberrant neuronal circuit functioning, subsequently leading to a readjustment in hypothalamic CRH and AVP synthesis and release [87]. Thus, in the case of antidepressant drug treatment and chronic rTMS, the neuro-endocrine endpoint (i.e. normalization of HPA system function via regulation of CRH and AVP gene expression) might be reached through different pathways.

Intracerebral Release Pattern of Arginine Vasopressin

As outlined above, specific local neurotransmitter/neuromodulator systems might be particular candidates for rTMS-induced changes in interneuronal communication. There is increasing evidence that neuropeptides are preferentially released and exert their main actions when neurons are strongly activated and under pathological conditions [88, 89]. Accordingly, hyperactivity of central neuropeptidergic circuits such as AVP and CRH neuronal systems is thought to play a causal role in the aetiology and symptomatology of affective disorders [88–90]. There is reason to believe that the brain AVP system can be considered a final common pathway in trait anxiety and depression-like behaviour [91]. In support of this, after prolonged stress, AVP is increasingly expressed and released from hypothalamic neurons in both humans and rodents [92, 93]. Similarly, a markedly increased synthetic activity of hypothalamic AVP neurons has been described in depressed patients [94]. In line with this, administration of a non-peptide AVP V1b receptor antagonist was shown to display anxiolytic and antidepressant-like effects in rodents [95]. The neuropeptide

AVP triggers a variety of central effects on neuro-endocrine, autonomic, emotional and cognitive functions and has been shown to exert behavioural effects such as increased anxiety following intracerebroventricular administration, and to increase CRH-induced ACTH secretion from pituitary corticotrope cells [90, 96]. In this context, it is of interest to note that AVP released into the portal blood is likely to become the primary secretagogue of ACTH in affective disorders, herewith contributing markedly to HPA system dysregulation [97, 98]. The observation that long-term rTMS of frontal brain regions in rats induced an attenuated HPA system response to stress may therefore be related to changes in intraparaventricular nucleus release of AVP [15, 20, 23]. Indeed, a continuous decrease in AVP release of up to 50% in response to acute rTMS was reported to occur in this nucleus [21]. Additional indirect evidence for AVP playing a role in affective disorders derives from the finding that fluoxetine treatment leads to a reduction in cerebrospinal fluid concentrations of AVP in patients with major depression [99]. In support of this, it was shown that long-term treatment with the antidepressant paroxetine is able to decrease hypothalamic AVP mRNA expression in rats [31, 32]. This phenomenon was accompanied by an increase in active stress coping and a normalization of HPA system regulation [31]. These findings further underline the hypothesis that the vasopressinergic system is likely to be critically involved in the behavioural and neuro-endocrine effects of antidepressant treatment [91].

Repetitive Transcranial Magnetic Stimulation-Induced Changes in Brain-Derived Neurotrophic Factor

Brain-derived neurotrophic factor (BDNF) belongs to the family of neurotrophins and was shown to be involved in survival and differentiation in specific areas of the central nervous system as well as in regulating neuronal connectivity and synaptic plasticity [100]. BDNF, which is expressed at high levels in the adult hippocampus, can be upregulated by electrical stimulation and plays a role in hippocampal long-term potentiation, a long-lasting increase in synaptic efficiency related to learning and memory [101]. Both long-term potentiation and long-term depression-like changes after rTMS have been monitored in the gerbil auditory cortex [102]. Moreover, rTMS has been demonstrated to enhance hippocampal long-term potentiation [103, 104].

Chronic rTMS treatment increased BDNF mRNA and protein level in the CA3 region of the hippocampal pyramidal cell layer and in the granule cell layer of the dentate gyrus [7]. Therefore, rTMS might be a stimulus for the release of endogenous BDNF comparable to the effect of direct electrical stimulation in neuronal cells [101]. It is noteworthy that after chronic rTMS treatment

BDNF mRNA and protein expression are increased in exactly the same brain regions as observed after electroconvulsive therapy and antidepressant drug treatment [105]. These findings suggest that a common molecular mechanism may underlie different antidepressant treatment strategies. This again might be achieved via attenuation of HPA system activity that occurs both in response to long-term rTMS and antidepressant drug treatment, as it has been shown that glucocorticoid and mineralocorticoid receptors participate in the control of neurotrophic factor gene expression [106].

Adult Neurogenesis

Accumulating evidence suggests a role of hippocampal neurogenesis in the pathophysiology of depression [107]. Adult neurogenesis is an extremely dynamic process that is regulated in both a positive and negative manner by neuronal activity and environmental factors [108]. Stress-induced structural remodelling in the adult hippocampus may provide a cellular basis for understanding the impairment of neural plasticity in depressive illness. Accordingly, reversal of structural remodelling might be a desirable goal for an antidepressant therapy. Proliferation and maturation of functional neurons have been demonstrated to occur at a significant rate in the adult hippocampus in many different mammalian species including humans [109]. Exposure to psychotropic drugs or stress regulates the rate of neurogenesis in adult brain, suggesting a possible role for neurogenesis in the pathophysiology and treatment of neurobiological illnesses such as depression and post-traumatic stress disorder [110]. In this context, the hypothesis relating stress hormone dysregulation to causality of depression is of interest [77]. In line with the above are the findings on chronic rTMS-induced changes in stress-induced ACTH and corticosterone plasma levels in rats providing evidence that rTMS of frontal brain regions attenuates the stress-induced activity of the HPA system (see above). In a study designed to examine the effects of concomitant rTMS treatment on plasma stress hormone levels and on neurogenesis in the hippocampal dentate gyrus of the adult rat during chronic psychosocial stress, rTMS (20 Hz) normalized the stress-induced elevation of plasma ACTH and corticosterone [15]. An important finding of this study is that the effect of rTMS on plasma stress hormone levels did not parallel the effects on hippocampal neurogenesis: rTMS normalized the stress-induced changes in HPA system activity but had no consistent effect on the stress-induced suppression of hippocampal neurogenesis. Recent studies demonstrated that single and multiple electroconvulsive shocks significantly and dose-dependently increased adult hippocampal neurogenesis in rats and it was hypothesized that this might be an important neurobiological element underlying the clinical effects of electroconvulsive treatment [111]. Similarly, treatment with various types of antidepressant drugs augmented neurogenesis [112]. It should be emphasized, however, that all these studies were conducted on otherwise undisturbed, non-stressed animals. Another possible explanation for the discrepancies in neurobiological findings between electroconvulsive shock, drug treatment and rTMS might be that these treatment strategies may have different effects on various neurobiological circuitries [87]. There is evidence suggesting that serotonin can regulate granule cell production [113]. Consistently, treatment with the serotonin reuptake inhibitor fluoxetine increased neurogenesis [112] and this increase is likely to be mediated, at least in part, by action at the 5-HT1A receptor [114]. Therefore, the findings that neither intrahippocampal release of serotonin [21] nor hippocampal 5-HT1A receptor number and affinity [67] are changed in response to rTMS (20 Hz) presumably also explain why rTMS had no stimulating effect on hippocampal cell proliferation in either stressed or unstressed animals.

Conclusion

An increasing amount of data testifies to the promising potential of rTMS in treating central nervous system disorders by modulating neuronal activity in brain areas involved in pathological processes. Though there are many caveats when trying to relate modulatory effects of rTMS in the rodent brain to rTMS effects in humans, the robust preclinical findings provide, at least in part, an explanation for the neurobiological mechanisms underlying the therapeutic effects reported in clinical trials. As such clinical effects are modest, translational psychiatry should now define which patient and treatment characteristics might lead to greater therapeutic effects with rTMS. In contrast to specificity-driven developments of novel drug actions, rTMS is likely to be a multitarget agent.

There is accumulating evidence that acute rTMS (20 Hz) of frontal brain regions leads to alterations in mesolimbic and mesostriatal release patterns of dopamine. Dopamine-active antidepressant treatment strategies may be of particular benefit in a subgroup of patients with a low level of dopamine function, as reflected by symptoms such as anhedonia, marked psychomotor retardation, concomitant Parkinson's disease or addiction. rTMS-induced modulation of dopaminergic neurotransmission in brain circuitries relevant to incentive motivation, e.g. might represent a new approach to the treatment of substance abuse-related disorders [16]. Accordingly, the identification of such patients with a putative deficit in dopaminergic neurotransmission related to psychopathology might lead to a better antidepressant efficacy of rTMS beyond the only moderate and rather short-lived therapeutic effects reported so far.

Acknowledgements

The transcranial magnetic stimulation studies at the Max Planck Institute of Psychiatry in Munich were supported by the German Federal Research Ministry within the promotional emphasis 'Competence Nets in Medicine' (Kompetenznetz Depression und Suizidalität; subproject 4.5, grant to M.E.K.) and by the Bavarian Research Ministry (Bayerischer Habilitationsförderpreis to M.E.K.). The author would like to acknowledge the excellent scientific work of Drs. Angelika Erhardt, Tobias Welt, Marianne B. Müller, Frauke Ohl, Mario Engelmann, Karl Ebner, Rainer Landgraf, Anke Post, Inge Sillaber and Nicola Toschi.

References

1 Padberg F, Zwanzger P, Keck ME, Kathmann N, Mikhaiel P, Ella R, Rupprecht P, Thoma H, Hampel H, Toschi N, Möller HJ: Repetitive transcranial magnetic stimulation (rTMS) in major depression: relation between efficacy and stimulation intensity. Neuropsychopharmacology 2002;27:638–645.

2 Siebner HR, Rothwell J: Transcranial magnetic stimulation: new insights into representational cortical plasticity. Exp Brain Res 2003;148:1–16.

3 Wassermann EM: Side effects of repetitive transcranial magnetic stimulation. Depress Anxiety 2000;12:124–129.

4 Keck ME, Pijnappels M, Schubert M, Colombo G, Curt A, Dietz V: Stumbling reactions in man: influence of corticospinal input. Electroencephalogr Clin Neurophysiol 1998;109:215–223.

5 Rossini PM, Barker AT, Berardelli A, Caramia MD, Caruso G, Cracco RQ, Dimitrijevic MR, Hallett M, Katayama Y, Lücking CH, Maertens de Noordhout AL, Marsden CD, Murray NMF, Swash M, Tomberg C: Non-invasive electrical and magnetic stimulation of the brain, spinal cord and roots: basic principles and procedures for routine clinical application. Electroencephalogr Clin Neurophysiol 1994;91:79–92.

6 Jennum P, Klitgaard H: Repetitive transcranial stimulations of the rat: effect of acute and chronic stimulations on pentylenetetrazole-induced clonic seizures. Epilepsy Res 1996;23:115–122.

7 Müller MB, Toschi N, Kresse AE, Post A, Keck ME: Long-term repetitive transcranial magnetic stimulation increases the expression of brain-derived neurotrophic factor and cholecystokinin mRNA, but not neuropeptide tyrosine mRNA in specific areas of rat brain. Neuropsychopharmacology 2000;23:205–215.

8 Luft AR, Kaelin-Lang A, Hauser TK, Cohen LG, Thakor NV, Hanley DF: Transcranial magnetic stimulation in the rat. Exp Brain Res 2001;140:112–122.

9 Hargreaves GA, McGregor IS, Sachdev PS: Chronic repetitive transcranial magnetic stimulation is antidepressant but not anxiolytic in rat models of anxiety and depression. Psychiatry Res 2005;137:113–121.

10 Padberg F, Möller HJ: rTMS: does it have potential in the treatment of depression? CNS Drugs 2003;17:383–403.

11 Loo C, Mitchell P, Sachdev P, McDarmont B, Parker G, Gandevia S: Double-blind controlled investigation of transcranial magnetic stimulation for the treatment of resistant major depression. Am J Psychiatry 1999;156:946–948.

12 Belmaker RH, Grisaru N: Magnetic stimulation of the brain in animal depression models responsive to ECS. J ECT 1998;14:194–205.

13 Lisanby SH, Datto CJ, Szuba MP: ECT and transcranial magnetic stimulation: past, present and future. Depress Anxiety 2002;12:115–117.

14 Post A, Muller MB, Engelmann M, Keck ME: Repetitive transcranial magnetic stimulation in rats: evidence for a neuroprotective effect in vitro and in vivo. Eur J Neurosci 1999;11:3247–3254.

15 Czéh B, Welt T, Fischer AK, Erhardt A, Schmitt W, Mueller MB, Toschi N, Fuchs E, Keck ME: Chronic psychosocial stress and concomitant repetitive transcranial magnetic stimulation: effects

on stress hormone levels and adult hippocampal neurogenesis. Biol Psychiatry 2002;52: 1057–1065.
16 Erhardt A, Sillaber I, Welt T, Müller MB, Singewald N, Keck ME: Repetitive transcranial magnetic stimulation increases the release of dopamine in the nucleus accumbens shell of morphine-sensitized rats during abstinence. Neuropsychopharmacology 2004;29:2074–2080.
17 Keck ME: The neurobiological basis of therapeutic use of repetitive transcranial magnetic stimulation (rTMS) in psychiatric disorders. Nervenheilkunde 2003;22:253–260.
18 Keck ME: Repetitive transcranial magnetic stimulation as a treatment strategy in psychiatric disorders – Neurobiological concepts. Clin Neurophysiol 2003;56:100–116.
19 Keck ME: Repetitive transkranielle Magnetstimulation (rTMS) – Anwendung bei Depression. Med Monatsschr Pharm 2003;26:227–232.
20 Keck ME, Engelmann M, Müller MB, Henninger MSH, Hermann B, Rupprecht R, Neumann I, Toschi N, Landgraf R, Post RM: Repetitive transcranial magnetic stimulation induces active coping strategies and attenuates the neuroendocrine stress response in rats. J Psychiatr Res 2000;34: 265–276.
21 Keck ME, Sillaber I, Ebner K, Welt T, Toschi N, Kaehler ST, Singewald N, Phillippu A, Elbel GK, Holsboer F, Landgraf R, Engelmann M: Acute transcranial magnetic stimulation of frontal brain regions selectively modulates the release of vasopressin, biogenic amines and amino acids in the rat brain. Eur J Neurosci 2000;12:3713–3720.
22 Keck ME, Welt T, Erhardt A, Müller MB, Sillaber I: Neuroendocrinological changes induced by transcranial magnetic stimulation (rTMS) – A focus on dopamine and vasopressin. Nervenheilkunde 2003;22:326–349.
23 Keck ME, Welt T, Post A, Müller MB, Toschi N, Wigger A, Landgraf R, Holsboer F, Engelmann M: Neuroendocrine and behavioral effects of repetitive transcranial magnetic stimulation in a psychopathological animal model are suggestive of antidepressant-like effects. Neuropsychopharmacology 2001;24:337–349.
24 Geyer MA, Markou A: Animal models of psychiatric disorders; in Bloom FE, Kupfer DJ (eds): Psychopharmacology: The Fourth Generation of Progress. New York, Raven Press, 1995, pp 787–798.
25 Geyer MA, Markou A: The role of preclinical models in the development of psychotropic drugs; in Davis KL, Charney DS, Coyle JT, Nemeroff CB (eds): Neuropsychopharmacology. The Fifth Generation of Progress. Philadelphia, Lippincott, Williams & Wilkins, 2002, pp 445–456.
26 Holsboer F: Animal models of mood disorders; in Charney DS, Nestler EJ, Bunney BS (eds): Neurobiology of Mental Illness. New York, Oxford University Press, 1999, pp 317–332.
27 Müller MB, Keck ME: Genetically engineered mice for studies of stress-related clinical conditions. J Psychiatr Res 2002;36:53–76.
28 Keck ME, Ohl F, Holsboer F, Müller MB: Listening to mutant mice: a spotlight on the role of CRF/CRF receptor systems in affective disorders. Neurosci Biobehav Rev 2005;29:867–889.
29 Landgraf R, Wigger A: High versus low anxiety-related behavior rats: an animal model of extremes in trait anxiety. Behav Genet 2002;32:301–314.
30 Keck ME, Sartori SB, Welt T, Muller MB, Ohl F, Holsboer F, Landgraf R, Singewald N: Differences in serotonergic neurotransmission between rats displaying high or low anxiety/depression-like behaviour: effects of chronic paroxetine treatment. J Neurochem 2005;92:1170–1179.
31 Keck ME, Welt T, Müller MB, Uhr M, Ohl F, Wigger A, Toschi N, Holsboer F, Landgraf R: Reduction of hypothalamic vasopressinergic hyperdrive contributes to clinically relevant behavioral and neuroendocrine effects of chronic paroxetine treatment in a psychopathological rat model. Neuropsychopharmacology 2003;28:235–243.
32 Keck ME, Wigger A, Welt T, Müller MB, Gesing A, Reul JMHM, Holsboer F, Landgraf R, Neumann I: Vasopressin mediates the response of the combined dexamethasone/CRH test in hyper-anxious rats: implications for pathogenesis of affective disorders. Neuropsychopharmacology 2002;26:94–105.
33 Cryan JF, Markou A, Lucki I: Assessing antidepressant activity in rodents: recent developments and future needs. Trends Pharmacol Sci 2002;23:238–245.
34 Zyss T, Gorka Z, Kowalska M, Vetulani J: Preliminary comparison of behavioral and biochemical effects of chronic transcranial magentic stimulation and electroconvulsive shock in rat. Biol Psychiatry 1997;42:920–924.

35 Sachdev P, McBride R, Loo C, Mitchell PM, Malhi GS, Croker V: Effects of different frequencies of transcranial magnetic stimulation (TMS) on the forced swim test model of depression in rats. Biol Psychiatry 2002;51:474–479.
36 Hedges DW, Massari C, Salyer DL, Lund TD, Hellewell JL, Johnson AC, Lephart ED: Duration of transcranial magnetic stimulation effects on the neuroendocrine stress response and coping behavior of adult male rats. Prog Neuropsychopharmacol Biol Psychiatry 2003;27:633–638.
37 Benmansour S, Cecchi M, Morilak DA, Gerhardt GA, Javors MA, Gould GG, Frazer A: Effects of chronic antidepressant treatments on serotonin transporter function, density, and mRNA level. J Neurosci 1999;19:10494–10501.
38 Kanno M, Matsumoto M, Togashi H, Yoshioka M, Mano Y: Effects of repetitive transcranial magnetic stimulation on behavioral and neurochemical changes in rats during an elevated plus-maze test. J Neurol Sci 2003;211:5–14.
39 Blier P, de Montigny C: Current advances and trends in the treatment of depression. Trends Pharmacol Sci 1994;15:220–226.
40 Sesack SR, Pickel VM: Prefrontal cortex efferents in the rat synapse on unlabeled neuronal targets of catecholamine terminals in the nucleus accumbens septi and on dopamine neurons in the ventral tegmental area. J Comp Neurol 1992;320:145–160.
41 Fibiger HC: Neurobiology of depression: focus on dopamine. Adv Biochem Psychopharmacol 1995;49:1–17.
42 Feldman RS, Meyer JS, Quenzer LF: Principles of Neuropsychopharmacology. Sunderland, Sinauer, 1997.
43 Taber MT, Das S, Fibiger HC: Cortical regulation of subcortical dopamine release: mediation via the ventral tegmental area. J Neurochem 1995;65:1407–1410.
44 You ZB, Tzschentke TM, Brodin E, Wise RA: Electrical stimulation of the prefrontal cortex increases cholecystokinin, glutamate, and dopamine release in the nucleus accumbens: an in vivo microdialysis study in freely moving rats. J Neurosci 1998;18:6492–6500.
45 Keck ME, Welt T, Muller MB, Erhardt A, Ohl F, Toschi N, Holsboer F, Sillaber I: Repetitive transcranial magnetic stimulation increases the release of dopamine in the mesolimbic and mesostriatal system. Neuropharmacology 2002;43:101–109.
46 Nestler EJ, Barrot M, DiLeone RJ, Eisch AJ, Gold SJ, Monteggia LM: Neurobiology of depression. Neuron 2002;34:13–25.
47 Cohen E, Bernado M, Masana J, Arrufat FJ, Navarro V, Valls-Solé J, Boget T, Barrantes N, Catarineu S, Font M, Lomena FJ: Repetitive transcranial magnetic stimulation in the treatment of chronic negative schizophrenia: a pilot study. J Neurol Neurosurg Psychiatry 1999;67:129–130.
48 Rollnik JD, Huber TJ, Mogk H, Siggelkow S, Kropp S, Dengler R, Emrich HM, Schneider U: High frequency repetitive transcranial magnetic stimulation of the dorsolateral prefrontal cortex in schizophrenic patients. Neuroreport 2000;11:4013–4015.
49 Di Chiara G: Nucleus accumbens shell and core dopamine: differential roles in associative learning and drug addiction. Behav Pharmacol 2002;13:481–482.
50 Di Chiara G: Cortical and limbic dopamine (on opiate addiction): do not mix before use! Trends Pharmacol Sci 1997;18:77–78.
51 Di Chiara G, Imperato A: Preferential stimulation of dopamine release in the nucleus accumbens by opiates, alcohol, and barbiturates: studies with transcerebral dialysis in freely moving rats. Ann NY Acad Sci 1986;473:367–381.
52 Maisonneuve IM, Warner LM, Glick SD: Biphasic dose-related effects of morphine on dopamine release. Drug Alcohol Depend 2001;65:55–63.
53 Nestler EJ: From neurobiology to treatment: progress against addiction. Nature Neurosci 2002;5:1076–1079.
54 Acquas E, Di Chiara G: Depression of mesolimbic dopamine transmission and sensitization to morphine during opiate abstinence. J Neurochem 1992;58:1620–1625.
55 Ahtee L, Attila LM, Carlson KR, Haikala H: Changes in brain monoamine metabolism during withdrawal from chronic oral self-administration of morphine and in response to a morphine challenge in the withdrawn state. J Pharmacol Exp Ther 1989;249:303–310.
56 Volkow ND, Fowler JS, Wang GJ: Role of dopamine in drug reinforcement and addiction in humans: results from imaging studies. Behav Pharmacol 2002;13:355–366.

57 Strafella AP, Paus T, Barrett J, Dagher A: Repetitive transcranial magnetic stimulation of the human prefrontal cortex induces dopamine release in the caudate nucleus. J Neurosci 2001;21: RC157.
58 Pogarell O, Koch W, Popperl G, Tatsch K, Jakob F, Zwanzger P, Mulert C, Rupprecht R, Möller HJ, Hegerl U, Padberg F: Striatal dopamine release after prefrontal repetitive transcranial magnetic stimulation in major depression: preliminary results of a dynamic [^{123}I] IBZM SPECT study. J Psychiatr Res 2006;40:307–314.
59 Funamizu H, Ogiue-Ikeda M, Mukai H, Kawato S, Ueno S: Acute repetitive transcranial magnetic stimulation reactivates dopaminergic system in lesion rats. Neurosci Lett 2005;383:77–81.
60 Ohnishi T, Hayashi T, Okabe S, Nonaka I, Matsuda H, Iida H, Imabayashi E, Watabe H, Miyake Y, Ogawa M, Teramoto N, Ohta Y, Ejima N, Sawada T, Ugawa Y: Endogenous dopamine release induced by repetitive transcranial magnetic stimulation over the primary motor cortex: an [^{11}C]raclopride positron emission tomography study in anesthetized macaque monkeys. Biol Psychiatry 2004;55:484–489.
61 Lomarev MP, Kanchana S, Bara-Jimenez W, Iyer M, Wassermann EM, Hallett M: Placebo-controlled study of rTMS for the treatment of Parkinson's disease. Mo Disord 2006;21:325–331.
62 Fregni F, Ono CR, Santos CM, Bermpohl F, Buchpiguel C, Barbosa ER, Marcolin MA, Pascual-Leone A, Valente KD: Effects of antidepressant treatment with rTMS and fluoxetine on brain perfusion in PD. Neurology 2006;66:1629–1637.
63 Levkovitz Y, Grisaru N, Segal M: Transcranial magnetic stimulation and antidepressive drugs share similar cellular effects in rat hippocampus. Neuropsychopharmacology 2001;25:608–616.
64 Levkovitz Y, Marx J, Grisaru N, Segal M: Long-term effects of transcranial magnetic stimulation on hippocampal reactivity to afferent stimulation. J Neurosci 1999;19:3198–3203.
65 Levkovitz Y, Segal M: Aging affects transcranial magnetic modulation of hippocampal evoked potentials. Neurobiol Aging 2001;22:255–263.
66 Mosimann UP, Marre SC, Werlen S, Schmitt W, Hess CW, Fisch HU, Schlaepfer TE: Antidepressant effects of rTMS in the elderly: correlation between effect size and coil-cortex distance. Arch Gen Psychiatry 2002;59:560–561.
67 Kole MHP, Fuchs E, Ziemann U, Paulus W, Ebert U: Changes in 5-HT1A and NMDA binding sites by a single rapid transcranial magnetic stimulation procedure in rats. Brain Res 1999;826:309–312.
68 Chalmers DT, Kwak SP, Mansour A, Akil H, Watson SJ: Corticosteroids regulate brain hippocampal 5-HT1A receptor mRNA expression. J Neurosci 1993;13:914–923.
69 Chaouloff F: Regulation of 5-HT receptors by corticosteroids: where do we stand? Fundam Clin Pharmacol 1955;9:219–233.
70 Hedges DW, Salyer DL, Higginbotham BJ, Lund TD, Hellewell JL, Ferguson D, Lephart ED: Transcranial magnetic stimulation (TMS) effects on testosterone, prolactin, and corticosterone in adult male rats. Biol Psychiatry 2002;51:417–421.
71 Ben-Shachar D, Gazawi H, Riboyad-Levin J, Klein E: Chronic repetitive transcranial magnetic stimulation alters alpha-adrenergic and 5-HT2 receptor characteristics in rat brain. Brain Res 1999;816:78–83.
72 Gur E, Lerer B, Dremencov E, Newman ME: Chronic repetitive transcranial magnetic stimulation induces subsensitivity of presynaptic serotonergic autoreceptor activity in rat brain. Neuroreport 2000;11:2925–2929.
73 Gur E, Lerer B, de Kar LDV, Newman ME: Chronic rTMS induces subsensitivity of post-synaptic 5-HT1A receptors in rat hypothalamus. Int J Neuropsychopharmacol 2004;7:335–340.
74 Tichomirowa MA, Keck ME, Schneider HJ, Paez-Pereda M, Renner U, Holsboer F, Stalla GK: Endocrine disturbances in depression. J Endocrinol Invest 2005;28:89–99.
75 Keck ME, Holsboer F: Hyperactivity of CRH neuronal circuits as a target for therapeutic interventions in affective disorders. Peptides 2001;22:835–844.
76 Binder EB, Salyakina D, Lichtner P, Wochnik GM, Ising M, Pütz B, Papiol S, DSeaman S, Lucae S, Kohli MA, Nickel T, Künzel HE, Fuchs B, Majer M, Pfennig A, Kern N, Brunner J, Modell S, Baghai T, Deiml T, Zill P, Bondy B, Rupprecht R, Messer T, Köhnlein O, Dabitz H, Brückl T, Mülller N, Pfister H, Lieb R, Muelllr JC, Lohmussar E, Strom TM, Bettecken T, Meitinger T, Uhr M, Rein T, Holsboer F, Muller-Myhsok B: Polymorphisms in FKBP5 are associated with increased

recurrence of depressive episodes and rapid response to antidepressant treatment. Nat Genet 2004;36:1319–1325.
77 Holsboer F: The corticosteroid receptor hypothesis of depression. Neuropsychopharmacology 2000;23:477–501.
78 Reul JMHM, Gesing A, Droste S, Stec ISM, Weber A, Bachmann C, Bilang-Bleuel A, Holsboer F, Linthorst ACE: The brain mineralocorticoid receptor: greedy for ligand, mysterious in function. Eur J Pharmacol 2000;405:235–249.
79 Holsboer F, Barden N: Antidepressants and hypothalamic-pituitary-adrenocortical regulation. Endocr Rev 1996;17:187–205.
80 de Kloet ER, Joels M, Holsboer F: Stress and the brain: from adaptation to disease. Nat Rev Neurosci 2005;6:463–475.
81 López JF, Chalmers DT, Littler KY, Watson SJ: Regulation of serotonin 1A, glucocorticoid, and mineralocorticoid receptor in rat and human hippocampus: implications for the neurobiology of depression. Biol Psychiatry 1998;43:547–573.
82 Holsboer F: Corticotropin-releasing hormone modulators and depression. Curr Opin Investig Drugs 2003;4:46–50.
83 Brady LS, Whitfield HJ, Fox RJ, Gold PW, Herkenham M: Long-term antidepressant administration alters corticotropin-releasing hormone, tyrosine hydroxylase, and mineralocorticoid receptor gene expression in rat brain. J Clin Invest 1991;87:831–837.
84 Seckl JR, Olsson T: Glucocorticoid hypersecretion and the age-impaired hippocampus: cause or effect? J Endocrinol 1995;145:201–211.
85 Ji RR, Schlaepfer TE, Aizenman CD, Epstein CM, Qiu D, Huang JC, Rupp F: Repetitive transcranial magnetic stimulation activates specific regions in rat brain. Med Sci 1998;95:15635–15640.
86 Diorio D, Viau V, Meaney M: The role of the medial prefrontal cortex (cingulate gyrus) in the regulation of hypothalamic-pituitary-adrenal response to stress. J Neurosci 1993;13:3839–3847.
87 Post A, Keck ME: Transcranial magnetic stimulation as a therapeutic tool in psychiatry: what do we know about the neurobiological mechanisms? J Psychiatr Res 2001;35:193–215.
88 Hökfelt T, Bartfai T, Bloom F: Neuropeptides: opportunities for drug discovery. Lancet Neurol 2003;2:463–472.
89 Hökfelt T, Broberger C, Xu ZQD, Sergeyev V, Ubink R, Diez M: Neuropeptides – An overview. Neuropharmacology 2000;39:1337–1356.
90 Landgraf R, Neumann ID: Vasopressin and oxytocin release within the brain: a dynamic concept of multiple and variable modes of neuropeptide communication. Front Neuroendocrinol 2004;25: 150–176.
91 Landgraf R, Holsboer F: The involvement of neuropeptides in evolution, signaling, behavioral regulation and psychopathology: focus on vasopressin. Drug Dev Res 2005;65:185–190.
92 Antoni FA: Vasopressinergic control of pituitary-adrenocorticotropin secretion comes of age. Front Neuroendocrinol 1993;14:76–122.
93 Keck ME, Hatzinger M, Wotjak C, Landgraf R, Holsboer F, Neumann ID: Ageing alters intrahypothalamic release patterns of vasopressin and oxytocin in rats. Eur J Neurosci 2000;12: 1487–1494.
94 Purba JS, Hoogendijk WJG, Hofman MA, Swaab DF: Increased number of vasopressin- and oxytocin-expressing neurons in the paraventricular nucleus of the hypothalamus in depression. Arch Gen Psychiatry 1996;53:137–143.
95 Griebel G, Simiand J, Serradeil-Le Gal C, Wagnon J, Pascal M, Scatton B, Maffrand JP, Soubrié P: Anxiolytic- and antidepressant-like effects of the non-peptide vasopressin V1b receptor antagonist, SSR149415, suggest an innovative approach for the treatment of stress-related disorders. Proc Natl Acad Sci USA 2002;99:6370–6375.
96 Engelmann M, Landgraf R, Wotjak CT: The hypothalamic-neurohypophysial system regulates the hypothalamic-pituitary-adrenal axis under stress: an old concept revisited. Front Neuroendocrinol 2004;25:132–149.
97 von Bardeleben U, Holsboer F, Stalla GK, Müller OA: Combined administration of human corticotropin-releasing factor and lysine vasopressin induces cortisol escape from dexamethasone suppression in healthy subjects. Life Sci 1985;37:1613–1618.

98 Holsboer F: The role of peptides in treatment of psychiatric disorders. J Neural Transm 2003;64:17–34.
99 De Bellis MD, Gold PW, Geracioti TDJ, Listwak SJ, Kling MA: Association of fluoxetine treatment with reductions in CSF concentrations of corticotropin-releasing hormone and arginine vasopressin in patients with major depression. Am J Psychiatry 1993;150:656–657.
100 Lewin GR, Barde YA: Physiology of neurotrophins. Ann Rev Neurosci 1996;19:289–317.
101 Balkowiec A, Katz DM: Activity-dependent release of endogenous brain-derived neurotrophic factor from primary sensory neurons detected by ELISA in situ. J Neurosci 2000;20:7417–7423.
102 Wang H, Wang X, Scheich H: LTD and LTP induced by transcranial magnetic stimulation in auditory cortex. Neuroreport 1996;7:521–525.
103 Ogiue-Ikeda M, Kawato S, Ueno S: The effect of repetitive transcranial magnetic stimulation on long-term potentiation in rat hippocampus depends on stimulus intensity. Brain Res 2003;993: 222–226.
104 Ahmed Z, Wieraszko A: Modulation of learning and hippocampal, neuronal plasticity by repetitive transcranial magnetic stimulation (rTMS). Bioelectromagnetics 2006;27:288–294.
105 Nibuya M, Morinobu S, Duman RS: Regulation of BDNF and trkB mRNA in the rat brainn by chronic electroconvulsive seizure and antidepressant drug treatments. J Neurosci 1995;15: 7539–7547.
106 Hansson AC, Cintra A, Belluardo N, Sommer W, Bhatnagar M, Bader M, Ganten D, Fuxe K: Gluco- and mineralocorticoid receptor-mediated regulation of neurotrophic factor gene expression in the dorsal hippocampus and the neocortex of the rat. Eur J Neurosci 2000;12:2918–2934.
107 Dranovsky A, Hen R: Hippocampal neurogenesis: regulation by stress and antidepressants. Biol Psychiatry 2006;59:1136–1143.
108 Gould E, Fuchs E: In vivo neurogenesis in the adult brain: regulation and functional implications. Eur J Neurosci 2000;12:2211–2214.
109 Van Praag H, Schinder AF, Christie BR, Toni N, Palmer TD, Gage FH: Functional neurogenesis in the adult hippocampus. Nature 2002;415:1030–1034.
110 Duman RS, Malberg JE, Thome J: Neural plasticity to stress and antidepressant treatment. Biol Psychiatry 1999;46:1181–1191.
111 Madsen TM, Treschow A, Bengzon J, Bolwig TG, Lindvall O, Tingström A: Increased neurogenesis in a model of ECT. Biol Psychiatry 2000;47:1043–1049.
112 Malberg JE, Eisch AJ, Nestler EJ, Duman RS: Chronic antidepressant treatment increases neurogenesis in adult rat hippocampus. J Neurosci 2000;20:9104–9110.
113 Brezun JM, Daszuta A: Depletion in serotonin decreases neurogenesis in the dentate gyrus and the subventricular zone of adult rats. Neuroscience 1999;89:999–1002.
114 Jacobs BL, Van Praag H, Gage FH: Adult brain neurogenesis and psychiatry: a novel theory of depression. Mol Psychiatry 2000;5:262–269.

Martin E. Keck, MD, PhD, MSc
Klinik Schlössli AG
Privatklinik für Psychiatrie und Psychotherapie
CH–8618 Oetwil am See/Zürich (Switzerland)
Tel. +41 44 929 82 45, Fax +41 44 929 84 50, E-Mail martin.keck@schloessli.ch

Marcolin MA, Padberg F (eds): Transcranial Brain Stimulation for Treatment of Psychiatric Disorders.
Adv Biol Psychiatr. Basel, Karger, 2007, vol 23, pp 35–52

Neuroimaging of Repetitive Transcranial Magnetic Stimulation Effects on the Brain

Mark S. George, Daryl E. Bohning, Xingbao Li, Ziad Nahas, Stewart Denslow, David Ramsey, Donna R. Roberts, Kevin Johnson, Raffaella Ricci, Jeffrey J. Borckardt

Brain Stimulation Laboratory and Center for Advanced Imaging Research, Departments of Psychiatry, Radiology and Neurology, Medical University of South Carolina, Charleston, S.C., USA

Abstract

Brain imaging can tell us a lot about how transcranial magnetic stimulation (TMS) affects the brain, and it can also help us guide and deliver TMS in more precise ways. For example, one can use structural or functional brain imaging to precisely position the TMS coil over the proper scalp position to interact with the brain. This chapter focuses on studies that have used brain imaging to understand exactly how TMS is influencing and affecting the brain. Researchers have now used the full quiver of imaging methods to address this issue. While there is still much more work to be done, studies to date reveal that TMS acts locally to change brain activity under the coil, with secondary, transynaptic effects. Different frequencies of stimulation divergently affect the brain, with some effects lasting beyond the acute stimulation. The intensity of stimulation matters, with effects following the known physics of TMS. Using brain imaging to better understand the translational neurobiological effects of TMS offers the promise of eventually using TMS in much more sophisticated ways to change brain function and treat illnesses. In this chapter, we overview this rapidly advancing field by posing a series of relatively simple questions, and responding to them informed by TMS and brain imaging studies.

How Deep into the Brain Does Transcranial Magnetic Stimulation Directly Stimulate?

This is one of the simplest questions one can ask regarding transcranial magnetic stimulation (TMS), but the answer is a little complex. The actual field

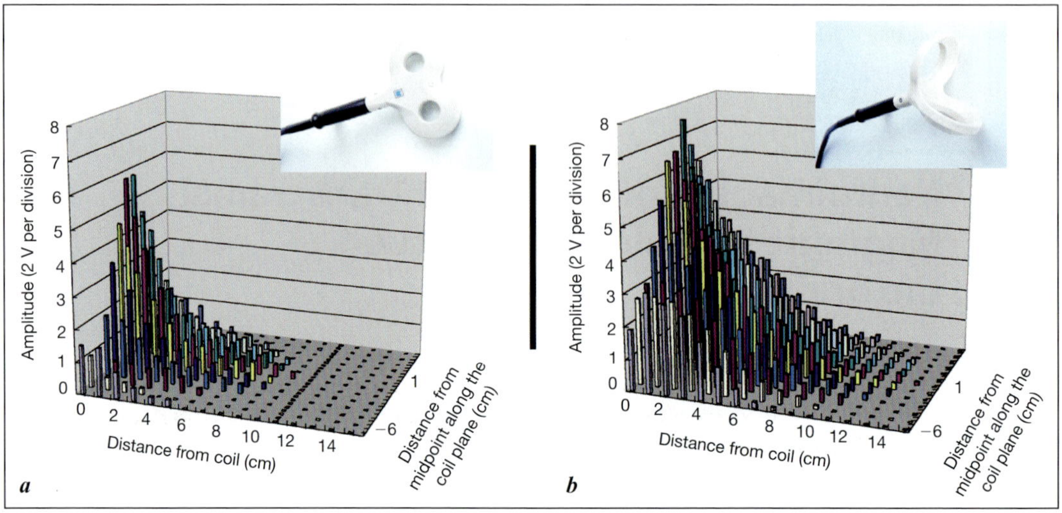

Fig. 1. These are graphical maps of the magnitude of induced electric fields as a function of the lateral and distal distance from the center of the standard flat figure-of-eight coil (***a***, pictured in the insert) and a larger double-cone coil (***b***, also pictured in the insert). These were generated by placing a copper wire coil at different parts of a grid and measuring the induced current. Note that the larger double-cone coil stimulates deeper into the brain, and is also wider (photo courtesy of the MUSC Brain Stimulation Laboratory).

shapes of different TMS coils are well known and can be measured and imaged away from the brain using arrays of sensors. Figure 1 shows an example of how one can calculate the magnetic field shape of simple and more complex coils outside of the brain.

Bohning et al. [1] discovered that one could use a modified TMS coil and a conventional MRI scanner to directly image the magnetic field produced by a TMS coil. This image, called an MRI phase map, accurately displays the TMS magnetic field [1]. Current theories hold however that the induced electrical field carries much of the neurobiologic effect of TMS, and thus imaging the magnetic field is only partially the answer to knowing where TMS is acting in the brain [2, 3]. However, new advances in MRI scanning might allow MRI also to image the TMS-induced electrical field – a development which would be enormously helpful in determining the neurobiological effects of TMS [4–6].

Does the Depth Change with Different Coils?

Yes. Figures 2 and 3 demonstrate the phase map produced by a flat figure-of-eight coil on the scalp. Note how the magnetic field drops off rapidly with

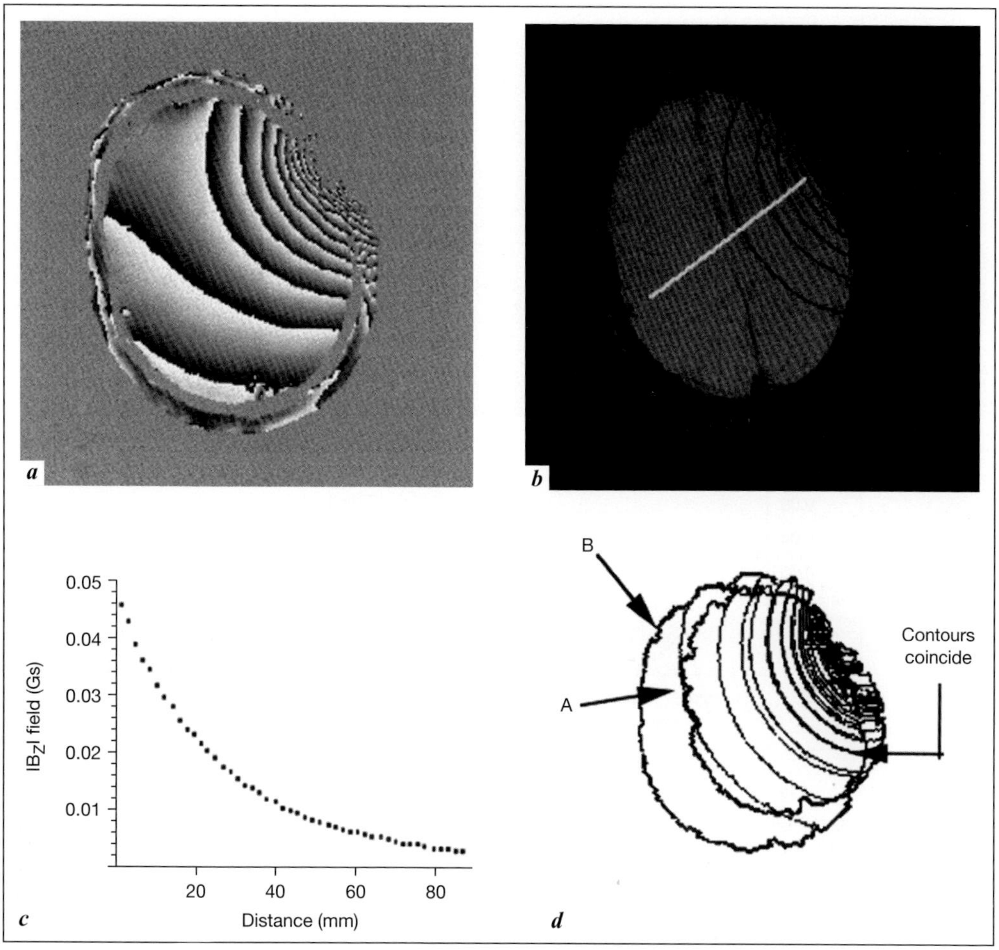

Fig. 2. Phase maps of a TMS coil over the temporal lobe and energized with a 50-mA DC current. ***a*** An MRI phase image of the brain. ***b*** A structural MRI brain scan has the magnitude from the phase map superimposed. ***c*** A plot of the TMS magnetic field intensity along the white line shown in (***b***). Note the sharp drop-off. ***d*** Multiple contour maps from different individuals are shown on the same image. Note that there is no difference from person to person, as the magnetic field induced by TMS is not affected by soft tissue.

distance from the coil. Thus, with most of the coils used today, TMS directly stimulates the cortex only about 2–3 cm away from the coil surface. Larger figure-of-eight coils, like the one pictured in figure 1, can stimulate deeper than others. Importantly, in this early study, Bohning et al. [1] also experimented with the idea of whether placing multiple coils on the scalp and stimulating them in phase

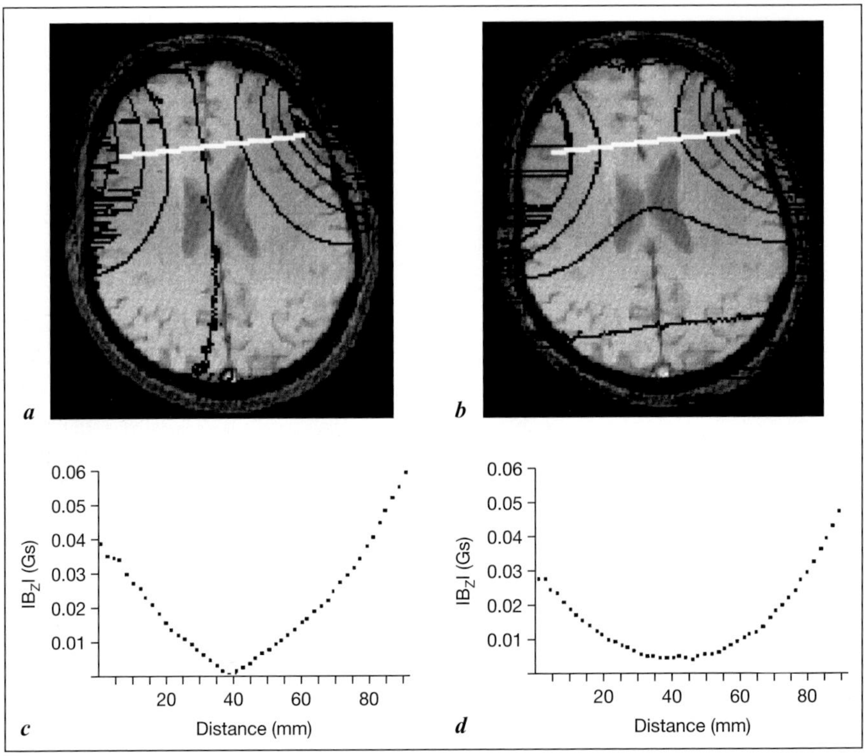

Fig. 3. Transverse images of the brain with the field intensity contours from two coils superimposed. ***a*** The coils have opposite polarity. ***b*** The coils have the same polarity. ***c, d*** The field intensity along the white lines above is shown. Note that when the coils have the same polarity, there is a small rise in TMS intensity in the center of the brain. Work like this raises the hope of eventually creating TMS devices that can focally stimulate deep in the brain (from Bohning et al. [1], reprinted with permission).

might summate stimulation deep in the brain. While this may work, it is still necessary to stimulate the superficial cortex under the skull with high amounts of magnetic field. That is, it is not easy to focus the TMS magnetic field such that you produce only stimulation of deep tissues, while sparing the superficial cortex. While there are groups working on building ever more powerful coils that can stimulate deeper, they do not spare the superficial cortex [7, 8].

How Do We Determine the Minimum Intensity Needed to Reach the Brain?

Without involving brain imaging, one can search for and find the scalp location over the motor cortex for the hand, and then determine the minimum stimulation needed to stimulate the hand, referred to as the motor threshold (MT). The MT is relatively stable for a given individual over time, but varies widely between individuals. Kozel et al. [9] used MRI to measure the scalp-to-cortex distance in healthy adults and then correlated this with each person's MT. Approximately 60% of the between-subject MT variation is due to differences in the scalp-to-cortex distance [9, 10]. As one would expect, more distance correlates with a higher MT.

But How Do We Determine the Amount Needed to Stimulate Nonmotor Areas, Where TMS Does Not Produce an Observable Response, and Thus There Is No Functional Threshold?

To begin to address this issue, Kozel et al. [9] acquired structural MRI scans in depressed subjects undergoing a depression treatment trial and measured the distance from the TMS coil (indicated by a marker or fiducial on the scan) to the closest edge of the prefrontal cortex [11]. This distance did not correlate with TMS antidepressant response. However, the distance did correlate with advancing age (the older the subject, the more space between the scalp and cortex) [9]. In that trial and others [12], TMS was not effective in treating older depressed subjects, and stimulating at 100% of MT, no one with a distance greater than 1.6 mm (or age greater than 50) responded. These MRI distance measurements suggested that one reason for TMS nonresponse in older depressed subjects might be that a higher intensity of stimulation is needed to reach the cortex that is further away from the coil. The correlation of poor antidepressant response with greater prefrontal atrophy has been confirmed in another clinical study [13], and then elaborated in a single photon emission computed tomography (SPECT) imaging study [14]. Using a formula developed by Daryl Bohning for a first approximation correction of the MT for cortex depth, one can calculate the MT, and the motor and prefrontal distance for each subject. Then one can confidently deliver, for each person, a TMS intensity over the prefrontal cortex equivalent, to first approximation, to that which causes movement in the subject's thumb when delivered over the motor cortex. Nahas et al. [15] did just that in a group of elderly depressed subjects, with good clinical response. Interestingly, no one needed greater than 120% of their MT to reach the prefrontal cortex.

What Do Imaging Studies Tell Us about TMS Safety?

MRI scans of depressed patients before and after a TMS treatment trial failed to find any radiographic evidence of TMS-induced changes, and careful measurement of the prefrontal volume failed to find a difference before and after treatment [16]. Diffusion tensor MRI allows one to examine the directional flow of water within the brain [4]. Diffusion tensor imaging (DTI) is therefore extremely sensitive to subtle brain trauma, and is used in the acute management and detection of stroke [17–19]. To investigate whether TMS changes diffusion, Li and colleagues initially performed DTI scans on 14 depressed patients before and then immediately after prefrontal TMS (100% MT, 1 Hz, 147 pulses). They then used region-of-interest analysis guided by phase maps to compare DTI measurements in the prefrontal cortex before and after TMS. They failed to find any significant changes. However, Mottaghy et al. [20] examined DTI before and after 1-Hz TMS (90% MT, 12 min) over the motor cortex, and found a 'temporary small restriction in diffusion' within the targeted left M1 [20, 21]. Further studies are needed and are ongoing to resolve these two differing studies, which have important implications for TMS safety.

Does TMS Cause Local Brain Changes? If so, What Are They?

The first combination of TMS and functional neuroimaging in real time was performed with fluorodeoxyglucose (FDG) PET in a patient before and after repetitive TMS (rTMS) treatment for refractory depression [22]. Conclusions from this single case study are limited. However, it clearly demonstrated the potential of combining TMS with functional imaging to begin to address clinical issues and understand what TMS is doing in the brain.

There have now been many formal TMS studies with FDG PET. For example, a study of 1-Hz stimulation over the motor cortex for the thumb showed decreased glucose uptake at the site of stimulation and in the contralateral motor cortex [23]. Stimulation was performed at 1 Hz because FDG takes 20 min to settle into neurons and is thus a composite picture of brain activity over 20 min. Stimulation at or around MT intensity at speeds faster than once per second carries the risk of a seizure. This paradoxical decrease in localized brain activity at the mirror or contralateral site during TMS has been confirmed by electrophysiology [24]. A similar study by this same group of slow (1 Hz) rTMS over the prefrontal cortex also found that TMS, compared to a baseline or sham condition, was associated with global reductions in blood flow, as well as localized reductions in activity in the left dorsolateral prefrontal cortex (the TMS site), and connected regions such as the caudate nucleus, the orbitofrontal cortex bilaterally, and the cerebellum [25]. This work implies that 1-Hz prefrontal stimulation in normal adults has profound brain effects both locally and remotely, perhaps explaining some of the more interesting clinical and research findings in mood regulation, obsessive-compulsive disorder, and working memory [25].

The FDG method has several limitations that detract somewhat from its utility in this area. The calculation of the models for determining the subtraction of one scan from the other is complex. The scanning technique also often requires an arterial line for rapid sampling. And finally, the final image is a summed picture of 20 min of brain activity. It is likely that TMS, which is not continuous but rather pulsatile, is having multiple different dynamic effects during that time. It likely produces increased activity immediately with stimulation, decreases during the rest time between TMS pulses, as well as dynamic changes across the 20 min. The advantages are that this method yields information about absolute brain metabolism (and not just blood flow) not possible with many other measures. Also, there is no concern about the TMS coil in the scanner causing artifact, as the TMS coil never enters the PET suite and is used only during tracer uptake away from the PET camera. After some disagreement in the literature [26, 27, 29–32], it appears that a TMS shield is not needed within the PET camera [33, 34].

Another imaging tool that allows for tracer injection away from the camera is perfusion SPECT [35]. In 8 healthy adults, George et al. [36] used perfusion SPECT, which is taken up in 30–40 s, to image cerebral blood flow (CBF) during fast (20 Hz) left dorsolateral prefrontal cortex rTMS. Compared to a control scan with sham TMS, they reported relative decreases under the coil site and in the anterior cingulate and orbitofrontal cortex. TMS produced relative increases in blood flow in the brainstem and the cerebellum. Perfusion SPECT can only yield information about brain changes relative to other brain regions, not absolute brain activity. The exact amount of time that the image represents is also unclear. This same group used SPECT to examine TMS-related changes in depressed subjects undergoing a treatment trial, and found TMS-induced changes in limbic activity, especially in TMS responders [37].

Oxygen (^{15}O) PET has a shorter time frame (approximately 1 min for tracer uptake) than ^{18}FDG PET (20–30 min). Paus et al. [27] were the first to publish a study combining ^{15}O PET and TMS and found that intermittent fast (10 Hz) rTMS over the frontal eye fields for 1 min caused dose-dependent increases in blood flow at the stimulation site and in the visual cortex. That is, when they increased the number of 10-Hz trains within the minute, blood flow increased. Surprisingly, when the investigators used the same rTMS parameters in the same subjects but shifted the coil to the motor cortex, they found a dose-dependent reduction in CBF [26]. In contrast, Fox et al. [38] found that slow (1 Hz) rTMS over the motor cortex caused increased CBF, although this was only in 4 subjects. These paradoxical findings may imply that results seen at the motor cortex cannot be applied to other brain regions. Alternatively, there may be a large individual variation in TMS effects on blood flow either because of differences in cortical excitability, direct TMS effects on blood vessel smooth muscle, or differences in gyral anatomy. Again, these PET images are averages of 1 min of activity where the researcher has been intermittently stimulating and pausing. Obviously, the net picture is a combination of increases during TMS and changes during rest.

In a most interesting study, with potentially far-reaching implications for using TMS in clinical treatment, Speer et al. [28] used ^{15}O PET to scan depressed patients before and after 10 days of prefrontal TMS treatment. Their cohort had some patients who received 1 Hz each day, while others received 20 Hz. Twenty-hertz rTMS over the left prefrontal cortex was associated only with increases in regional CBF (rCBF). Significant increases in rCBF across the group of all 10 patients were located in the prefrontal cortex (L > R), the cingulate gyrus (L >> R), and the left amygdala, as well as the bilateral insula, basal ganglia, uncus, hippocampus, parahippocampus, thalamus, and cerebellum. In contrast, 1-Hz rTMS was associated only with decreases in rCBF. Significant decreases in flow were noted in small areas of the right prefrontal cortex, left medial temporal cortex, left basal ganglia, and left amygdala. The changes in mood following the two rTMS frequencies were inversely related ($r = -0.78$, $p < 0.005$, $n = 10$) such that individuals who improved with one frequency worsened with the other. These data indicate that 2 weeks of daily 20-Hz rTMS over the left prefrontal cortex at 100% MT induce persistent increases in rCBF in bilateral frontal, limbic, and paralimbic regions implicated in depression, whereas 1-Hz rTMS produces more circumscribed decreases (including in the left amygdala). These data demonstrate frequency-dependent, opposite effects of high- and low-frequency rTMS on local and distant regional brain activity that may have important ramifications for clinical use of rTMS.

In another landmark study, Strafella et al. [39] used ligand PET and showed that TMS over the motor cortex caused dopamine release in the ipsilateral caudate nucleus. This study demonstrates the ability of focal electrical stimulation to cause site-specific neurochemical changes in distant regions of the brain.

A promising, but also technically challenging, imaging modality for TMS is combining TMS and functional MRI (fMRI). Bohning et al. [40] first demonstrated the capability of interleaving TMS and blood flow imaging [blood-oxygen-level-dependent (BOLD) fMRI] with good spatial and temporal resolution. This technique was initially thought impossible by many, due to concerns about introducing a focal TMS magnetic field (1–2 T) inside a clinical MRI scanner. This group found that this technique, with the right precautions, is both feasible and safe. At least two research groups now have devised systems for interleaving TMS with fMRI, which is also feasible at higher MRI scanner field strengths (2.0 and 3.0 T) [40–51]. Figure 4 shows a group map of depressed subjects while being stimulated over the left prefrontal cortex, with areas of TMS-induced activation superimposed in color. Note that as the TMS machine is alternately triggered at 1 Hz for 7 s and then is turned off, regional brain activity changes both underneath the coil, and in deeper limbic regions.

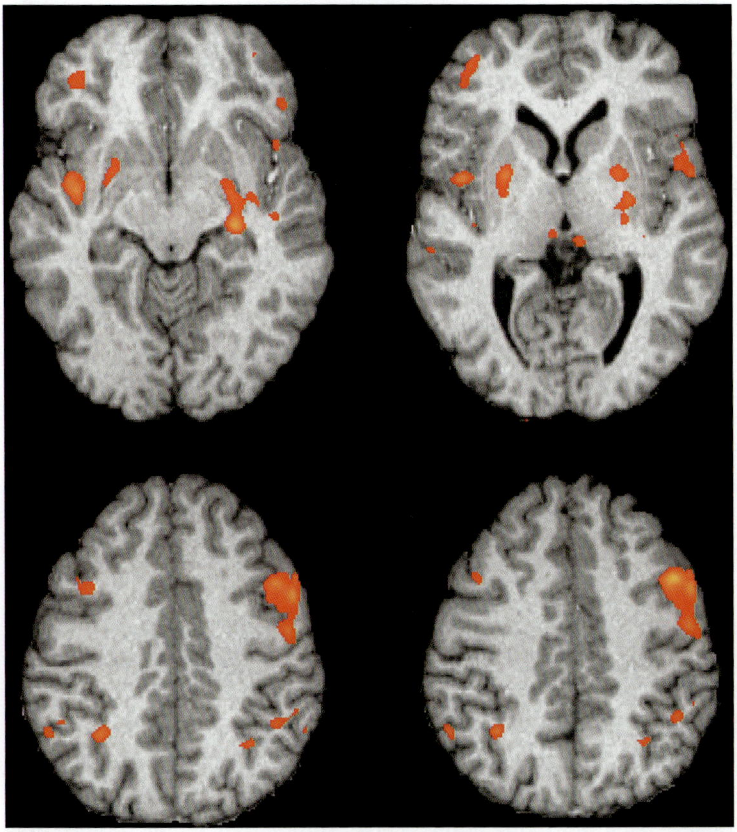

Fig. 4. Transverse images of MRI scans at different depths. Superimposed in color are the brain regions that were significantly activated during left prefrontal TMS in 9 medication-free depressed patients. Note the activation in the left (right-side of image) prefrontal cortex, directly underneath the coil. Also note the increased activation in other connected areas, including the orbitofrontal cortex and insula. Imaging studies such as this one demonstrate that TMS has both an immediate local effect in the brain directly under the coil, as well as secondary effects in connected regions (from Li et al. [82], reprinted with permission).

Work to date has shown that interleaved TMS/fMRI is sensitive enough to detect subtle differences in brain blood flow response that result from changes in TMS intensity [46, 52]. Additionally, directly comparing blood flow in the motor cortex caused by TMS or by volition shows a similarity between TMS and normal movement. For example, the peak area of blood flow change is the same for TMS and normal movement (within 2 mm) [44]. Also, stimulating at around 1 Hz and just at the MT activates roughly the same amount of brain tissue, and to the same degree. Thus, although many have the perception that TMS is causing supraphysiologic changes in the brain, these fMRI studies imply that TMS at these parameters is acting remarkably like normal physiology [53–55].

Thus, by combining TMS and imaging, the field of functional imaging can now begin to directly address causal issues in the field of brain-behavior relationships. However, the distribution of functions within the brain is quite complex and there may be only a few behaviors and even fewer regions where there is a direct one-to-one necessary relationship. Our brain structure and function developed incrementally through evolution and there are multiple redundant circuits for many behaviors [56–59]. Thus, although combined TMS and imaging will allow the field to ask the questions of direct necessary causation, it is likely that many behaviors are modulated by multiple regions in circuits, and that stimulation of one node in the circuit will cause complex changes both in behavior and brain activity in other areas of the circuit. Nevertheless, combined TMS/imaging will likely help understand the activity in distributed circuits as well, although perhaps not with the same causal rigor.

How Do We Know What Is Due to Direct TMS, and What Is Due to a Ripple Effect of the TMS on Other Brain Systems?

When TMS stimulates brain regions, they immediately send signals to connected areas, and then behaviors occur that are due not to the immediate TMS impulse, but secondarily to the induced effects. This thorny problem first presented itself with the initial TMS/fMRI studies described above. Some speculated that the blood flow changes seen with TMS were not due to direct stimulation, but were rather due to TMS causing the thumb to move, and then sensory feedback back into the brain. Thus, some argued, the blood flow changes attributed to TMS were really due to the TMS-induced sensation [48]. Through a series of elegant studies, it now appears that, in fact, the initial studies were correct and TMS alone causes a direct observable local increase in brain activity [49, 50].

Can We Position the TMS Coil Based on Images of Brain Structure or Function?

One of the major problems confronting TMS research, especially when stimulating outside of primary motor or visual pathways, is trying to determine exactly where one is stimulating in the brain [60–64]. In many TMS studies, the placement of the TMS coil has been determined by referencing the stimulation a certain distance from a functionally determined spot, such as the motor area for the thumb, or by choosing an anatomical landmark (e.g. distance from the lateral canthus of the eye), or by using a variant of the EEG electrode placement system [65]. These techniques serve to standardize TMS placement, but it is well known that different individuals have widely varying brain sizes and morphology. In addition to differences in brain structure, the functional location of behaviors varies even more across different individuals, especially for behaviors other than simple movement or vision. Thus in general, except for motor and visual studies where external monitoring of TMS effects may be possible, researchers have struggled to invent better methods for positioning the TMS coil.

There are currently several different systems for positioning a TMS coil based on a subjects' structural MRI scan. A widely used system is Brainsight, developed at McGill University in Montreal, Canada [26, 66]. There are other systems for performing this same function either in a clinical laboratory [67, 68] or inside the MRI scanner [69]. Initially one might think that the ideal way to determine where to place the TMS coil would be to invisibly peal away the scalp and skull and directly position the TMS coil on specific gyri. In fact, most neurosurgery departments now routinely employ MRI-guided presurgical mapping systems. These systems allow one to perform a brain MRI scan on a patient, with markers in key areas, and then place the MRI scan in a computer workstation. Next, with the subject sitting in a chair with a head holder, one can move an attached stereotactic wand to a position on the skull that is directly over a brain region. Conversely, one can position the wand on the skull and the system will electronically display the brain regions under the wand on the computer terminal. This method can reliably determine where stimulation will occur. However, it is unclear at present how necessary this degree of coil positioning is for many TMS research and clinical applications. As mentioned above, gyral anatomy and morphology varies a great deal between individuals. Additionally, it is not trivial, even with the brain fully exposed, to agree on specific gyri across individuals. Finally, as noted above, even when the problems with structural differences are resolved, the location of different functions within the brain also varies. So even stimulating the same anatomical spot across individuals does not guarantee that one is stimulating the same functional location or equivalent. A different approach uses probabilistic coil placement. This adjusts for differences in skull size and shape, but only loosely guarantees that the TMS coil is positioned over the part of an individual's brain involved in performing a task. Some systems using this approach are relatively simple and straightforward to perform in a clinical setting, and eliminate the need for a brain MRI scan [70].

Finally, the most sophisticated method involves having the person perform a task within the scanner, and then determining the specific functional location, and finally placing the TMS coil on the scalp location designed to stimulate this region. However, it is not trivial to determine, within an individual, the precise location involved in complex tasks [71]. Johnson et al. [71] scanned 25 right-handed healthy men twice while they performed a working memory task and discovered a large amount of within-individual variance over several scans. Scientists should exercise caution in using individual maps of cognitive brain function for TMS targeting. With higher field strength MRI scanners, and multichannel acquisition coils, there has been rapid progress recently in using fMRI to determine an individual's functional anatomy (e.g. see Kozel et al. [72]) and the next few years should see improvements in this area for research studies. Whether the clinical applications of TMS would require individual MRI-guided application is still an unanswered question.

An additional important unanswered question to be addressed over the next decade is whether there are specific regions of the prefrontal cortex that might prove more effective in TMS as a treatment for depression. For example, one would think that stimulation over a gyrus would be more clinically effective than placement over a sulcus. Additionally important is whether stimulation over particular Brodmann regions, or different aspects of the prefrontal cortex (e.g. medial, lateral, anterior), is more effective than others. The current probabilistic approach to coil placement for depression treatment was developed and adopted initially in 1995 [22, 64]. Herwig et al. [70, 73] in Munich elegantly demonstrated the limitations of this approach. They found that in some individuals, particularly those with large skulls, or where their motor strip is posterior, the 5-cm rule results in stimulation of the premotor and not prefrontal cortex. It is likely that more sophisticated and flexible approaches to coil positioning and individual adjustment will be needed to optimize TMS as a treatment for depression and other neuropsychiatric illnesses. To accommodate such different approaches in interleaved TMS/fMRI research applications, our laboratory has developed an MRI-guided TMS coil positioner/holder [42]. This device uses MR structural images acquired at the beginning of the study to determine the correct settings of the device for TMS stimulation of a particular location in the brain, based either on the subject's brain anatomy, or a location corresponding to the subject's brain as seen in probabilistic space.

When We Position the Coil Over the Motor Cortex, Where Exactly Are We Stimulating in the Brain?

An important background neuroscience question in attempting to validate various TMS placement methods is *whether TMS is stimulating the same brain regions that are normally involved in carrying out a task.* Numerous studies have been done in a retrospective fashion comparing the skull locations where TMS found an effect with the known structural neuroanatomy, or with changes observed on a functional image. Several initial studies demonstrated that the TMS-determined motor area for the thumb was close to the area that PET or fMRI scanning also revealed was responsible for thumb movement [74, 75]. These studies were reassuring in that the optimal TMS scalp location that caused thumb movement was located over the same cortex that was also implicated by more conventional functional imaging. However, the actual story may be a bit more complicated. For example, using a specially designed MRI-guided TMS coil positioner/holder [42] which allowed millimeter accuracy in coil positioning, Denslow et al. [76] at the Medical University of South Carolina assessed the variation in location and intensity of BOLD contrast associated with movements induced by TMS or volition relative to TMS coil placement. They scanned 11 healthy adults three times each at 1.5 T. Interleaved with fMRI, 1-Hz TMS was applied over the motor cortex and volition alternated with TMS during the scans. The intrasubject standard deviations in BOLD locations ranged between 3 and 6 mm, allowing localization to subregions of the motor strip. Interestingly, the placement of the TMS coil relative to the motor cortex anatomy varied more than did the location of the BOLD response, with a consistent anterior displacement of the coil compared to where one would have predicted. There were no significant differences between TMS and volition BOLD locations or intensities. The high repeatability of the location of TMS-induced BOLD activation suggested that TMS-fMRI stimulation could be used as a precise tool in the investigation of cortical mechanisms. The similarity between volition and TMS suggests that TMS may act through 'natural' brain movement circuits. Locations of the center of the TMS coil and its projection to the cortex, calculated from settings on the TMS holder, showed that while the locations were generally over the crown of the precentral gyrus, they clearly tended to be anterior to the location of the majority of Brodmann's area 4 on the posterior bank of the central sulcus. These results demonstrate that TMS stimulation, at 1 Hz and 110% MT for 21 s inducing twitch of the contralateral thumb, leads to BOLD activation that varies little in anatomical location or intensity over repeated scans. The level of variance in location observed in this study sets a benchmark for what level of precision can be expected in the determination of anatomical sites of BOLD activity resulting from TMS.

The mean location of BOLD activation in the motor strip was approximately 10 ± 4 mm interior to the cortical surface, or about 5 mm below the locations found by others. These results also differ from the results of Epstein et al. [77] who concluded that the point of stimulation occurs at a depth of about 6 mm. Epstein et al. [77] did not measure a BOLD location but instead estimated the stimulus site based on electric field strength patterns from different coils. These differing results may imply that the point of initial triggering by the TMS-generated field is different than the point of maximum BOLD response. This situation might occur if the form of the BOLD response region was at least partially dependent on the particular arborization of the microvasculature and draining veins, which are the source of the BOLD signal [78–80]. It is also reasonable to suggest that TMS may initially trigger only axonal spiking depolarization rather than synaptic activity. Axonal spiking requires only small amounts of energy and thus may not produce a BOLD contrast increase. The signal from an initial spiking event might then activate more energy-intensive, synaptic activity in an area of the motor cortex somewhat displaced from the initial location of depolarization, or an entirely separate cortical, subcortical or spinal location.

Conclusion

By combining TMS with imaging one can both aid in understanding how TMS is affecting the brain, as well as perhaps explain how the brain mediates behavior. This field is advancing rapidly. All the necessary tools are in place now for sophisticated functional imaging studies where TMS is used to clinch whether a particular region is responsible for a behavior under study. MRI offers promise with the proven ability to guide where to place the TMS coil, as well as to confirm what the magnetic field is at any given spot, and then to image changes in brain blood flow with stimulation. It is at least possible that in the near future a modified MRI scanner might be able to both image brain structure and function, and then to also stimulate the brain, perhaps even reaching deep structures with a combination of TMS coils in a deep array [7, 81]. This MRI/TMS machine would have powerful research applications, and might even transform TMS therapeutics – allowing one to tailor the stimulation within an individual to regions of hypo- or hyperactivity. Before that dream can be realized, much work needs to be done with all aspects of TMS and imaging. This area offers much promise.

References

1 Bohning DE, Pecheny AP, Epstein CM, Speer AM, Vincent DJ, Dannels W, George MS: Mapping transcranial magnetic stimulation (TMS) fields in vivo with MRI. Neuroreport 1997;8:2535–2538.

2 Wagner TA, Zahn M, Grodzinsky AJ, Pascual-Leone A: Three-dimensional head model simulation of transcranial magnetic stimulation. IEEE Trans Biomed Eng 2004;51:1586–1598.

3 Wagner T, Gangitano M, Romero R, Theoret H, Kobayashi M, Anschel D, Ives J, Cuffin N, Schomer D, Pascual-Leone A: Intracranial measurement of current densities induced by transcranial magnetic stimulation in the human brain. Neurosci Lett 2004;354:91–94.

4 Le Bihan D, Mangin JF, Poupon C, Clark CA, Pappata S, Molko N, Chabriat H: Diffusion tensor imaging: concepts and applications. J Magn Reson Imaging 2001;13:534–546.

5 Baumer T, Rothwell JC, Munchau A: Functional connectivity of the human premotor and motor cortex explored with TMS. Suppl Clin Neurophysiol 2003;56:160–169.

6 Roth BJ, Momen S, Turner R: Algorithm for the design of magnetic stimulation coils. Med Biol Eng Comput 1994;32:214–216.

7 Roth Y, Zangen A, Voller B, Hallett M: Transcranial magnetic stimulation of deep brain regions: evidence for efficacy of the H-coil. Clin Neurophysiol 2005;116:775–779.

8 Roth Y, Zangen A, Hallett M: A coil design for transcranial magnetic stimulation of deep brain regions. J Clin Neurophysiol 2002;19:361–370.

9 Kozel FA, Nahas Z, deBrux C, Molloy M, Lorberbaum JP, Bohning D, Risch SC, George MS: How coil-cortex distance relates to age, motor threshold, and antidepressant response to repetitive transcranial magnetic stimulation. J Neuropsychiatry Clin Neurosci 2000;12:376–384.

10 McConnell KA, Nahas Z, Shastri A, Lorberbaum JP, Kozel FA, Bohning DE, George MS: The transcranial magnetic stimulation motor threshold depends on the distance from coil to underlying cortex: a replication in healthy adults comparing two methods of assessing the distance to cortex. Biol Psychiatry 2001;49:454–459.
11 George MS, Nahas Z, Molloy M, Speer AM, Oliver NC, Li XB, Arana GW, Risch SC, Ballenger JC: A controlled trial of daily left prefrontal cortex TMS for treating depression. Biol Psychiatry 2000;48:962–970.
12 Figiel GS, Epstein C, McDonald WM, Amazon-Leece J, Figiel L, Saldivia A, Glover S: The use of rapid-rate transcranial magnetic stimulation (rTMS) in refractory depressed patients. J Neuropsychiatry Clin Neurosci 1998;10:20–25.
13 Mosimann UP, Marre SC, Werlen S, Schmitt W, Hess CW, Fisch HU, Schlaepfer TE: Antidepressant effects of repetitive transcranial magnetic stimulation in the elderly: correlation between effect size and coil-cortex distance. Arch Gen Psychiatry 2002;59:560–561.
14 Nahas Z, Teneback HC, Kozel A, Speer AM, DeBrux C, Molloy M, Stallings L, Spicer KM, Arana G, Bohning DE, Risch SC, George MS: Brain effects of TMS delivered over prefrontal cortex in depressed adults: role of stimulation frequency and coil-cortex distance. J Neuropsychiatry Clin Neurosci 2001;13:459–470.
15 Nahas Z, Li X, Kozel FA, Mirski D, Memoun M, Miller K, Yamanaka K, Anderson B, Chae JH, Bohning DE, Mintzer J, George MS: Safety and benefits of distance-adjusted prefrontal transcranial magnetic stimulation in depressed patients 55–75 years of age: a pilot study. Depress Anxiety 2004;19:249–256.
16 Nahas Z, DeBrux C, Chandler V, Lorberbaum JP, Speer AM, Molloy MA, Liberatos C, Risch SC, George MS: Lack of significant changes on magnetic resonance scans before and after 2 weeks of daily left prefrontal repetitive transcranial magnetic stimulation for depression. J ECT 2000;16:380–390.
17 Zivan JA: Diffusion-weighted MRI for diagnosis and treatment of ischemic stroke. Ann Neurol 1997;41:567–568.
18 Koroshetz WJ, Gonzalez G: Diffusion-weighted MRI: an ECG for 'brain attack'? Ann Neurol 1997;41:565–566.
19 Lutsep HL, Albers GW, deCrespigny A, Kamat GN, Marks MP, Moseley ME: Clinical utility of diffusion-weighted magnetic resonance imaging in the assessment of ischemic stroke. Ann Neurol 1997;41:574–580.
20 Mottaghy FM, Gangitano M, Horkan C, Chen Y, Pascual-Leone A, Schlaug G: Repetitive TMS temporarily alters brain diffusion. Neurology 2003;60:1539–1541.
21 Duning T, Rogalewski A, Steinstraeter O, Kugel H, Jansen A, Breitenstein C, Knecht S: Repetitive TMS temporarily alters brain diffusion. Neurology 2004;62:2144 (author reply 2144–2145, erratum 2146).
22 George MS, Wassermann EM, Williams WA, Callahan A, Ketter TA, Basser P, Hallett M, Post RM: Daily repetitive transcranial magnetic stimulation (rTMS) improves mood in depression. Neuroreport 1995;6:1853–1856.
23 Wassermann EM, Kimbrell TA, George MS, Danielson AL, Herscovitch P, Hallett M, Post RM: Local and distant changes in cerebral glucose metabolism during repetitive transcranial magnetic stimulation (rTMS). Neurology 1997;48:A107–P102.049.
24 Chae JH, Nahas Z, Wassermann E, Li X, Sethuraman G, Gilbert D, Sallee FR, George MS: A pilot safety study of repetitive transcranial magnetic stimulation (rTMS) in Tourette's syndrome. Cogn Behav Neurol 2004;17:109–117.
25 Kimbrell TA, Dunn RT, George MS, Danielson AL, Willis MW, Repella JD, Benson BE, Herscovitch P, Post RM, Wassermann EM: Left prefrontal-repetitive transcranial magnetic stimulation (rTMS) and regional cerebral glucose metabolism in normal volunteers. Psychiatry Res 2002;115:101–103.
26 Paus T, Jech R, Thompson CJ, Comeau R, Peters T, Evans AC: Transcranial magnetic stimulation during positron emission tomography: a new method for studying connectivity of the human cerebral cortex. J Neurosci 1997;17:3178–3184.
27 Paus T, Jech R, Thompson CJ, Comeau R, Peters T, Evans AC: Dose-dependent reduction of cerebral blood flow during rapid-rate transcranial magnetic stimulation of the human sensorimotor cortex. J Neurophysiol 1997;79:1102–1107.

28 Speer AM, Kimbrell TA, Wassermann EM, et al: Opposite effects of high and low frequency rTMS on regional brain activity in depressed patients. Biol Psychiatr 2000;48:1133–1141.

29 Paus T, Wolforth M: Transcranial magnetic stimulation during PET: reaching and verifying the target site. Hum Brain Mapp 1998;6:399–402.

30 Paus T, Jech R, Thompson CJ, Comeau R, Peters T, Evans AC: Dose-dependent reduction of cerebral blood flow during rapid-rate transcranial magnetic stimulation of the human sensorimotor cortex. J Neurophysiol 1998;79:1102–1107.

31 Paus T: Imaging the brain before, during, and after transcranial magnetic stimulation. Neuropsychologia 1999;37:219–224.

32 Paus T: Integration of transcranial magnetic stimulation and brain imaging. Biol Psychiatry 2001;49:6S–21S.

33 Lancaster JL, Narayana S, Wenzel D, Luckemeyer J, Roby J, Fox P: Evaluation of an image-guided, robotically positioned transcranial magnetic stimulation system. Hum Brain Mapp 2004;22:329–340.

34 Lee JS, Narayana S, Lancaster J, Jerabek P, Lee DS, Fox P: Positron emission tomography during transcranial magnetic stimulation does not require micro-metal shielding. Neuroimage 2003;19: 1812–1819.

35 George MS, Ring HA, Costa DC, Ell PJ, Kouris K, Jarritt P: Neuroactivation and Neuroimaging with SPET. London, Springer, 1991.

36 George MS, Stallings LE, Speer AM, Spicer KM, Vincent DJ, Bohning DE, Cheng KT, Molloy M, Teneback CC, Risch SC: Prefrontal repetitive transcranial magnetic stimulation (rTMS) changes relative perfusion locally and remotely. Hum Psychopharmacol 1999;14:161–170.

37 Teneback CC, Nahas Z, Speer AM, Molloy M, Stallings LE, Spicer KM, Risch SC, George MS: Changes in prefrontal cortex and paralimbic activity in depression following two weeks of daily left prefrontal TMS. J Neuropsychiatry Clin Neurosci 1999;11:426–435.

38 Fox P, Ingham R, George MS, Mayberg HS, Ingham J, Roby J, Martin C, Jerabek P: Imaging human intra-cerebral connectivity by PET during TMS. Neuroreport 1997;8:2787–2791.

39 Strafella AP, Paus T, Fraraccio M, Dagher A: Striatal dopamine release induced by repetitive transcranial magnetic stimulation of the human motor cortex. Brain 2003;126:2609–2615.

40 Bohning DE, Shastri A, Nahas Z, Lorberbaum JP, Andersen SW, Dannels WR, Haxthausen EU, Vincent DJ, George MS: Echoplanar BOLD fMRI of brain activation induced by concurrent transcranial magnetic stimulation. Invest Radiol 1998;33:336–340.

41 Bohning DE, Denslow S, Bohning PA, Lomarev MP, George MS: Interleaving fMRI and rTMS. Suppl Clin Neurophysiol 2003;56:42–54.

42 Bohning DE, Denslow S, Bohning PA, Walker JA, George MS: A TMS coil positioning/holding system for MR image-guided TMS interleaved with fMRI. Clin Neurophysiol 2003;114: 2210–2219.

43 Bohning DE, Shastri A, Lomarev MP, Lorberbaum JP, Nahas Z, George MS: BOLD-fMRI response vs transcranial magnetic stimulation (TMS) pulse-train length: testing for linearity. J Magn Reson Imaging 2003;17:279–290.

44 Bohning DE, Shastri A, McGavin L, McConnell KA, Nahas Z, Lorberbaum JP, Roberts DR, George MS: Motor cortex brain activity induced by 1-Hz transcranial magnetic stimulation is similar in location and level to that for volitional movement. Invest Radiol 2000;35:676–683.

45 Bohning DE, Shastri A, Wassermann EM, Ziemann U, Lorberbaum JP, Nahas Z, Lomarev MP, George MS: BOLD-fMRI response to single-pulse transcranial magnetic stimulation (TMS). J Magn Reson Imaging 2000;11:569–574.

46 Bohning DE, Shastri A, McConnell KA, Nahas Z, Lorberbaum JP, Roberts DR, Teneback C, Vincent DJ, George MS: A combined TMS/fMRI study of intensity-dependent TMS over motor cortex. Biol Psychiatry 1999;45:385–394.

47 Baudewig J, Siebner HR, Bestmann S, Tergau F, Tings T, Paulus W, Frahm J: Functional MRI of cortical activations induced by transcranial magnetic stimulation (TMS). Neuroreport 2001;12:3543–3548.

48 Bestmann S, Baudewig J, Siebner HR, Rothwell JC, Frahm J: Is functional magnetic resonance imaging capable of mapping transcranial magnetic cortex stimulation? Suppl Clin Neurophysiol 2003;56:55–62.

49 Bestmann S, Baudewig J, Siebner HR, Rothwell JC, Frahm J: Subthreshold high-frequency TMS of human primary motor cortex modulates interconnected frontal motor areas as detected by interleaved fMRI-TMS. Neuroimage 2003;20:1685–1696.

50 Bestmann S, Baudewig J, Siebner HR, Rothwell JC, Frahm J: Functional MRI of the immediate impact of transcranial magnetic stimulation on cortical and subcortical motor circuits. Eur J Neurosci 2004;19:1950–1962.

51 Siebner HR, Lee L, Bestmann S: Interleaving TMS with functional MRI: now that it is technically feasible how should it be used? Clin Neurophysiol 2003;114:1997–1999.

52 Nahas Z, Lomarev M, Roberts DR, Shastri A, Lorberbaum JP, Teneback C, McConnell K, Vincent DJ, Li X, George MS, Bohning DE: Unilateral left prefrontal transcranial magnetic stimulation (TMS) produces intensity-dependent bilateral effects as measured by interleaved BOLD fMRI. Biol Psychiatry 2001;50:712–720.

53 Denslow S, Lomarev M, Bohning DE, Mu Q, George MS: A high resolution assessment of the repeatability of relative location and intensity of transcranial magnetic stimulation-induced and volitionally induced blood oxygen level-dependent response in the motor cortex. Cogn Behav Neurol 2004;17:163–173.

54 Denslow S, Lomarev M, George MS, Bohning DE: Cortical and subcortical brain effects of transcranial magnetic stimulation (TMS)-induced movement: an interleaved TMS/functional magnetic resonance imaging study. Biol Psychiatry 2005;57:752–760.

55 Denslow S, Bohning DE, Bohning PA, Lomarev MP, George MS: An increased precision comparison of TMS-induced motor cortex BOLD fMRI response for image-guided versus function-guided coil placement. Cogn Behav Neurol 2005;18:119–127.

56 Maclean PD: The limbic system and its hippocampal formation: studies in the animals and their possible application to man. J Neurosurg 1954;11:29–44.

57 Maclean PD: Culminating developments in the evolution of the limbic system: the thalamocingulate division; in Doane BK, Livingston KE (eds): The Limbic System: Functional Organization and Clinical Disorders. New York, Raven Press, 1986.

58 MacLean PD: The Triune Brain in Evolution: Role in Paleocerebral Functions. New York, Plenum Press, 1990.

59 MacLean PD: Introduction: perspectives on cingulate cortex in the limbic system; in Vogt BA, Gabriel M (eds): Neurobiology of Cingulate Cortex and Limbic Thalamus: A Comprehensive Handbook. Boston, Birkhäuser, 1993, pp 1–19.

60 George MS: Tickling the brain: the emerging new science of electrical brain stimulation. Sci Am 2003;289:66–73.

61 George MS, Wassermann EM, Williams WA, Callahan A, Ketter TA, Basser P, Hallett M, Post RM: Daily repetitive transcranial magnetic stimulation (rTMS) improves mood in depression. Neuroreport 1995;6:1853–1856.

62 George MS, Wassermann EM, Kimbrell T, Speer AM, Stallings L, Roberts D, Vincent DJ, Beale M, Cheng K, Spicer KM: An overview of initial studies combining conventional functional imaging (PET, SPECT, fMRI) with transcranial magnetic stimulation (TMS) to actively probe brain-behavior relationships. J Neuropsychiatry Clin Neurosci 1997;9:131.

63 George MS, Wassermann EM, Williams WE, Kimbrell TA, Little JT, Hallett M, Post RM: Mood improvements following daily left prefrontal repetitive transcranial magnetic stimulation in patients with depression: a placebo-controlled crossover trial. Am J Psychiatry 1997;154: 1752–1756.

64 George MS, Wassermann EM, Williams WA, Steppel J, Pascual-Leone A, Basser P, Hallett M, Post RM: Changes in mood and hormone levels after rapid-rate transcranial magnetic stimulation (rTMS) of the prefrontal cortex. J Neuropsychiatry Clin Neurosci 1996;8:172–180.

65 Kahkonen S, Komssi S, Wilenius J, Ilmoniemi RJ: Prefrontal transcranial magnetic stimulation produces intensity-dependent EEG responses in humans. Neuroimage 2005;24:955–960.

66 Peters T, Davey B, Munger P, Comeau R, Evans A, Oliver A: Three-dimensional multi-modal image guidance for neurosurgery. IEEE Trans Med Imaging 1996;15:121–128.

67 Smith DT, Jackson SR, Rorden C: Transcranial magnetic stimulation of the left human frontal eye fields eliminates the cost of invalid endogenous cues. Neuropsychologia 2005;43:1288–1296.

68 Neggers SF, Langerak TR, Schutter DJ, Mandl RC, Ramsey NF, Lemmens PJ, Postma A: A stereotactic method for image-guided transcranial magnetic stimulation validated with fMRI and motor-evoked potentials. Neuroimage 2004;21:1805–1817.

69 Bohning DE, Denslow S, Bohning PA, Walker JA, George MS: A TMS coil positioning/holding system for MR image-guided TMS interleaved with fMRI. Clin Neurophysiol 2003;114: 2210–2219.

70 Herwig U, Satrapi P, Schonfeldt-Lecuona C: Using the international 10–20 EEG system for positioning of transcranial magnetic stimulation. Brain Topogr 2003;16:95–99.

71 Johnson KA, Mu Q, Yamanaka K, Mishory A, Koola J, Hill S, Horner MD, Nahas Z, Bohning DE, George MS: Repeatability of within-individual blood oxygen level-dependent functional magnetic resonance imaging maps of a working memory task for transcranial magnetic stimulation targeting Neurosci Imaging 2004;1:95–111.

72 Kozel FA, Johnson KA, Mu Q, Grenesko EL, Laken SJ, George MS: Detecting deception using functional magnetic resonance imaging. Biol Psychiatry 2005;58:605–613.

73 Herwig U, Padberg F, Unger J, Spitzer M, Schonfeldt-Lecuona C: Transcranial magnetic stimulation in therapy studies: examination of the reliability of 'standard' coil positioning by neuronavigation. Biol Psychiatry 2001;50:58–61.

74 Wassermann EM, Wang B, Zeffiro TA, Sadato N, Pascual-Leone A, Toro C, Hallett M: Locating the motor cortex on the MRI with transcranial magnetic stimulation and PET. Neuroimage 1996;3:1–9.

75 Roberts DR, Vincent DJ, Speer AM, Bohning DE, Cure J, Young J, George MS: Multi-modality mapping of motor cortex: comparing echoplanar BOLD fMRI and transcranial magnetic stimulation. Short communication. J Neural Transm 1997;104:833–843.

76 Denslow S, Bohning DE, Bohning PA, Lomarev MP, George MS: An increased precision comparison of TMS-induced motor cortex BOLD fMRI response for image-guided versus function-guided coil placement. Cogn Behav Neurol 2005;18:119–126.

77 Epstein CM, Schwartzenberg DG, Davey KR, Sudderth DB: Localizing the site of magnetic brain stimulation in humans. Neurology 1990;40:666–670.

78 Menon RS, Ogawa S, Hu X, Strupp JP, Anderson P, Ugurbil K: BOLD based functional MRI at 4 tesla includes a capillary bed contribution: echo-planar imaging correlates with previous optical imaging using intrinsic signals. Magn Reson Med 1995;33:453–459.

79 Logothetis NK, Pauls J, Augath M, Trinath T, Oeltermann A: Neurophysiological investigation of the basis of the fMRI signal. Nature 2001;412:150–157.

80 Weiskopf N, Veit R, Erb M, Mathiak K, Grodd W, Goebel R, Birbaumer N: Physiological self-regulation of regional brain activity using real-time functional magnetic resonance imaging (fMRI): methodology and exemplary data. Neuroimage 2003;19:577–586.

81 Hallett M: Transcranial magnetic stimulation and the human brain. Nature 2000;406:147–150.

82 Li X, Nahas Z, Kozel FA, Anderson B, Bohning DE, George MS: Acute left prefrontal transcranial magnetic stimulation in depressed patients is associated with immediately increased activity in prefrontal cortical as well as subcortical regions. Biol Psychiatry 2004;55:882–890.

Mark S. George, MD
502 N, IOP, 67 President St.
Medical University of South Carolina
Charleston, SC 29425 (USA)
Tel. +1 843 876 5142, Fax +1 843 792 5702, E-Mail georgem@musc.edu

Marcolin MA, Padberg F (eds): Transcranial Brain Stimulation for Treatment of Psychiatric Disorders.
Adv Biol Psychiatr. Basel, Karger, 2007, vol 23, pp 53–83

Efficacy and Safety of Prefrontal Repetitive Transcranial Magnetic Stimulation in Affective Disorders

Frank Padberg[a], *Nicola Grossheinrich*[a], *Oliver Pogarell*[a], *Hans-Jürgen Möller*[a], *Felipe Fregni*[b]

[a]Department of Psychiatry and Psychotherapy, Ludwig-Maximilian University Munich, Munich, Germany; [b]Department of Neurology, Beth Israel Deaconess Medical Center, Harvard Medical School, Boston, Mass., USA

Abstract

For more than a decade, repetitive transcranial magnetic stimulation (rTMS) has been investigated as therapeutic intervention in mental diseases. Depression was the first psychiatric disorder where rTMS was applied and is still a major application with more than 30 published placebo-controlled trials showing on average a moderate antidepressant efficacy. Large multicenter trials have been published very recently or are still under way which will finally answer many of the open questions in this field. It is important not to look at the available data just in terms of general antidepressant efficacy, but to differentiate the efficacy data regarding distinct applications as treatment of therapy-resistant depression, primary treatment of depression eventually combined with specific pharmacological and nonpharmacological interventions, bipolar depression or situations where depression occurs as comorbid disorder (e.g. after stroke). The application of rTMS in moderately therapy-resistant depression is close to a general approval allowing the method to be introduced into clinical practice, whereas other applications still require solid evidence of efficacy. Moreover, future studies need to clarify how rTMS acts on the specific pathophysiology of depression. The main mechanism of action is believed to be linked to neuronal networks which are dysfunctional in depression and can be externally stimulated by focal prefrontal rTMS. However, rTMS also exerts effects on various neurotransmitter systems. It leads to striatal dopamine release and modulates serotonergic and glutamatergic neurotransmission, and may influence hypothalamic-pituitary-adrenal axis activity. Future research will follow these tracks by differentiating real and specific vs. real and nonspecific vs. placebo effects associated with rTMS treatment. Finally, the huge potential of methodological development (e.g. theta burst rTMS, deep rTMS) hopefully leading to optimized treatment protocols has to be emphasized.

Major goals of current research in affective disorders include treating therapy-resistant patients, preventing chronic conditions and relapse of depressive episodes in unipolar depression as well as manic or mixed episodes in bipolar patients. This has recently generated tremendous interest not only in the spectrum of established pharmacological approaches including atypical antipsychotics and anticonvulsants, but also in the proposal of novel principles of pharmacological treatment, e.g. substance P antagonists or corticotropin-releasing hormone (CRH) receptor antagonists, and nonpharmacological, biophysical approaches such as transcranial magnetic stimulation (TMS) [1, 2], vagus nerve stimulation (VNS) [3], deep brain stimulation (DBS) [4] and most recently transcranial direct current stimulation [5].

Barker et al. [6] originally introduced TMS in 1985 as a noninvasive tool to electromagnetically stimulate the primary motor cortex in humans. More recently, repetitive TMS (rTMS) has become a powerful research tool in neurophysiology and cognitive neuroscience [1, 7]. Pilot studies have suggested a possible application of rTMS as a therapeutic tool in various neurological and psychiatric disorders [1, 2, 8], based on the assumption that targeted stimulation of dysfunctional corticosubcortical circuits are involved in the pathophysiology of these conditions. Generally, two different rTMS modalities have been applied in previous intervention studies: low-frequency (LF) rTMS with stimulation frequencies $\leq$1 Hz and high-frequency (HF) rTMS with frequencies $\geq$5 Hz. LF and HF rTMS are proposed to exert opposite effects on cortical excitability, i.e. LF rTMS reduces and HF rTMS increases excitability [9]. Thus, it is hypothesized that rTMS allows to modulate regional cortical activity in the direction intended to compensate temporary changes of brain activity in affective disorders revealed by functional neuroimaging studies. This review attempts to evaluate existing preclinical and clinical studies in answering the question of whether rTMS may be a useful treatment in the spectrum of affective disorders.

Effects on Mood and Emotions

Marked emotional reactions observed in single patients and volunteers participating in early single-pulse studies have triggered research on rTMS-induced modulation of mood and emotions in healthy volunteers. Theoretically, prefrontal rTMS could alter measures of mood and emotions in a similar fashion as it may transiently influence experimental parameters in neurocognitive paradigms. Three pilot studies demonstrated transient effects of rTMS applied to the dorsolateral prefrontal cortex (DLPFC) on mood self-rating [10–12]. These studies provided data supporting the so-called valence model of emotions, i.e. the left hemisphere is believed to mediate positive, the right hemisphere to mediate negative emotions [13]. However, observed changes in self-reported mood were generally subtle and only based on self-rating. The majority of recent studies has failed to replicate such clearly lateralized effects of both HF rTMS [14–18] and LF rTMS [19, 20]. Only Barrett et al. [21] observed a decline in mood after left prefrontal HF rTMS; however, this study was not sham-controlled. This means that the initial hypothesis of lateralized mood effects induced by rTMS has not been substantiated to date. Generally, individual emotional reactions strongly varied between individuals, and occasionally impressive reactions to rTMS were observed, e.g. single subjects developed hypomanic states [17]. It is not clear whether such effects are genuine effects of rTMS on mood or rather based on the suggestive character of these experiments. Thus, other brain regions and aspects of emotions need to be investigated as recently done by Schutter and van Honk [22] who observed a selective improvement of memory for happy faces after LF rTMS of the left orbitofrontal cortex. Studies in healthy subjects have shown multifold effects of prefrontal rTMS on more objective experimental paradigms such as facial expression analysis, electroencephalogram and neuroendocrine parameters, e.g. concentrations of the thyroid-stimulating hormone [15, 18, 23, 24]. Therefore, observational approaches and neurobiological measures should be used in addition to measures of self-reported mood to explore suitable hypotheses in future studies.

Early Studies in Major Depression

In the 1990s, several independent groups from the USA, Germany, Austria and Israel started simultaneously investigating rTMS as an antidepressant treatment [25–29]. Single-pulse stimulators were used in the majority of initial studies, triggered at frequencies of 0.3 Hz or less, together with large circular coils [25, 27–29]. Treatment was of short duration (5 days), and only one of these studies included treatment under placebo conditions comparing a supra- and subthreshold condition [29]. In this trial patients were only randomized to the real rTMS groups and a placebo group was added later. Antidepressant effects were assumed in most of these pilot studies, however, the effect sizes were not impressive.

Proof of Concept and Antidepressant Efficacy

Considering the basic hypothesis that rTMS normalizes regional brain activity at cortical sites which show changes in depressed subjects, one would

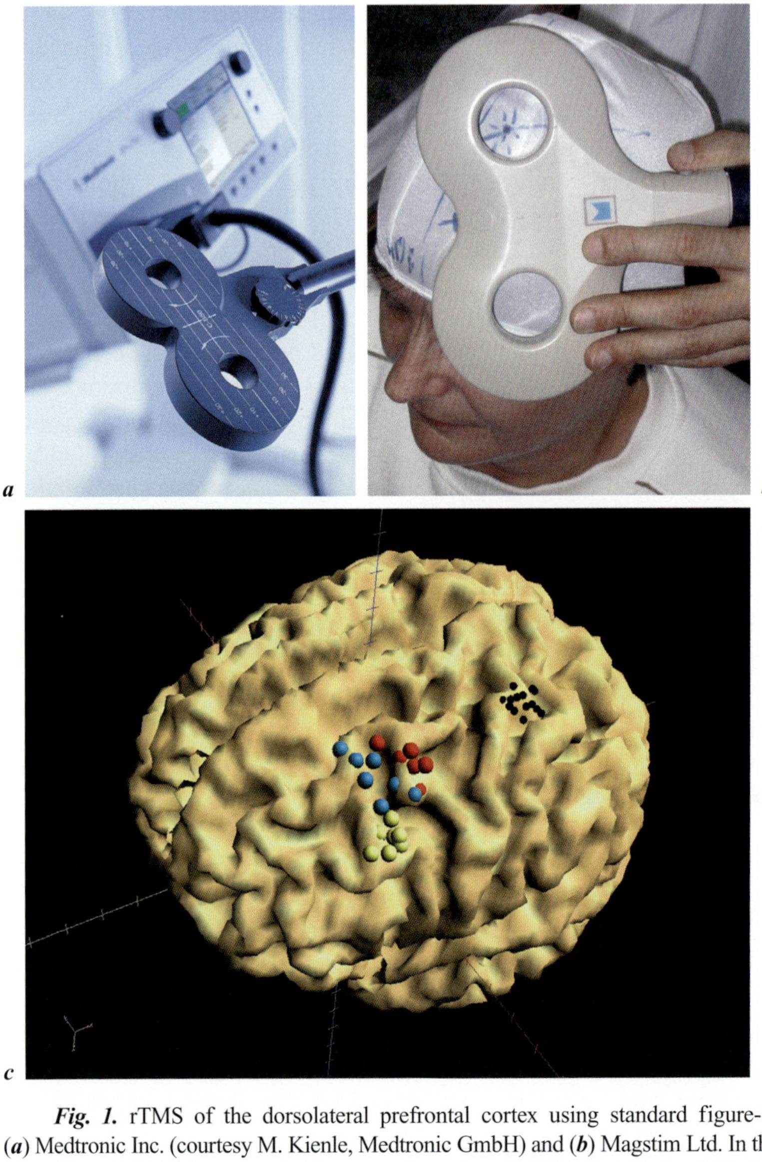

Fig. 1. rTMS of the dorsolateral prefrontal cortex using standard figure-8 coils by (***a***) Medtronic Inc. (courtesy M. Kienle, Medtronic GmbH) and (***b***) Magstim Ltd. In the majority of studies rTMS has been applied in repeated sessions (1,000 to 3,000 stimuli/day) once daily during working days and the total duration of treatment has varied between 2 and 6 weeks. The most common coil position targets the left dorsolateral prefrontal cortex by measuring 5 cm anterior (on the skull surface) to the optimal position for evoking a motor evoked potential in hand muscles. ***c*** A considerable variability occurs with this approach, as demonstrated applying neuronavigated rTMS. The small black dots indicate the optimal sites for abductor pollicis brevis muscle stimulation over the motor cortex, i.e. the region around the lateral edge of the

expect that proof of concept studies are available supporting this notion. However, very few studies compared rTMS of different cortex regions with otherwise identical parameters. Figure 1 shows the typical stimulation position applying a standard procedure for positioning the coil over the left DLPFC which results in a considerable anatomical variability [30]. In other studies, HF rTMS was applied over the right DLPFC resulting also in significant antidepressant effects [31–35]. Thus, the two options of left prefrontal HF and right prefrontal LF rTMS are usually discussed as complementary treatment approaches based on the idea that regional brain activity within the left and right prefrontal cortices is dysregulated in opposite directions. Few trials [36–38] investigated whether rTMS-associated effects on depressive symptoms vary as a function of baseline cortical activity at the stimulation site. Kimbrell et al. [37] observed that response to both HF and LF rTMS indeed varied with regional glucose metabolism of DLPFC at baseline, i.e. patients who showed a reduced metabolism improved after HF rTMS and patients who showed an increased metabolism improved after LF rTMS. Herwig et al. [38] investigated whether rTMS directed to hypometabolic areas using a neuronavigation device is superior to rTMS just applied over the prefrontal cortex and not directed specifically. In this study, no difference was found between both strategies supporting the primary hypothesis. Similarly, Garcia-Toro et al. [36] found no additional advantage of focusing rTMS on functionally altered cortex regions identified by single photon emission tomography. In both studies, however, the sample size was far too small to exclude a type II error as reason for these negative findings. Thus, a 'proof of concept trial' in a larger sample is still clearly needed.

To date, however, more than 30 individual randomized, placebo-controlled clinical trials including over 900 patients suffering from major depressive episodes have been conducted investigating the safety and efficacy of rTMS as antidepressant intervention [31–34, 38–64]. In the majority of these trials, significant placebo/real rTMS differences have been observed with antidepressant effects ranging from modest to substantial. Due to the methodological limitations of many of these trials such as rather small sample sizes, difficulties in controlling placebo rTMS and short observation periods, the current view about its efficacy is more sober after the initial enthusiasm has ceased. Several meta-analyses (table 1) have been conducted [65–70] supporting the

hand knob. The larger dots indicate the rostral coil positions over the different Brodman areas: red = BA 6, blue = BA 6/8 and 8, yellow = BA 8/9 and 9. Talairach coordinates before and after 'standard positioning' of the coil are visualized in an individual surface rendered MRI of the brain (white matter segmentation), which was transformed into Talairach space. Reprinted from Herwig et al. [30] with kind permission from Elsevier Science.

Table 1. Overview of meta-analyses of studies investigating rTMS in depression

Meta-analysis	Trials	Patients	Comparison of rTMS parameters	Comparison of MD subtypes	Effect sizes	Conclusions
McNamara et al. [70]	5	81	no	no	NNT = 2.3*	beneficial effects in depression
Holtzheimer et al. [68]	12	ND	yes (site)	no	WMD = 0.81/0.89*	real rTMS statistically superior to sham rTMS
Burt et al. [65]	16	377	yes (LF vs. HF rTMS)	no	d_{pooled} = 0.67*	statistically robust effect favoring real rTMS, effect sizes heterogeneous
Martin et al. [69]	12	217	yes (site and frequency)	no	SMD = −0.35* (left HF rTMS, only after 2 weeks)	low-quality trials, insufficient evidence
Couturier [66]	6	91	only left prefrontal HF rTMS, no	no	WMD = −1.1, n.s.	no significant difference between real and sham rTMS, low power of trials
Herrmann and Ebmeier [67]	33	877	only left prefrontal HF rTMS, yes (intensity, frequency, number of stimuli)	no	d_{pooled} = 0.71*	real rTMS more effective than sham rTMS, great variability and no significant predictors either due to insufficient power or to nonspecific effects of rTMS on depression

* = Statistically significant difference between real and sham rTMS; MD = major depression; ND = not determined; NNT = number needed to treat; SMD = standardized mean difference; WMD = weighted mean difference.

antidepressant efficacy of rTMS, but clinical effects are not strong and the clinical significance may be questionable. The most recent meta-analysis [67] included 33 individual trials with 877 patients and found rTMS to be more effective than sham rTMS, with a large effect size of 0.71 (fig. 2). The average

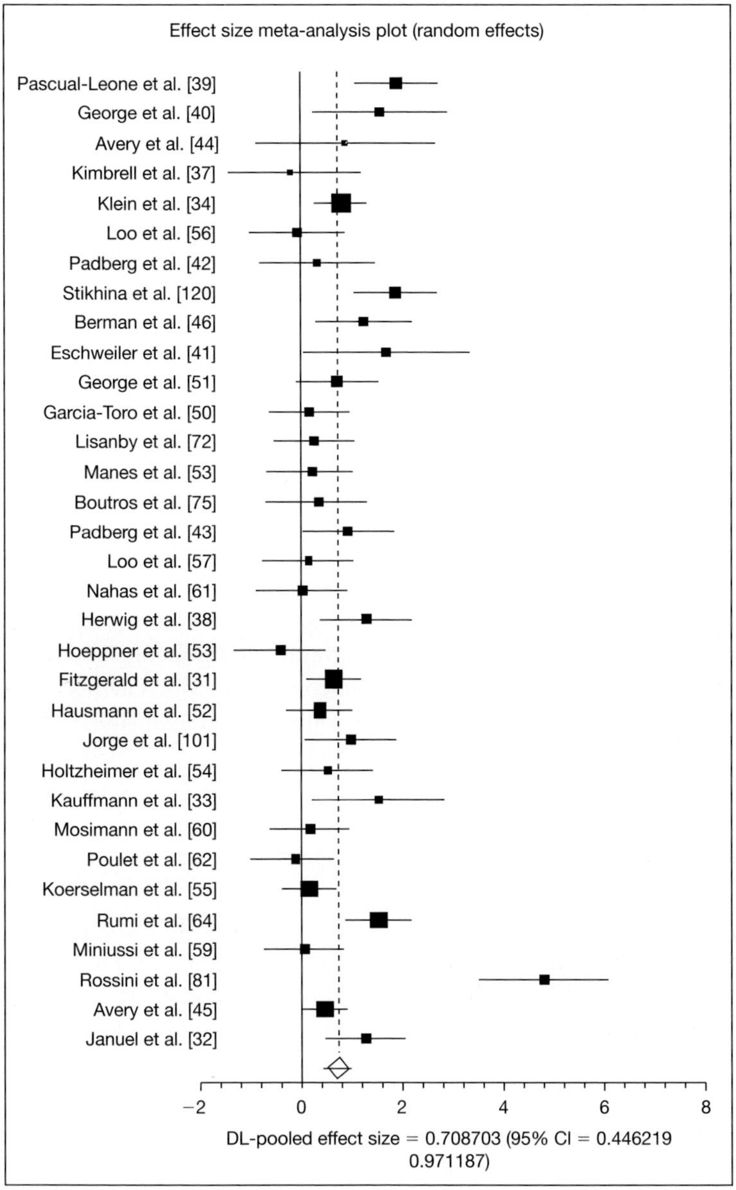

Fig. 2. Forest plot of 33 rTMS treatment trials in depression. Reprinted from Herrmann and Ebmeier [67], copyright 2006, Physicians Postgraduate Press, with kind permission from K. Ebmeier, Oxford, UK and the publisher.

Table 2. Potential applications of rTMS in affective disorders

Primary treatment of MDE: combined treatment with antidepressants or monotherapy
Treatment of therapy-resistant MDE: add-on or monotherapy
Treatment of subtypes of depression: e.g. bipolar depression and others (psychotic, melancholic, atypical, SAD)
Treatment of comorbid depression: organic brain diseases, addiction, PTSD, schizophrenia
Treatment on mania
Treatment of patients 'at risk' during pharmacotherapy (medical comorbidity, pregnancy)
Maintenance treatment, prevention of MDE and manic episodes

MDE = Major depressive episode; PTSD = posttraumatic stress disorder; SAD = seasonal affective disorder.

reduction of depression scores after active rTMS was 33.6% compared to 17.4% after sham rTMS. As trials showed a substantial variability, it was not possible to identify a particularly efficacious protocol. This was in contrast to a previous critical review [71] that suggested several patient factors and treatment parameters predicting a better clinical outcome of rTMS. The best prediction of a clinical response was achieved when stimulation intensities ≥90% of the resting motor threshold (MT) were applied [67].

Differential Use in the Affective Disorder Spectrum

It is important to emphasize that specific applications of rTMS in depressive disorders need to be investigated by trials specifically designed for the respective hypotheses. Table 2 shows a list of such applications and the following sections, as well as subsequent chapters of this book will address the specific use in these conditions.

rTMS Combined with Antidepressant Pharmacotherapy as First-Line Intervention

New antidepressant treatment strategies that promise to speed up and increase primary response rates in depression are of great interest. Combining rTMS with other antidepressant interventions, e.g. pharmacotherapy, psychotherapy or sleep deprivation early in the treatment of a depressive episode aims at this goal. Several studies have addressed this question in a placebo-controlled manner and combined HF rTMS treatment with selective serotonin reuptake inhibitors, tricyclic antidepressants and novel-acting agents. Garcia-Toro et al. [50] and Lisanby et al. [72] failed to show a significant difference between real rTMS and sham rTMS, each combined with sertraline for a treatment period of 2 weeks. Similarly, Hausmann et al. [52] did not observe a significant difference between different real rTMS approaches and sham treatment combined with citalopram, milnacipran, mirtazapine or reboxetine for a 2-week period. More recently, Rumi et al. [64] successfully combined 5-Hz left prefrontal rTMS with amitriptyline which was started 7 days prior to the course of rTMS treatment in 46 patients. The total treatment was longer (4 weeks vs. 2 weeks) compared to previous studies. Rossini et al. [63] reported superior efficacy of 15-Hz left prefrontal rTMS combined with venlafaxine, sertraline or citalopram compared to sham rTMS. Very recently, the first multicenter trial addressing this combined treatment approach has been conducted in Germany and Austria [73]. One hundred and twenty-seven patients with moderate to severe major depressive episodes were recruited at seven study sites. The patients were newly started on antidepressant treatment with either mirtazapine or venlafaxine following a standardized titration protocol. Simultaneously, patients were randomized to active or sham rTMS (10 Hz, 110% MT intensity, 2,000 stimuli per day), and treated for 3 weeks with a 3-week follow-up period. After 3 weeks, response rates in both treatment groups were about 31%. Only at the follow-up visit real rTMS was slightly superior to sham rTMS (48% responders after real rTMS vs. 37% after sham rTMS) without reaching statistical significance. Thus, the question is still not answered, whether rTMS may be successfully used as primary treatment with or without other antidepressant interventions. Nonpharmacological approaches are also of interest in this respect; for example, rTMS has been reported to extend the treatment effects of partial sleep deprivation for several days [74].

rTMS in Therapy-Resistant Depression

rTMS was originally regarded as a potential substitute for electroconvulsive therapy (ECT). Therefore, the majority of previous trials has been conducted in rather pharmacotherapy-resistant or even refractory patients [39–43, 45, 46, 48, 49, 51, 57–59, 75]. Treatment-resistant patients show lower response rates, which is generally the case for antidepressant interventions including other novel, nonpharmacological approaches, e.g. VNS [3]. It is however an advantage in small controlled trials that placebo response rates are also lower, thus making it easier to demonstrate differences between real and sham rTMS with a small sample size.

Whereas in most studies investigators applied rTMS basically as an add-on treatment to a stable medication [34, 39–43, 45, 48, 49, 56], few trials have only included medication-free patients who received rTMS monotherapy [51, 58].

Aside from differences in patient characteristics, a major confounding factor for the varying effect sizes could be the huge variation of stimulation parameters across studies. Dosing parameters of rTMS include frequency, intensity, stimulation site, number of stimuli, and duration of treatment. All of these may influence the efficacy. Basically all studies were conducted using different stimulation parameters. Several studies attempted to compare different rTMS conditions [31, 39, 42, 43, 48, 51, 52, 76, 77]. However, larger dose-finding trials for HF rTMS have not been conducted to date. Recently, Fitzgerald et al. [35] compared two frequencies (1 vs. 2 Hz) in a sample of 130 subjects and did not observe a difference in terms of therapeutic efficacy.

We have previously investigated whether stimulation intensity affects the antidepressant efficacy of rTMS in 31 patients suffering from a medication-resistant major depressive episode [43]. We randomly assigned patients to three groups, who then underwent 10 sessions of 10 Hz rTMS over a 2-week period under the following conditions: (1) MT intensity, (2) subthreshold intensity, and (3) sham rTMS (MT intensity with the stimulation coil angled at 90°). Results indicated that antidepressant efficacy increased in a linear fashion over all three groups (best response after rTMS at MT intensity: 30% reduction of the Hamilton Depression Rating Scale (HDRS) score from baseline). Thus, there is preliminary evidence that the antidepressant efficacy of rTMS depends on the stimulation intensity. This finding coincides with evidence from a recent fMRI study [78] that demonstrates intensity-dependent effects on brain activity in healthy volunteers and secondly, with research in elderly depressed patients where a disproportionate frontal atrophy and the resulting decrease of the magnetic field strength at the prefrontal cortex are associated with lower antidepressant efficacy [79, 80]. More recently, our findings were essentially confirmed by Rossini et al. [81] who compared rTMS with 100% MT intensity, 80% MT intensity and sham rTMS and observed a significant difference between treatment groups favoring a higher stimulation intensity.

Fitzgerald et al. [31] were the first who directly compared left HF rTMS and right LF rTMS with sham treatment. Both real rTMS groups improved significantly over 2 weeks compared to the sham rTMS group and improvement was continued if subjects underwent real rTMS during weeks 3 and 4. Thus, this study provided first support for extending rTMS in order to increase response and remission rates. Recently, Avery et al. [45] have reported data of 68 patients with medication-resistant major depression with a response rate of 31% (vs. 6% after sham rTMS) and a remission rate of 20% (vs. 3% after sham rTMS) after 15 sessions of 10 Hz rTMS during a 4-week period. The difference between real and sham rTMS groups reached the magnitude of verum placebo differences for response and remission rates in meta-analyses of antidepressnat drug trials [82].

A very recent US multicenter trial compared real and sham rTMS in a large sample of 325 outpatients (23 trial sites) suffering from a major depressive episode [83]. Inclusion criteria were: HDRS score $>$20, item 1 $>$ 2, treatment resistance defined by failure to respond to at least 1 and no more than 4 antidepressant trials during the current episode (average 1.6 trials), and duration of the current episode $\leq$3 years. It was clinically appropriate to discontinue the current antidepressant medication, i.e. patients were medication free during the trial. Psychotic and bipolar patients were excluded. The treatment was conducted using the Neuronetics Model 210B Therapy System investigational device at aggressive stimulation parameters (120% MT intensity or highest tolerable dosage, 10 Hz, 3,000 stimuli/day) and extended for 6 weeks. HDRS scores rapidly declined already during the first 2 weeks and significantly differed after 4 and 6 weeks of treatment. Response ($HDRS_{24}$) rates were 19% after 4 weeks of real rTMS (vs. 12% after sham rTMS; significant) and 24% (vs. 15%; significant) after 6 weeks, and the respective remission rates ($HDRS_{24}$ score $<$11) were 9% (vs. 8%; not significant) after 4 weeks and 17% (vs. 8%; significant) after 6 weeks. These data were compared to the results of the Sequenced Treatment Alternatives to Relieve Depression (STAR*D) trials where similar baseline and outcome measures were applied in order to allow further interpretation of rTMS efficacy in relation to antidepressant pharmacotherapy [84]. It was concluded that remission rates after rTMS compare to those seen in equally treatment-resistant patients in the STAR*D reports.

Several groups investigated whether more intense stimulation protocols show improved antidepressant efficacy in therapy-resistant patients [48, 52, 57]. Two of these studies [52, 57] failed to show an (improved) efficacy of bilateral rTMS (left prefrontal HF combined with right prefrontal LF rTMS [52], bilateral prefrontal HF rTMS [57]). In contrast, Fitzgerald et al. [48] found a clinically meaningful effect of left prefrontal HF (10 Hz, 750 stimuli/day) combined with right prefrontal LF (1 Hz, 420 stimuli/day) rTMS which was superior to sham rTMS. However, there was no comparison with a standard unilateral rTMS. Generally, longer treatment periods are currently suggested extending the 1- to 2-week treatment in the early studies to 4–6 weeks' protocols [31, 48, 83, 85].

In summary, evidence from numerous small trials, meta-analyses and one large randomized controlled trial support the use of rTMS in depressed subjects who exhibit a moderate degree of treatment resistance. It is of interest that the most robust body of evidence regarding the action of rTMS on neurotransmitter systems points to an action on the dopaminergic system resulting in dopamine release in mesostriatal and mesolimbic regions. Very recently, our group [86] observed a reduction of iodobenzamide (IBZM) binding to striatal

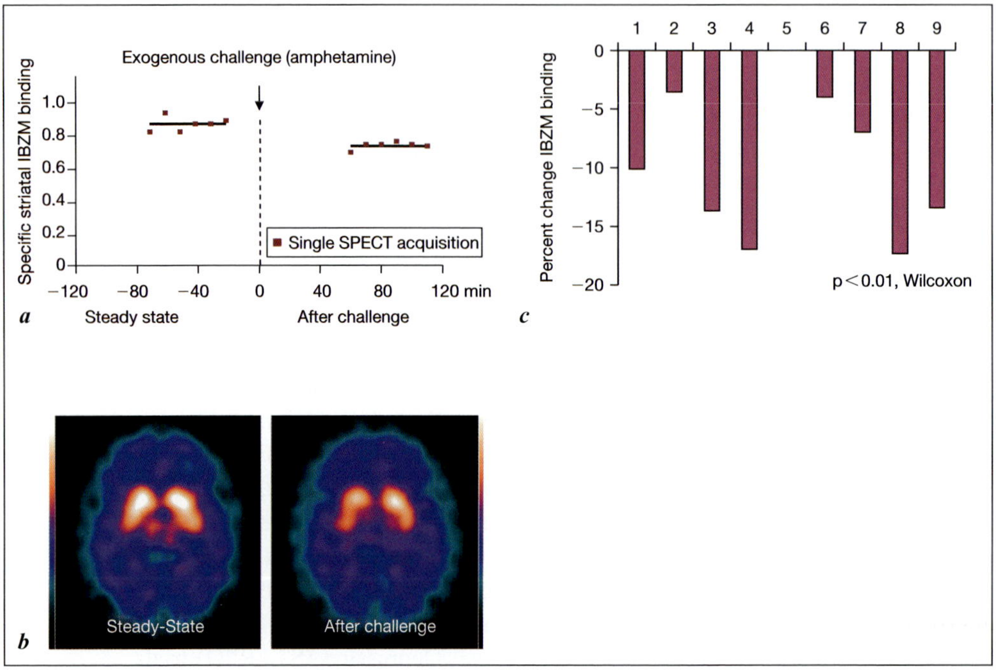

Fig. 3. ***a*** Striatal dopamine release in a dynamic [^{123}I] iodobenzamide (IBZM) single photon emission computed tomography (SPECT) challenge paradigm modified from Laruelle et al. [121]. [^{123}I]-IBZM is given as bolus injection immediately followed by a constant infusion. Two hours after the radiotracer bolus injection an equilibrium is observed, which represents a steady state between radioligand binding and dissociation in the presence of endogenous dopamine. At this time-point the first baseline SPECT is performed. After the first scan, an exogenous dopaminergic stimulation (challenge with amphetamine or rTMS) is applied, followed by a second SPECT scan. After challenge a decrease of specific striatal IBZM binding in the same subject for the six consecutive frames of each SPECT acquisition pre and post challenge is observed (courtesy Dr. Walter Koch). ***b*** Single IBZM-SPECT scans (transaxial slices) of a subject before and after dopaminergic challenge. ***c*** After acute left prefrontal rTMS (10 Hz, 3,000 stimuli/session, 100% MT) a mean reduction of specific IBZM binding by 9.6% was found (data of nine investigations in depressed patients).

D_2/D_3 receptors in antidepressant-free depressed subjects following very similar stimulation parameters (10 Hz, 3,000 stimuli/session, 100% MT) as applied in the US multicenter trial (fig. 3). This change reached the magnitude observed after a single dose of 0.3 mg/kg α-amphetamine. These findings converge with the recent discussion regarding the role of dopamine in major depression and the use of dopaminergic agents (e.g. bupropion and amineptine) in treatment-resistant depressive states.

rTMS in Bipolar Depression

Management of depression in the context of bipolar disorders poses a major clinical problem. Although antidepressant properties have been reported, many mood stabilizers such as the anticonvulsants carbamazepine and valproic acid are not particularly effective in bipolar depression. The use of antidepressant medication during the depressed phase may counterproductively increase a patient's cycle frequency. In several studies investigating the efficacy of rTMS in major depressive episodes also bipolar patients were included. However, separate data of these patients are not available and switches to manic states have been reported [87].

In the first study of rTMS in bipolar depression, Dolberg et al. [47] compared active and sham rTMS in 20 patients. Half of them received 10 sessions, half of them 20 sessions as add-on intervention. In the real rTMS group, HDRS scores decreased from 22 to 15.7 after 2 weeks and to 17.4 after 4 weeks. In the sham group, HDRS scores dropped from 25.5 to 21.3 (2 weeks) and to 13.8 4 weeks). A significant difference between both groups was apparent after 2 weeks and lost after 4 weeks. Due to the lack of a more detailed description of the patient sample and additional interventions, these data are difficult to interpret.

Nahas et al. [61] investigated rTMS in 23 depressed bipolar patients (12 diagnosed with bipolar I disorder in a depressed state, 9 with bipolar II disorder in a depressed state, 2 with bipolar I disorder in mixed states). In two groups, patients were randomly assigned to receive either left prefrontal rTMS (5 Hz, 110% MT, 8 s on, 22 s off, over 20 min) or placebo each weekday morning for 2 weeks. The patients tolerated the stimulation well, exhibiting no significant adverse events and no induction of mania. There was no statistically significant difference between the two groups regarding the number of responders and remitters and the mean change of the HDRS score from baseline over 2 weeks. Compared to sham rTMS, real rTMS produced a trend towards greater improvement in daily subjective mood ratings after treatment. Interestingly, 7 patients of this acute study were followed during weekly maintenance treatment with rTMS for up to 1 year [88]. Three subjects completed the full 1-year period and preserved an average HDRS score of 13 during the whole period. Two of these subjects had no relapses and 1 subject had once a relapse, but quickly responded to a 2-week acute-phase treatment and recovered. The other 4 subjects had multiple relapses despite weekly rTMS and were not able to complete the full year of the maintenance study. Thus, there is preliminary evidence that rTMS can also be used successfully as maintenance treatment in individual patients. Though rTMS is an acute intervention compared to VNS or DBS, maintenance rTMS may be clinically useful and should be differentially tested in future trials.

rTMS in Mania

An early pilot study compared right vs. left prefrontal 20 Hz rTMS and found that right prefrontal treatment was superior to left prefrontal treatment [89]. This finding reflects the valence hypothesis of emotional regulation which has often been involved in early rTMS research [13]. However, the same group of researchers failed to replicate their findings [90]. In the replication study, no difference was observed between right prefrontal rTMS and sham rTMS in 19 patients with moderate mania. Later, case reports and two open trials were published reporting successful treatment of mania with rTMS applied add-on to psychopharmacological treatment [91, 92]. Moreover, an experimental model of amphetamine-induced mania-like behavior has been investigated in animals and humans in order to further explore the antimanic action of 20- to 25-Hz rTMS. In rats, Shaldivin et al. [93] found that 2 and 7 daily rTMS sessions significantly reduced the activity of amphetamine, whereas twice-daily treatment for 7 days enhanced hyperactivity in this model. In healthy volunteers, no change in the psychostimulant action of 0.15 mg/kg amphetamine was observed after right prefrontal stimulation [94]. In summary, these findings do not support the use of rTMS for treating mania and this approach needs to be carefully reconsidered based on changes of regional brain function observed in bipolar disorders [95].

rTMS in Other Depressive Disorders

rTMS treatment might have a therapeutic benefit not only for major depression, but also for depression associated with neurological disorders, such as Parkinson's disease (PD) and stroke. Although depression in neurological conditions is associated with a significant impact on quality of life, it is poorly managed and one of the main reasons is the lack of satisfactory therapies as antidepressants are often inadequate due to side effects and drug interactions.

There are two main advantages for using rTMS for the treatment of depression in neurological disorders: (1) rTMS is associated with few adverse events (see review in Machii et al. [96]) and does not interact with drugs commonly used for the treatment of neurological disorders – this is particularly important for PD patients that usually take several medications that have drug interactions with antidepressants. (2) rTMS may be applied to treat both the underlying neurological disease and psychiatric symptoms. For instance, rTMS treatment for depression in PD patients has been reported to improve mood and motor function simultaneously [97]. Additionally, other techniques of brain stimulation have shown concurrent effects on neurological and psychiatric symptoms, such as ECT for PD patients with depression [98], and VNS for patients with epilepsy and depression [99].

Initial studies have been conducted to evaluate the antidepressant effects of rTMS in PD [97, 100] and stroke [101], and, in addition, rTMS treatment could be useful for depression in epilepsy and Alzheimer's disease.

Two studies have explored the question of whether rTMS treatment for depression in PD is effective. The first open trial by Dragasevic et al. [97] showed that LF rTMS of the left and right prefrontal cortices results in a significant improvement of depression and motor function. After this study, Fregni et al. [100] performed a randomized, double-blind, controlled study to evaluate the effects of HF rTMS on mood in patients with PD. This study showed that 10 consecutive sessions of rTMS lead to a similar antidepressant effect as that induced by fluoxetine lasting for at least 2 months. This study also showed a cognitive improvement after treatment that was further explored by Boggio et al. [102].

Similar positive results were obtained for the treatment of depression in stroke. Jorge et al. [101] showed that 10 sessions of real rTMS (10 Hz, 110% of the MT), as compared with sham stimulation, significantly reduce depressive symptoms and are associated with a trend toward a cognitive improvement.

Finally, rTMS has been shown to decrease the frequency of seizures [103] and to induce a significant improvement of some aspects of cognition in patients with major depression [104]. Thus, it is conceivable to hypothesize that this therapy might be suited to treat depression in epilepsy and in dementia syndromes, such as Alzheimer's disease. Further trials need to be performed to evaluate the clinical utility of rTMS for the treatment of depression in these neurological disorders.

Special Issues

Duration of Effects and Maintenance

It remains to be clarified, whether subsequent antidepressant treatment is necessary to stabilize the clinical response after rTMS. A deterioration of depressive symptoms within 3 weeks after 1 week of rTMS treatment was reported by Pascual-Leone et al. [39].

We [106] conducted a follow-up study on drug-free patients participating in an open rTMS trial over 2 weeks. They underwent 10 rTMS sessions (10 Hz, left prefrontal stimulation at 100% MT intensity) and received subsequent standardized antidepressant medication with mirtazapine (either monotherapy or combined with carbamazepine or lithium) for an additional 4 weeks. The interval between the last rTMS and the first day of pharmacotherapy varied between 1 and 5 days. A significant increase in the HDRS score of rTMS responders was observed after treatment interruption following rTMS. The length of the interval without treatment was correlated with the degree of deterioration. However, during subsequent mirtazapine treatment this deterioration subsided and the further clinical course was stabilized. This observation corresponds with the outcome in the combined dexamethasone suppression/CRH test, where no effect of rTMS on CRH-induced ACTH and cortisol release was observed [107] which suggests a high risk for relapse after improvement of depressive symptoms.

Maintenance treatment with rTMS has been used successfully in single patients and open trials showing favorable long-term outcomes after maintenance schedules of 0.5–2 rTMS sessions/week. However, this method has its drawbacks, as it is more time-consuming for patients and psychiatrists than pharmacotherapy.

Predictors of Antidepressant Response after rTMS

A number of studies have demonstrated that rTMS induces a significant antidepressant effect with few, usually mild adverse effects. However, other studies fail to show such benefits of rTMS treatment in depressed patients. This variability could be explained by the random variability of the 'true' rTMS effect, particularly because most published rTMS studies to date are small and lack adequate statistical power; or alternatively by different patient characteristics. Therefore, it is important to recognize the predictors of the antidepressant response to rTMS treatment.

In a recent study, Fregni et al. [108] pooled data from 6 clinical trials performed at different institutions to investigate the predictors of the antidepressant response to rTMS treatment based on patient and treatment characteristics. A regression model was performed to analyze whether the items of the HDRS, age, gender, psychiatric and drug history and rTMS parameters were associated with the antidepressant response as indexed by the HDRS score.

The only variables that remained in the model were age, treatment refractoriness, item 17 of the HDRS and gender. This model showed that only age and medication refractoriness were significant predictors when the multivariate analysis was performed. Moreover, these two variables were significant in additional models and remained significant after adjusting for other potential confounders. Therefore, younger and nonrefractory patients seem to respond better to rTMS antidepressant treatment. Importantly, the significant variables remained significant after adjusting for the study site. This is particularly important as heterogeneity from different studies is expected.

These results are in accordance with previous studies which showed that elderly patients had a poorer response to rTMS. In an open study with 56 patients,

Figiel et al. [109] showed that the antidepressant response rate was higher for younger (less than age 65) compared to older patients – 56 vs. 23%. In addition, two other studies have reported that elderly patients less satisfactorily respond to rTMS [58, 60]. Nahas et al. [110] hypothesized that this lack of effect in the elderly is due to frontal atrophy and conducted a pilot study that showed that rTMS treatment adjusted for prefrontal atrophy in terms of stimulation intensity is more effective than standard rTMS.

Regarding the smaller effect in patients with more refractory depression, this finding seems to be intuitive, as patients refractory to antidepressants might have a more chronic form of depression and may be more resistant to antidepressant interventions in general. In fact, medication resistance also decreases the effect sizes of ECT [111]. Although we showed that age and refractoriness are significant predictors of the antidepressant response, other predictors such as depression subtype and depression severity should be further studied in prospective large cohorts as our study included trials that used different methodologies, such as differences in rTMS parameters and patient populations.

Safety

The notion that rTMS is safe and well tolerated by patients within a range of parameters defined according to a consensus [112] can be substantiated by an extensive body of data. After 10 days of daily prefrontal rTMS in depressed patients, there was no sign of structural changes on MR scans [113]. There was no deterioration in neuropsychologic performance, no significant mean changes in auditory threshold, and no significant electroencephalogram abnormality after 2–4 weeks of rTMS shown in safety studies [32, 42, 45, 104, 114–116]. Table 3 provides a synopsis of neuropsychological findings in clinical studies investigating rTMS in depressed subjects. Thus, there seem to be no adverse effects on cognition as observed after ECT. If patients with contraindications are excluded (e.g. implanted electronic devices, previous history of seizures), meaningful side effects include physical discomfort on the scalp during and headache after rTMS. Moreover, rare single cases of rTMS-associated seizures have been reported since 1998 when safety guidelines were published limiting stimulation parameters [112, 117]. The risk of a seizure may be increased by higher frequencies and intensities, longer train duration, short intertrain intervals and concomitant medication. However, these cases have to be regarded in the light of many thousands of subjects who have undergone rTMS to date. A very recent overview of published rTMS trials also including systematically collected safety data from a leading brain stimulation laboratory

Table 3. Neuropsychological assessment in clinical studies investigating rTMS as treatment in major depressive episodes

Study	n	Design	Medication	Stimulation site	Stimulus parameters				Measures	Findings
					frequency Hz	intensity (MT%)	stimuli per day	total number of stimuli		
Padberg et al. [42]	18	parallel, random-ized, sham-controlled	stable medication or drug-free	left DLPFC	10 or 0.3	90	250	1,250	Verbal learning task	Significant improvement in verbal memory after 10-Hz rTMS
Triggs et al. [122]	10	open	drug-free	left DLPFC	20	80	2,000	20,000	MMSE, Hopkins Verbal Learning Test digit span, COWA, BNT	No impairment, significant improvement in COWA test scores after rTMS
Little et al. [123]	16	cross-over, random-ized, sham-controlled	drug-free or mood stabilizers	left DLPFC	1 or 20	80	800	8,000	Buschke Selective Reminding Test, memory cards, COWA, CPT	No impairment; improvement on list recall ($p < 0.05$) 1 week after rTMS
Loo et al. [115]	18	parallel, random-ized, sham-controlled	stable medication or drug-free	left DLPFC	10	110	1,500	15,000–20,000	MMSE, digit span, RAVLT, VPAL, COWA, RT, AMI	No impairment; no association between changes in neuropsycho-logic scores and

										clinical course; no differences between sham and real groups
Speer et al. [77]	18	cross-over, random-ized, sham-controlled	drug-free or valproate or carba-mazepine	left DLPFC	1 or 20	100	1,600	16,000	Memory tests (see Little et al. [123] above), CPT, COWA	No major changes in test scores (for both the 1-Hz and 20-Hz group); improvement trends on some tests; no correlation with clinical improvement
Moser et al. [104]	19	parallel, random-ized, sham-controlled	drug-free	left DLPFC	20	80	800	4,000	Trial Making Test A and B, WAIS-R Digit Symbol, Stroop Test, COWA, BNT, sentence repetition, Rey Auditory Verbal Learning, Judgement of Line Orientation	Higher digit symbol scores after real rTMS, improvement in Trail Making Test B
Shajahan et al. [124]	15	parallel, random-ized, sham-controlled	stable medication	left DLPFC	5 or 10 or 20	80	500	5,000	Stress Arousal Inventory, Auditory Verbal Learning, Wechsler	No changes

Table 3. (continued)

Study	n	Design	Medication	Stimulation site	Stimulus parameters				Measures	Findings
					frequency Hz	intensity (MT%)	stimuli per day	total number of stimuli		
									Memory Scale, Digit Symbol Substitution Test, Traffic Light Test	
Martis et al. [116]	15	open	drug-free	left DLPFC	10	110	1,000	4,000–20,000	Attention/mental speed, working memory/executive function, memory, fine motor speed	No impairment; significant improvement (baseline-post) in 3 of 4 domains; improvement not related to clinical change
Loo et al. [57]	19	parallel, random-ized, sham-controlled	stable medication	left and right DLPFC (bilateral)	15	90	1,800	27,000	MMSE, measure of psychomotor retardation (CORE) Controlled Oral Word Association Test, Expanded	Improvement after sham rTMS after sham rTMS after real rTMS in Tower of London, no differences between groups

									Paired Associates Test, Rey Auditory Verbal Learning, Tower of London, visual learning, visual paired associates learning	over time after correction for multiple comparisons
O'Connor et al. [125]	28	open (ECT vs. rTMS)	drug-free	left DLPFC	10	90	1,600	16,000	Rey Auditory Verbal Learning, Letter Number Sequencing Task, Transient News Events Test	Mild improvement in Letter Number Sequencing Task and Transient News Events Test
Hoeppner et al. [53]	30	parallel, random-ized, sham-controlled	stable medication	left DLPFC (20 Hz), right DLPFC (1 Hz)	20 vs. 1	90 (20 Hz), 110 (1 Hz)	800 (20 Hz), 120 (1 Hz)	8,000 (20 Hz), 1,200 (1 Hz)	Motor Agitation and Retardation Scale, D2 test	Significant improvement of slight motor retardation after real rTMS
Hausmann et al. [114]	41	parallel, random-ized, sham-controlled	new antide-pressant starting day 1 of rTMS	left DLPFC (20 Hz), right DLPFC (1 Hz)	20 vs. 20 plus 1	100 (20 Hz), 120 (1 Hz)	2,000 (20 Hz), 2,600 (20 Hz plus 1 Hz)	20,000 (20 Hz), 26,000 (20 Hz plus 1 Hz)	Münchner verbaler Gedächtnistest, Trail Making Test, Stroop Test, Verbal Fluency Test	Improvement in Stroop and Trail Making Test performance after real rTMS, but no difference between real and sham rTMS groups

Table 3. (continued)

Study	n	Design	Medication	Stimulation site	Stimulus parameters				Measures	Findings
					frequency Hz	intensity (MT%)	stimuli per day	total number of stimuli		
Avery et al. [45]	68	parallel, randomized, double-blind	stable medication or drug-free	left DLPFC	10	110	1,600	24,000	MMSE, Rey Auditory Verbal Learning, Digit Symbol Test, Digit Span Test, Trail Making Test, Controlled Word Association Test, Color Stroop Test, Galveston Orientation and Amnesia Test	No differences between real and sham rTMS
Schulze-Rauschenbach et al. [126]	30	open (ECT vs. rTMS)	stable medication	left DLPFC	10	100	400–600	mean: 10 sessions	MMSE, Trail Making Test, Digit span, letter-number span, word fluency, Auditory Verbal Learning Test, Memory for Persons Test, autobiographical memory	rTMS superior to ECT in anterograde verbal memory, two retrograde memory parameters and memory self-assessment. Subject's rating of memory significantly

									interview, four-card task of the Rivermead Behavioral Memory Test, Squire Subjective Memory Questionnaire	improved after rTMS (correlation with self-rating of depression)
Januel et al. [32]	27	parallel, random-ized, double-blind	drug-free	right DLPFC	1	90	120	1,200	Grober and Buschke's Test (for verbal memory), Stroop Test, Trail Making Test, auditory and visual attention span, Cardebat's fluency, visuospatial reasoning	No significant differences after rTMS in either group
Kuroda et al. [127]	9	open	fluvoxamine	left DLPFC	10	100	1,000	10,000	MMSE, Wechsler Memory Scale-Revised, Trail Making Test, Everyday Memory Checklist	Improvement of verbal memory function

AMI = Autobiographical memory interview; BNT = Boston naming test; COWA = Controlled word association; CPT = Continuous performance test; MMSE = Mini mental state examination; RAVLT = Rey auditory verbal learning test; RT = Reaction time; VPAL = Visual paired associates learning; WAIS-R = Wechsler adult intelligence scale-revised; MT = Motor threshold.

in the USA concluded that rTMS to nonmotor areas appears to be safe with few, generally mild adverse effects [96].

Particular attention, however, should be paid to the detection of psychiatric side effects and the possibility should be mentioned to the patients before obtaining their informed consent for participation in rTMS studies. Case reports showed that bipolar patients treated with rTMS for depression may be at risk of switching to manic states [87]. We have reported the case of a depressed patient who newly developed psychotic symptoms during left prefrontal HF rTMS and who never had experienced such symptoms before [118].

Conclusions and Perspectives

In addition to its importance as an experimental research tool in neuroscience, rTMS has been established among novel nonpharmacological treatment strategies for major depression. As supported by neuroimaging data, long-term rTMS modulates neuronal circuits involved in the pathophysiology of depression. Preclinical studies have shown dopaminergic and serotonergic effects, among others, as well as an attenuation of the hypothalamic-pituitary-adrenal response to stress, which is hypothesized to occur at hippocampal and hypothalamic levels. The majority of clinical trials demonstrate significant antidepressant effects as compared to sham conditions, with optimal parameters yet to be identified. Recent evidence from a large US multicenter trial supports the antidepressant efficacy of rTMS in therapy-resistant depression and will presumably stimulate a wider use of rTMS in clinical practice. Other specific clinical applications of rTMS require further testing either in specifically selected patient populations or through the use of specific study designs. Moreover, a wide range of methodological developments such as neuronavigated rTMS, a new generation of powerful magnetic stimulators, novel stimulation protocols (e.g. theta burst stimulation), new stimulation coils (e.g. H-coils) and the combined application of rTMS together with transcranial direct current stimulation will allow to further improve today's rTMS interventions in the future [119].

References

1 George MS, Lisanby SH, Sackeim HA: Transcranial magnetic stimulation. Arch Gen Psychiatry 1999;56:300–311.

2 Padberg F, Goldstein-Müller B, Zwanzger P, Möller HJ: Prefrontal cortex stimulation as antidepressant treatment: mode of action and clinical effectiveness of rTMS. Clin Neurophysiol 2003;56:406–432.

3 Sackeim HA, Rush AJ, George MS, Marangell LB, Husain MM, Nahas Z, Johnson CR, Seidman S, Giller C, Haines S, Simpson RKJ, Goodman RR: Vagus nerve stimulation (VNS) for treatment-resistant depression: efficacy, side effects, and predictors of outcome. Neuropsychopharmacology 2001;25:713–728.
4 Mayberg HS, Lozano AM, Voon V, McNeely HE, Seminowicz D, Hamani C, Schwalb JM, Kennedy SH: Deep brain stimulation for treatment-resistant depression. Neuron 2005;45: 651–660.
5 Fregni F, Boggio P, Nitsche M, Marcolin M, Rigonatti S, Pascual-Leone A: Treatment of major depression with transcranial direct current stimulation. Bipolar Disord 2006;8:203–205.
6 Barker AT, Jalinous R, Freeston IL: Noninvasive magnetic stimulation of human motor cortex. Lancet 1985;ii:1106–1107.
7 Hallett M: Transcranial magnetic stimulation: a tool for mapping the central nervous system. Electroencephalogr Clin Neurophysiol Suppl 1996;46:43–51.
8 Hoffman RE, Cavus I: Slow transcranial magnetic stimulation, long-term depotentiation, and brain hyperexcitability disorders. Am J Psychiatry 2002;159:1093–1102.
9 Fitzgerald PB, Fountain S, Daskalakis ZJ: A comprehensive review of the effects of rTMS on motor cortical excitability and inhibition. Clin Neurophysiol 2006;117:2584–2596.
10 Dearing MJ: Mood effects of prefrontal repetitive high-frequency TMS in healthy volunteers. CNS Spectr 1997;2:53, 68.
11 George MS, Wassermann EM, Williams WA, Steppel J, Pascual-Leone A, Basser P, Hallett M, Post RM: Changes in mood and hormone levels after rapid-rate transcranial magnetic stimulation (rTMS) of the prefrontal cortex. J Neuropsychiatry Clin Neurosci 1996;8:172–180.
12 Pascual-Leone A, Catalá MD, Pascual-Leone A: Lateralized effect of rapid-rate transcranial magnetic stimulation of the prefrontal cortex on mood. Neurology 1996;46:499–502.
13 George MS, Speer AM, Wassermann EM, Kimbrell TA, William WA, Kellner CH, Risch SC, Stallings L, Post RM: Repetitive TMS as a probe of mood in health and disease. CNS Spectr 1997;2:39–44.
14 Baeken C, Leyman L, De Raedt R, Vanderhasselt MA, D'Haenen H: Lack of impact of repetitive high frequency transcranial magnetic stimulation on mood in healthy female subjects. J Affect Disord 2006;90:63–66.
15 Cohrs S, Tergau F, Riech S, Kastner S, Paulus W, Ziemann U, Ruether E, Hajak G: High-frequency repetitive transcranial magnetic stimulation delays rapid eye movement sleep. Neuroreport 1998;9: 3439–3443.
16 Mosimann UP, Rihs TA, Engeler J, Fisch H, Schlaepfer TE: Mood effects of repetitive transcranial magnetic stimulation of left prefrontal cortex in healthy volunteers. Psychiatry Res 2000;94: 251–256.
17 Nedjat S, Folkerts HW: Induction of a reversible state of hypomania by rapid-rate transcranial magnetic stimulation over the left prefrontal cortex. J ECT 1999;15:166–168.
18 Padberg F, Juckel G, Praessl A, Zwanzger P, Mavrogiorgou P, Hegerl U, Hampel H, Moeller H-J: Facial expressions and mood after transcranial magnetic stimulation of the prefrontal cortex. J Neuropsychiatry Clin Neurosci 2001;13:206–212.
19 Grisaru N, Bruno R, Pridmore S: Effect on the emotions of healthy individuals of slow repetitive transcranial magnetic stimulation applied to the prefrontal cortex. J ECT 2001;17:184–189.
20 Jenkins J, Shajahan PM, Lappin JM, Ebmeier KP: Right and left prefrontal transcranial magnetic stimulation at 1 Hz does not affect mood in healthy volunteers. BMC Psychiatry 2002;2:1.
21 Barrett J, Della-Maggiore V, Chouinard PA, Paus T: Mechanisms of action underlying the effect of repetitive transcranial magnetic stimulation on mood: behavioral and brain imaging studies. Neuropsychopharmacology 2004;29:1172–1189.
22 Schutter DJ, van Honk J: Increased positive emotional memory after repetitive transcranial magnetic stimulation over the orbitofrontal cortex. J Psychiatry Neurosci 2006;31:101–104.
23 Cohrs S, Tergau F, Korn J, Becker W, Hajak G: Suprathreshold repetitive transcranial magnetic stimulation elevates thyroid-stimulating hormone in healthy male subjects. J Nerv Ment Dis 2001;189:393–397.
24 Schutter DJ, van Honk J, d'Alfonso AA, Postma A, de Haan EH: Effects of slow rTMS at the right dorsolateral prefrontal cortex on EEG asymmetry and mood. Neuroreport 2001;12:445–447.

25 Conca A, Koppi S, Koenig P, Swoboda E, Krecke N: Transcranial magnetic stimulation: a novel antidepressive strategy? Neuropsychobiology 1996;34:204–207.
26 George MS, Wassermann EM, Williams WA, Callahan A, Ketter TA, Basser P, Hallett M, Post RM: Daily left prefrontal repetitive transcranial magnetic stimulation (rTMS) improves mood in depression. Neuroreport 1995;6:1–6.
27 Grisaru N, Yarovslavsky U, Abarbanel J, Lamberg T, Belmaker RH: Transcranial magnetic stimulation in depression and schizophrenia. Eur Neuropsychopharmacol 1994;4:287–288.
28 Hoeflich G, Kasper S, Hufnagel A, Ruhrmann S, Moeller H-J: Application of transcranial magnetic stimulation in treatment of drug-resistant major depression. Hum Psychopharmacol 1993;8:361–365.
29 Kolbinger HM, Hoeflich G, Hufnagel A, Moeller H-J, Kasper S: Transcranial magnetic stimulation (TMS) in the treatment of major depression – A pilot study. Hum Psychopharmacol 1995;10:305–310.
30 Herwig U, Padberg F, Unger J, Spitzer M, Schonfeldt-Lecuona C: Transcranial magnetic stimulation in therapy studies: examination of the reliability of 'standard' coil positioning by neuronavigation. Biol Psychiatry 2001;50:58–61.
31 Fitzgerald PB, Brown TL, Marston NA, Daskalakis ZJ, De Castella A, Kulkarni J: Transcranial magnetic stimulation in the treatment of depression: a double-blind, placebo-controlled trial. Arch Gen Psychiatry 2003;60:1002–1008.
32 Januel D, Dumortier G, Verdon CM, Stamatiadis L, Saba G, Cabaret W, Benadhira R, Rocamora JF, Braha S, Kalalou K, Vicaut PE, Fermanian J: A double-blind sham controlled study of right prefrontal repetitive transcranial magnetic stimulation (rTMS): therapeutic and cognitive effect in medication free unipolar depression during 4 weeks. Prog Neuropsychopharmacol Biol Psychiatry 2006;30:126–130.
33 Kauffmann CD, Cheema MA, Miller BE: Slow right prefrontal transcranial magnetic stimulation as a treatment for medication-resistant depression: a double-blind, placebo-controlled study. Depress Anxiety 2004;19:59–62.
34 Klein E, Kreinin I, Chistyakov A, Koren D, Mecz L, Marmur S, Ben-Shachar D, Feinsod M: Therapeutic efficacy of right prefrontal slow repetitive transcranial magnetic stimulation in major depression. Arch Gen Psychiatry 1999;56:315–320.
35 Fitzgerald PB, Huntsman S, Gunewardene R, Kulkarni J, Daskalakis ZJ: A randomized trial of low-frequency right-prefrontal-cortex transcranial magnetic stimulation as augmentation in treatment-resistant major depression. Int J Neuropsychopharmacol 2006;7:1–12.
36 Garcia-Toro M, Salva J, Daumal J, Andres J, Romera M, Lafau O, Echevarria M, Mestre M, Bosch C, Collado C, Ibarra O, Aguirre I: High (20-Hz) and low (1-Hz) frequency transcranial magnetic stimulation as adjuvant treatment in medication-resistant depression. Psychiatry Res 2006;146:53–57.
37 Kimbrell TA, Little JT, Dunn RT, Frye MA, Greenberg BD, Wassermann EM, Repella JD, Danielson AL, Willis MW, Benson BE, Speer AM, Osuch E, George MS, Post RM: Frequency dependence of antidepressant response to left prefrontal repetitive transcranial magnetic stimulation (rTMS) as a function of baseline cerebral glucose metabolism. Biol Psychiatry 1999;46:1603–1613.
38 Herwig U, Lampe Y, Juengling FD, Wunderlich A, Walter H, Spitzer M, Schonfeldt-Lecuona C: Add-on rTMS for treatment of depression: a pilot study using stereotaxic coil-navigation according to PET data. J Psychiatr Res 2003;37:267–275.
39 Pascual-Leone A, Rubio B, Pallardó F, Catalá MD: Rapid-rate transcranial magnetic stimulation of left dorsolateral prefrontal cortex in drug-resistant depression. Lancet 1996;348:233–237.
40 George MS, Wassermann EM, Kimbrell TA, Little JT, Williams WE, Danielson AL, Greenberg BD, Hallett M, Post RM: Mood improvement following daily left prefrontal repetitive transcranial magnetic stimulation in patients with depression: a placebo-controlled crossover trial. Am J Psychiatry 1997;154:1752–1756.
41 Eschweiler GW, Wegerer C, Schlotter W, Spandl C, Stevens A, Bartels M, Buchkremer G: Left prefrontal activation predicts therapeutic effects of repetitive transcranial magnetic stimulation (rTMS) in major depression. Psychiatry Res 2000;99:161–172.
42 Padberg F, Zwanzger P, Thoma H, Kathmann N, Haag C, Greenberg BD, Hampel H, Moeller H-J: Repetitive transcranial magnetic stimulation (rTMS) in pharmacotherapy-refractory major depression: comparative study of fast, slow and sham rTMS. Psychiatry Res 1999;88:163–171.

43 Padberg F, Zwanzger P, Keck ME, Kathmann N, Mikhaiel P, Ella R, Rupprecht P, Thoma H, Hampel H, Toschi N, Moeller H-J: Repetitive transcranial magnetic stimulation (rTMS) in major depression: relation between efficacy and stimulation intensity. Neuropsychopharmacology 2002;27:638–645.

44 Avery DH, Claypoole K, Robinson L, Neumaier JF, Dunner DL, Scheele L, Wilson L, Roy-Byrne P: Repetitive transcranial magnetic stimulation in the treatment of medication-resistant depression: preliminary data. J Nerv Ment Dis 1999;187:114–117.

45 Avery DH, Holtzheimer PE 3rd, Fawaz W, Russo J, Neumaier J, Dunner DL, Haynor DR, Claypoole KH, Wajdik C, Roy-Byrne P: A controlled study of repetitive transcranial magnetic stimulation in medication-resistant major depression. Biol Psychiatry 2006;59:187–194.

46 Berman RM, Narasimhan M, Sanacora G, Miano AP, Hoffman RE, Hu XS, Charney DS, Boutros NN: A randomized clinical trial of repetitive transcranial magnetic stimulation in the treatment of major depression. Biol Psychiatry 2000;47:332–337.

47 Dolberg OT, Dannon PN, Schreiber S, Grunhaus L: Transcranial magnetic stimulation in patients with bipolar depression: a double blind, controlled study. Bipolar Disord 2002;4 (suppl 1):94–95.

48 Fitzgerald PB, Benitez J, de Castella A, Daskalakis ZJ, Brown TL, Kulkarni J: A randomized, controlled trial of sequential bilateral repetitive transcranial magnetic stimulation for treatment-resistant depression. Am J Psychiatry 2006;163:88–94.

49 Garcia-Toro M, Mayol A, Arnillas H, Capllonch I, Ibarra O, Crespi M, Mico J, Lafau O, Lafuente L: Modest adjunctive benefit with transcranial magnetic stimulation in medication-resistant depression. J Affect Disord 2001;64:271–275.

50 Garcia-Toro M, Pascual-Leone A, Romera M, Gonzalez A, Mico J, Ibarra O, Arnillas H, Capllonch I, Mayol A, Tormos JM: Prefrontal repetitive transcranial magnetic stimulation as add on treatment in depression. J Neurol Neurosurg Psychiatry 2001;71:546–548.

51 George MS, Nahas Z, Molloy M, Speer AM, Oliver NC, Li XB, Arana GW, Risch SC, Ballenger JC: A controlled trial of daily left prefrontal cortex TMS for treating depression. Biol Psychiatry 2000;48:962–970.

52 Hausmann A, Kemmler G, Walpoth M, Mechtcheriakov S, Kramer-Reinstadler K, Lechner T, Walch T, Deisenhammer EA, Kofler M, Rupp CI, Hinterhuber H, Conca A: No benefit derived from repetitive transcranial magnetic stimulation in depression: a prospective, single centre, randomised, double blind, sham controlled 'add on' trial. J Neurol Neurosurg Psychiatry 2004;75: 320–322.

53 Hoeppner J, Schulz M, Irmisch G, Mau R, Schlafke D, Richter J: Antidepressant efficacy of two different rTMS procedures. High frequency over left versus low frequency over right prefrontal cortex compared with sham stimulation. Eur Arch Psychiatry Clin Neurosci 2003;253: 103–109.

54 Holtzheimer PE 3rd, Russo J, Claypoole KH, Roy-Byrne P, Avery DH: Shorter duration of depressive episode may predict response to repetitive transcranial magnetic stimulation. Depress Anxiety 2004;19:24–30.

55 Koerselman F, Laman DM, van Duijn H, van Duijn MA, Willems MA: A 3-month, follow-up, randomized, placebo-controlled study of repetitive transcranial magnetic stimulation in depression. J Clin Psychiatry 2004;65:1323–1328.

56 Loo CK, Mitchell P, Sachdev P, McDarmont B, Parker G, Gandevia S: Double-blind controlled investigation of transcranial magnetic stimulation for the treatment of resistant major depression. Am J Psychiatry 1999;156:946–948.

57 Loo CK, Mitchell PB, Croker VM, Malhi GS, Wen W, Gandevia SC, Sachdev PS: Double-blind controlled investigation of bilateral prefrontal transcranial magnetic stimulation for the treatment of resistant major depression. Psychol Med 2003;33:33–40.

58 Manes F, Jorge R, Morcuende M, Yamada T, Paradiso S, Robinson RG: A controlled study of repetitive transcranial magnetic stimulation as a treatment of depression in the elderly. Int Psychogeriatr 2001;13:225–231.

59 Miniussi C, Bonato C, Bignotti S, Gazzoli A, Gennarelli M, Pasqualetti P, Tura GB, Ventriglia M, Rossini PM: Repetitive transcranial magnetic stimulation (rTMS) at high and low frequency: an efficacious therapy for major drug-resistant depression? Clin Neurophysiol 2005;116:1062–1071.

60 Mosimann UP, Schmitt W, Greenberg BD, Kosel M, Muri RM, Berkhoff M, Hess CW, Fisch HU, Schlaepfer TE: Repetitive transcranial magnetic stimulation: a putative add-on treatment for major depression in elderly patients. Psychiatry Res 2004;126:123–133.
61 Nahas Z, Kozel FA, Li X, Anderson B, George MS: Left prefrontal transcranial magnetic stimulation (TMS) treatment of depression in bipolar affective disorder: a pilot study of acute safety and efficacy. Bipolar Disord 2003;5:40–47.
62 Poulet E, Brunelin J, Boeuve C, Lerond J, D'Amato T, Dalery J, Saoud M: Repetitive transcranial magnetic stimulation does not potentiate antidepressant treatment. Eur Psychiatry 2004;19: 382–383.
63 Rossini D, Magri L, Lucca A, Giordani S, Smeraldi E, Zanardi R: Does rTMS hasten the response to escitalopram, sertraline, or venlafaxine in patients with major depressive disorder? A double-blind, randomized, sham-controlled trial. J Clin Psychiatry 2005;66:1569–1575.
64 Rumi DO, Gattaz WF, Rigonatti SP, Rosa MA, Fregni F, Rosa MO, Mansur C, Myczkowski ML, Moreno RA, Marcolin MA: Transcranial magnetic stimulation accelerates the antidepressant effect of amitriptyline in severe depression: a double-blind placebo-controlled study. Biol Psychiatry 2005;57:162–166.
65 Burt T, Lisanby SH, Sackeim HA: Neuropsychiatric applications of transcranial magnetic stimulation: a meta analysis. Int J Neuropsychopharmacol 2002;5:73–103.
66 Couturier JL: Efficacy of rapid-rate repetitive transcranial magnetic stimulation in the treatment of depression: a systematic review and meta-analysis. J Psychiatry Neurosci 2005;30:83–90.
67 Herrmann LL, Ebmeier KP: Factors modifying the efficacy of transcranial magnetic stimulation in the treatment of depression: a review. J Clin Psychiatry 2006;67:1870–1876.
68 Holtzheimer PE 3rd, Russo J, Avery DH: A meta-analysis of repetitive transcranial magnetic stimulation in the treatment of depression. Psychopharmacol Bull 2001;35:149–169.
69 Martin JL, Barbanoj MJ, Schlaepfer TE, Thompson E, Perez V, Kulisevsky J: Repetitive transcranial magnetic stimulation for the treatment of depression. Systematic review and meta-analysis. Br J Psychiatry 2003;182:480–491.
70 McNamara B, Ray JL, Arthurs OJ, Boniface S: Transcranial magnetic stimulation for depression and other psychiatric disorders. Psychol Med 2001;31:1141–1146.
71 Gershon AA, Dannon PN, Grunhaus L: Transcranial magnetic stimulation in the treatment of depression. Am J Psychiatry 2003;160:835–845.
72 Lisanby SH, Pascual-Leone A, Sampson SM, Boylan LS, Burt T, Sackeim HA: Augmentation of sertraline antidepressant treatment with transcranial magnetic stimulation. Biol Psychiatry 2002;49:81S.
73 Herwig U, Spitzer M, Eschweiler G, Fallgatter AJ, Hajak G, Heiden A, Hoeppner J, Padberg F, Abler B, Eichhammer P, Grossheinrich N, Kammer T, Langguth B, Laske C, Plewnia C, Schulz M, Unterecker S, Schoenfeldt-Lecuona C: Antidepressant transcranial magnetic stimulation – Results from the first multi-center trial (abstract). Biol Psychiatry 2006;59:97S.
74 Eichhammer P, Kharraz A, Wiegand R, Langguth B, Frick U, Aigner JM, Hajak G: Sleep deprivation in depression stabilizing antidepressant effects by repetitive transcranial magnetic stimulation. Life Sci 2002;70:1741–1749.
75 Boutros NN, Gueorguieva R, Hoffman RE, Oren DA, Feingold A, Berman RM: Lack of a therapeutic effect of a 2-week sub-threshold transcranial magnetic stimulation course for treatment-resistant depression. Psychiatry Res 2002;113:245–254.
76 Isenberg K, Downs D, Pierce K, Svarakic D, Garcia K, Jarvis M, North C, Kormos TC: Low frequency rTMS stimulation of the right frontal cortex is as effective as high frequency rTMS stimulation of the left frontal cortex for antidepressant-free, treatment-resistant depressed patients. Ann Clin Psychiatry 2005;17:153–159.
77 Speer AM, Repella JD, Figueras S, Deminan NK, Kimbrell TA, Wasserman EM, Post RM: Lack of adverse cognitive effects on 1 Hz and 20 Hz repetitive transcranial magnetic stimulation at 100% of motor threshold over left prefrontal cortex in depression. J ECT 2001;17:259–263.
78 Nahas Z, Lomarev M, Roberts DR, Shastri A, Lorberbaum JP, Teneback C, McConnell K, Vincent DJ, Li X, George MS, Bohning DE: Unilateral left prefrontal transcranial magnetic stimulation (TMS) produces intensity-dependent bilateral effects as measured by interleaved BOLD fMRI. Biol Psychiatry 2001;50:712–720.

79 Kozel FA, Nahas Z, deBrux C, Molloy M, Lorberbaum JP, Bohning D, Risch SC, George MS: How coil-cortex distance relates to age, motor threshold, and antidepressant response to repetitive transcranial magnetic stimulation. J Neuropsychiatry Clin Neurosci 2000;12:376–384.
80 Mosimann U, Marré SC, Werlen S, Schmitt W, Hess CW, Fisch HU, Schlaepfer TE: Antidepressant effects of repetitive transcranial magnetic stimulation in the elderly: correlation between effect size and coil-cortex distance. Arch Gen Psychiatry 2002;59:560–561.
81 Rossini D, Lucca A, Zanardi R, Magri L, Smeraldi E: Transcranial magnetic stimulation in treatment-resistant depressed patients: a double-blind, placebo-controlled trial. Psychiatry Res 2005;137:1–10.
82 Thase ME: Effectiveness of antidepressants: comparative remission rates. J Clin Psychiatry 2003;64(suppl 2):3–7.
83 O'Reardon JP: Repetitive transcranial magnetic stimulation (rTMS) at 10 Hz in the treatment of pharmacoresistant major depression – Results from a controlled multicenter clinical trial. APA Annu Meet, Toronto, 2006.
84 Fava M, Rush AJ, Wisniewski SR, Nierenberg AA, Alpert JE, McGrath PJ, Thase ME, Warden D, Biggs M, Luther JF, Niederehe G, Ritz L, Trivedi MH: A comparison of mirtazapine and nortriptyline following two consecutive failed medication treatments for depressed outpatients: a STAR*D report. Am J Psychiatry 2006;163:1161–1172.
85 Grunhaus L, Dannon PN, Schreiber S, Dolberg OH, Amiaz R, Ziv R, Lefkifker E: Repetitive transcranial magnetic stimulation is as effective as electroconvulsive therapy in the treatment of nondelusional major depressive disorder: an open study. Biol Psychiatry 2000;47:314–324.
86 Pogarell O, Koch W, Popperl G, Tatsch K, Jakob F, Zwanzger P, Mulert C, Rupprecht R, Moller HJ, Hegerl U, Padberg F: Striatal dopamine release after prefrontal repetitive transcranial magnetic stimulation in major depression: preliminary results of a dynamic [123I] IBZM SPECT study. J Psychiatr Res 2006;40:307–314.
87 Ella R, Zwanzger P, Stampfer R, Preuss U, Mueller-Siecheneder F, Moeller H-J, Padberg F: Switch to mania after slow rTMS of the right prefrontal cortex. J Clin Psychiatry 2002;63:249.
88 Li X, Nahas Z, Anderson B, Kozel FA, George MS: Can left prefrontal rTMS be used as a maintenance treatment for bipolar depression? Depress Anxiety 2004;20:98–100.
89 Grisaru N, Chudakov B, Yaroslavsky Y, Belmaker RH: Transcranial magnetic stimulation in mania: a controlled study. Am J Psychiatry 1998;155:1608–1610.
90 Kaptsan A, Yaroslavsky Y, Applebaum J, Belmaker RH, Grisaru N: Right prefrontal TMS versus sham treatment of mania: a controlled study. Bipolar Disord 2003;5:36–39.
91 Michael N, Erfurth A: Treatment of bipolar mania with right prefrontal rapid transcranial magnetic stimulation. J Affect Disord 2004;78:253–257.
92 Saba G, Rocamora JF, Kalalou K, Benadhira R, Plaze M, Lipski H, Januel D: Repetitive transcranial magnetic stimulation as an add-on therapy in the treatment of mania: a case series of eight patients. Psychiatry Res 2004;128:199–202.
93 Shaldivin A, Kaptsan A, Belmaker RH, Einat H, Grisaru N: Transcranial magnetic stimulation in an amphetamine hyperactivity model of mania. Bipolar Disord 2001;3:30–34.
94 Clark L, McTavish SF, Harmer CJ, Mills KR, Cowen PJ, Goodwin GM: Repetitive transcranial magnetic stimulation to right prefrontal cortex does not modulate the psychostimulant effects of amphetamine. Int J Neuropsychopharmacol 2000;3:297–302.
95 Blumberg HP, Krystal JH, Bansal R, Martin A, Dziura J, Durkin K, Martin L, Gerard E, Charney DS, Peterson BS: Age, rapid-cycling, and pharmacotherapy effects on ventral prefrontal cortex in bipolar disorder: a cross-sectional study. Biol Psychiatry 2006;59:611–618.
96 Machii K, Cohen D, Ramos-Estebanez C, Pascual-Leone A: Safety of rTMS to non-motor cortical areas in healthy participants and patients. Clin Neurophysiol 2006;117:455–471.
97 Dragasevic N, Potrebic A, Damjanovic A, Stefanova E, Kostic VS: Therapeutic efficacy of bilateral prefrontal slow repetitive transcranial magnetic stimulation in depressed patients with Parkinson's disease: an open study. Mov Disord 2002;17:528–532.
98 Kennedy R, Mittal D, O'Jile J: Electroconvulsive therapy in movement disorders: an update. J Neuropsychiatry Clin Neurosci 2003;15:407–421.
99 George MS, Nahas Z, Bohning DE, Kozel FA, Anderson B, Chae JH, Lomarev M, Denslow S, Li X, Mu C: Vagus nerve stimulation therapy: a research update. Neurology 2002;59:S56–S61.

100 Fregni F, Santos CM, Myczkowski ML, Rigolino R, Gallucci-Neto J, Barbosa ER, Valente KD, Pascual-Leone A, Marcolin MA: Repetitive transcranial magnetic stimulation is as effective as fluoxetine in the treatment of depression in patients with Parkinson's disease. J Neurol Neurosurg Psychiatry 2004;75:1171–1174.

101 Jorge RE, Robinson RG, Tateno A, Narushima K, Acion L, Moser D, Arndt S, Chemerinski E: Repetitive transcranial magnetic stimulation as treatment of poststroke depression: a preliminary study. Biol Psychiatry 2004;55:398–405.

102 Boggio PS, Fregni F, Bermpohl F, Mansur CG, Rosa M, Rumi DO, Barbosa ER, Odebrecht Rosa M, Pascual-Leone A, Rigonatti SP, Marcolin MA, Araujo Silva MT: Effect of repetitive TMS and fluoxetine on cognitive function in patients with Parkinson's disease and concurrent depression. Mov Disord 2005;20:1178–1184.

103 Fregni F, Thome-Souza S, Bermpohl F, Marcolin MA, Herzog A, Pascual-Leone A, Valente KD: Antiepileptic effects of repetitive transcranial magnetic stimulation in patients with cortical malformations: an EEG and clinical study. Stereotact Funct Neurosurg 2005;83:57–62.

104 Moser DJ, Jorge RE, Manes F, Paradiso S, Benjamin ML, Robinson RG: Improved executive functioning following repetitive transcranial magnetic stimulation. Neurology 2002;58:1288–1290.

105 Dannon PN, Dolberg OT, Schreiber S, Grunhaus L: Three- and six-month outcome following courses of either ECT or rTMS in a population of severely depressed individuals – Preliminary report. Biol Psychiatry 2002;51:687–690.

106 Schuele C, Zwanzger P, Baghai T, Mikhaiel P, Thoma H, Moeller H-J, Rupprecht R, Padberg F: Effects of antidepressant pharmacotherapy after repetitive transcranial magnetic stimulation in major depression: an open follow-up study. J Psychiatr Res 2003;37:145–153.

107 Zwanzger P, Baghai TC, Padberg F, Ella R, Minov C, Mikhaiel P, Schuele C, Thoma H, Rupprecht R: The combined dexamethasone-CRH test before and after repetitive transcranial magnetic stimulation (rTMS) in major depression. Psychoneuroendocrinology 2003;28:376–385.

108 Fregni F, Marcolin MA, Myczkowski M, Amiaz R, Hasey G, Rumi DO, Rosa M, Rigonatti SP, Camprodon J, Walpoth M, Heaslip J, Grunhaus L, Hausmann A, Pascual-Leone A: Predictors of antidepressant response in clinical trials of transcranial magnetic stimulation. Int J Neuropsychopharmacol 2005;23:1–14.

109 Figiel GS, Epstein C, McDonald WM, Amazon-Leece J, Figiel L, Saldivia A, Glover S: The use of rapid-rate transcranial magnetic stimulation (rTMS) in refractory depressed patients. J Neuropsychiatry Clin Neurosci 1998;10:20–25.

110 Nahas Z, Li X, Kozel FA, Mirzki D, Memon M, Miller K, Yamanaka K, Anderson B, Chae JH, Bohning DE, Mintzer J, George MS: Safety and benefits of distance-adjusted prefrontal transcranial magnetic stimulation in depressed patients 55–75 years of age: a pilot study. Depress Anxiety 2004;19:249–256.

111 UK ECT Review Group: Efficacy and safety of electroconvulsive therapy in depressive disorders: a systematic review and meta-analysis. Lancet 2003;361:799–808.

112 Wassermann EM: Risk and safety of repetitive transcranial magnetic stimulation: report and suggested guidelines from the International Workshop on the Safety of Repetitive Transcranial Magnetic Stimulation, June 5–7, 1996. Electroencephalogr Clin Neurophysiol 1998;108:1–16.

113 Nahas Z, DeBrux C, Chandler V, Lorberbaum JP, Speer AM, Molloy MA, Liberatos C, Risch SC, George MS: Lack of significant changes on magnetic resonance scans before and after 2 weeks of daily prefrontal repetitive transcranial magnetic stimulation for depression. J ECT 2000;16:380–390.

114 Hausmann A, Pascual-Leone A, Kemmler G, Rupp CI, Lechner-Schoner T, Kramer-Reinstadler K, Walpoth M, Mechtcheriakov S, Conca A, Weiss EM: No deterioration of cognitive performance in an aggressive unilateral and bilateral antidepressant rTMS add-on trial. J Clin Psychiatry 2004;65:772–782.

115 Loo CK, Sachdev PS, Elsayed H, McDarmont BN, Mitchell PB, Wilkinson M, Parker G, Gandevia SC: Effects of a 2- to 4-week course of repetitive transcranial magnetic stimulation (rTMS) on neuropsychological functioning, electroencephalogram and auditory threshold in depressed patients. Biol Psychiatry 2001;49:615–623.

116 Martis B, Alam D, Dowd SM, Hill SK, Sharma RP, Rosen C, Pliskin N, Martin E, Carson V, Janicak PG: Neurocognitive effects of repetitive transcranial magnetic stimulation in severe major depression. Clin Neurophysiol 2003;114:1125–1132.

117 Conca A, Konig P, Hausmann A: Transcranial magnetic stimulation induces 'pseudoabsence seizure'. Acta Psychiatr Scand 2000;101:246–248.
118 Zwanzger P, Ella R, Keck ME, Rupprecht R, Padberg F: Occurrence of delusions during repetitive transcranial magnetic stimulation (rTMS) in major depression. Biol Psychiatry 2002;51:602–603.
119 Lang N, Siebner HR, Ernst D, Nitsche MA, Paulus W, Lemon RN, Rothwell JC: Preconditioning with transcranial direct current stimulation sensitizes the motor cortex to rapid-rate transcranial magnetic stimulation and controls the direction of after-effects. Biol Psychiatry 2004;56:634–639.
120 Stikhina NI, Lyskov EB, Lomarev MP, Aleksanian ZA, Mikhailov VO, Medvedev SV: [Transcranial magnetic stimulation in neurotic depression]. Zh nevrol Psikhiatr Im S S Korsakova 1999;99:26–29.
121 Laruelle M, Abi-Dargham A, van Dyck CH, Gil R, D'Souza CD, Erdos J, McCance E, Rosenblatt W, Fingado C, Zoghbi SS, Baldwin RM, Seibyl JP, Krystal JH, Charney DS, Innis RB: Single photon emission computerized tomography imaging of amphetamine-induced dopamine release in drug-free schizophrenic subjects. Proc Natl Acad Sci USA 1996;93:9235–9240.
122 Triggs WJ, McCoy KJM, Greer R, Rossi F, Bowers D, Kortenkamp S, Nadeau SE, Heilman KM, Goodman WK: Effects of left frontal transcranial magnetic stimulation on depressed mood, cognition, and corticomotor threshold. Biol Psychiatry 1999;45:1440–1446.
123 Little JT, Kimbrell TA, Wassermann EM: Cognitive effects of 1- and 20-hertz repetitive transcranial magnetic stimulation in depression: preliminary report. Neuropsychiatry Neuropsychol Behav Neurol 2000;13:119–124.
124 Shajahan PM, Glabus MF, Steele JD, Doris AB, Anderson K, Jenkins JA, Gooding PA, Ebmeier KP: Left dorso-lateral repetitive transcranial magnetic stimulation affects cortical excitability and functional connectivity, but does not impair cognition in major depression. Prog Neuropsychopharmacol Biol Psychiatry 2002;26:945–954.
125 O'Connor M, Brenninkmeyer C, Morgan A, Bloomingdale K, Thall M, Vasile R, Pascual-Leone A: Relative effects of repetitive transcranial magnetic stimulation and electroconvulsive therapy on mood and memory: a neurocognitive risk-benefit analysis. Cogn Behav Neurol 2003;16:118–127.
126 Schulze-Rauschenbach SC, Harms U, Schlaepfer TE, Maier W, Falkai P, Wagner M: Distinctive neurocognitive effects of repetitive transcranial magnetic stimulation and electroconvulsive therapy in major depression. Br J Psychiatry 2005;186:410–416.
127 Kuroda Y, Motohashi N, Ito H, Ito S, Takano A, Nishikawa T, Suhara T: Effects of repetitive transcranial magnetic stimulation on [^{11}C]raclopride binding and cognitive function in patients with depression. J Affect Disord 2006;95:35–42.

Priv. Doz. Dr. med. Frank Padberg
Department of Psychiatry and Psychotherapy, Ludwig-Maximilian University Munich
Nussbaumstrasse 7
DE–80336 Munich (Germany)
Tel. +49 89 5160 5879, Fax +49 89 5160 5882, E-Mail padberg@med.uni-muenchen.de

Marcolin MA, Padberg F (eds): Transcranial Brain Stimulation for Treatment of Psychiatric Disorders.
Adv Biol Psychiatr. Basel, Karger, 2007, vol 23, pp 84–96

Repetitive Transcranial Magnetic Stimulation in Augmentation of Antidepressant Drugs

Demetrio Ortega Rumi[a], *Andreas Conca*[c], *Uwe Herwig*[d], *Wagner Farid Gattaz*[b], *Marco Antonio Marcolin*[a]

[a]Institute of Psychiatry, University of São Paulo, and [b]Laboratory of Neuroscience, Department of Psychiatry, Faculty of Medicine, University of São Paulo, São Paulo, Brazil; [c]Department of Psychiatry I, Regional Hospital of Rankweil, Rankweil, Austria; [d]Department of Psychiatry Research and Psychogeriatric Medicine, Psychiatric University Hospital, Zurich, Switzerland

Abstract

Repetitive transcranial magnetic stimulation (rTMS) is a new technology which holds promise as a treatment in neuropsychiatry. Drugs and psychotherapy are inadequate for relieving depressive symptoms in a substantial portion of severely depressed patients. In that patient group, neurostimulation techniques such as rTMS could be useful. Augmentation and combination strategies are commonly employed to address this problem, but there are few randomized, controlled studies to guide treatment choice. This article presents an overview of currently available rTMS techniques for depression, including its use as an add-on therapy reviewing also its efficacy and safety.

Unipolar depression is one of the most burdening disorders worldwide [1]. While many effective treatments are available, this disorder is often underdiagnosed and undertreated. Primary care providers should strongly consider the presence of depression in their patients; studies suggest a high prevalence of affective disorders among patients seeking medical attention in the office setting. Unipolar depression is a disorder with significant potential morbidity and mortality, contributing as it does to suicide, medical illness, disruption in interpersonal relationships, substance abuse, and lost working time. Depression plays a role in 50–90% of the suicide attempts, dependent on applied criteria, while the death rate from suicide among those with affective disorders can exceed 15%. Studies also show that unipolar depression contributes to higher mortality and morbidity in the context of other medical illnesses, such as myocardial infarction, and that successful treatment of the depressive episode improves medical and surgical outcomes [1–4].

Potential complications of depression may develop across the biopsychosocial spectrum. Other adverse outcomes may arise from attempts at self-injury, untreated medical conditions, or physical decline due to inanition. Medical and surgical prognosis and recovery are also affected adversely by concurrent depression [1–4].

Regarding the psychosocial aspects, depression, particularly when chronic or untreated, can contribute to unemployment or failure in school, social isolation, substance abuse, and marital/family dysfunction [1–4].

The published success rates of pharmacological interventions for major depression are less than ideal. Approximately 50% of depressed patients do not respond to a trial of a particular antidepressant [5], and as many as 20% of patients do not respond to any antidepressant medication [6]. Additionally, the latency of onset of improvement has a marked clinical impact. When medication is augmented with psychotherapy, response rates range from about 45 to 90% at best [7–9]. The purpose of this review is to evaluate the role of combined psychological and pharmacological therapies in minimizing relapse and recurrence and to analyze the current status of other options recently mentioned for the treatment of depression. It does not refer to the acute response (see the review by Hollon et al. [8]) and for patients with treatment-resistant depression, especially those with psychotic features or a high risk of suicide, other therapeutic options must be considered and, if available, pursued [7–9].

Challenges in Antidepressant Augmentation

Basically, the augmentation strategies have 3 main goals:

(1) acceleration of the drug efficacy and reaction if refractory to therapy;
(2) add-on therapy (adding a new mechanism of action);
(3) complementary therapy (enhancing the preexisting mechanism of action).

Medication for depression, or pharmacotherapy, usually requires a 4- to 6-week time frame. This allows for observation in order to find out if the antidepressant medication is appropriate, i.e. if it is working and does not have unbearable unwanted side effects on a patient. Up to two thirds of depressed patients receiving pharmacotherapy experience some form of improvement. Many patients also experience dose-dependent undesired side effects from these medications which may include: dizziness, sedation, peripheral anticholinergic side effects, weight gain, sexual dysfunction, neurological and cardiovascular side effects, insomnia and anxiety among others [7].

It is a paradox of current clinical practice that some of the most common augmentation strategies in depression are also those with the least controlled evidence. Despite extensive data on the use of adjunctive lithium or thyroid hormone in refractory depression, these approaches are not the most favored by practitioners. The popularity and the use of adjunctive bupropion, psychostimulants, atypical antipsychotics, modafinil, buspirone, lamotrigine, estrogen and mifepristone as augmentors is supported by limited open and controlled evidence, but is not yet fully substantiated by randomized, controlled studies.

Biological Treatments for Depression

Considering the scenario of depression mentioned above, safety and short- or long-term tolerability issues regarding drug therapy, time to achieve response and the imperious need to improve the results of the current pharmacological treatments of depression, some new evolving therapeutic modalities, which hold promise for patients with refractory depression, have been studied and tested in order to augment the action of the antidepressant drugs generally employed. These new therapeutic approaches are based on neurostimulation which is a physical intervention that utilizes either electric current or magnetic field to stimulate the brain. The various techniques used include electroconvulsive therapy (ECT), repetitive transcranial magnetic stimulation (rTMS), magnetic seizure therapy, vagus nerve stimulation and deep brain stimulation. Although ECT has been in use for many decades, the technique is still being refined and improved [9]. The other, more novel neurostimulation treatments have been developed more recently and have efficacy profiles that are widely considered less well established than that of ECT [9, 10]. Although the mechanisms of antidepressant action of ECT are unknown, recent data indicate that the production of a generalized convulsion alone is not sufficient to treat depression; the quality and thus the effect of the ECT seizure on regional brain function are also important in determining the therapeutic benefit [11, 12]. These data are consistent with evidence from functional neuroimaging studies that have implicated prefrontal, temporal, and limbic structures in depression.

Transcranial Magnetic Stimulation

TMS has been developed as a new tool to explore brain-behavior relationships noninvasively for potential therapeutic application [13]. It involves placing a copper winded coil on the scalp, which causes cortical neurons just below the skull to depolarize in response to a short pulse of electric current which generates an electromagnetic field reaching the cortex. A single electromagnetic pulse, which generates a field of approximately 1–2 T 1–2 cm below the coil, will cause a cluster of neurons to discharge and repetitive pulses can cause neurons to repeatedly discharge [14]. At higher frequencies (>1 Hz), information processing in the respective cortical region may be disturbed [15]. For example, rTMS over frontotemporal areas may block speech production [16] and over the left dorsolateral prefrontal cortex (LDLPFC) it may affect working memory [17]. TMS, as observed by positron emission tomography, is supposed to cause modifications in cortical metabolism and changes in regional cortical blood flow and to interrupt the regional neural activity in the cortex [18, 19]. These phenomena are also observed at sites far from the stimulus, showing that the effects of TMS propagate to other parts of the brain [19]. Besides modulating the response of the contralateral motor cortex (for instance the stimulus over the left prefrontal cortex has been shown to increase the release of dopamine in the ipsilateral caudate nucleus [19–21]), TMS might alter gene expression patterns, for example the activation of c-*fos* expression in the thalamic paraventricular nucleus. This implies that the effect of TMS does not depend on the direction of the magnetic stimulus or on the integrity of neural circuits, suggesting that it might alter gene expression directly by a mechanism independent of the generation of action potentials [18, 20].

TMS for Depression: Current Status

TMS as a Stand-Alone Therapy

Some findings supporting the clinical efficacy of excitatory rTMS to the left prefrontal cortex and, although less well studied, inhibitory rTMS to the right prefrontal cortex have provided a functional correlate to data from imaging and lesion studies suggesting that lateralized alterations in brain activity might play a role in depressive symptoms. Another important aspect is that these data have been contributed for additional understanding of the physiologic effects of TMS and have provided clues to the pathophysiology of depression. Furthermore, evidence linking regional brain activity to treatment responsiveness and the paradoxical response of some patients have allowed research groups to identify two metabolically distinct populations that have different responses to excitatory and inhibitory treatment frequencies [20].

Antidepressant effects of fast rTMS of the LDLPFC have been demonstrated in the majority of previous controlled studies [21–27] although some investigators found only marginal or no significant effects when compared with sham rTMS [28–33]. Despite the range of stimulation intensities in prior studies, solid conclusions regarding the relationship between efficacy and intensity were impeded by:

(1) the lack of a direct comparison between different intensities;
(2) the problem that studies widely varied with respect to other stimulation parameters (e.g. frequency, number of stimuli) and clinical characteristics of patient samples.

Previous trials demonstrated that short courses of rTMS produced a modest benefit in groups of patients seen in the mean scores on the Hamilton Depression Rating Scale (HDRS), although remission of depression in individual patients was rare. However, refinements in TMS methods have led to improvements on these initial results. According to a review by Gershon et al. [34], 41% of 139 patients treated with high-frequency rTMS (HF-rTMS) to the left prefrontal cortex achieved either a 50% decrease in their HDRS scores or a final score of 7 or less. More recent trials have pointed to the longer treatment course (more than 10 days), more magnetic pulses (10,000–30,000), increased field intensity (100–110%) motor threshold (MT), the absence of psychosis, younger age, and previous TMS responsiveness as likely contributors to treatment success, even when rTMS is the only antidepressant therapy, and have produced results with rTMS that are comparable to those of ECT.

The largest sham-controlled study to date of HF-rTMS, performed by Avery et al. [35] as a treatment for medication-resistant depression, showed that the response rates and remission rates are higher in the TMS group compared with the sham group. The active TMS group had a significantly greater response rate, i.e. 30.6% (11/35), compared with 6.1% (2/33) in the sham group (Fisher's $p = 0.008$, effect size = 0.69), as well as a significantly greater remission rate, i.e. 20.0% (7/35), compared with 3.0% (1/33) in the sham group (Fisher's $p = 0.033$, effect size = 0.58). The baseline clinical characteristics of the 68 patients with major depression treated with TMS were as follows: 31% received some concomitant antidepressant drug and 27% were included in the sham stimulation group; however, different drugs were given, which could result in various kinds of responses. A similar situation was reported for the treatment with benzodiazepines. Sometimes such findings have been misinterpreted because sham TMS, which was intended to be a placebo, might be partially active. However, improved sham conditions that minimize physiologic effects have been described lately. In most studies, and when the aggregate data are tested, real rTMS is superior to sham TMS. These results are encouraging; however, two important queries need clarification before including this promising empiric approach in our current therapeutic armamentarium. The first is systematic investigation of better and adequate treatment parameters such as intensity, duration, and the number of magnetic pulses. All of them should be tested and analyzed separately. Methods to accurately target TMS on the basis of mapping of brain anatomy by MRI have been described [36]. It will be useful to test whether anatomical accuracy really enhances clinical efficacy. Patient parameters, both clinical and physiologic, are even less well explored and deserve systematic investigation as well. Another priority is larger-scale studies whose outcome measure is clinical remission. Large multicenter trials or smaller ones that are sufficiently similar to permit meta-analysis could prove (or disprove) the clinical efficacy of TMS. If data from such studies support the clinical value of TMS, it would then be possible to define a clinical role for TMS and to address the issues of whether TMS is most useful as an adjunct or stand-alone therapy, whether it is as effective as current first-line therapies, and whether maintenance TMS is beneficial.

Add-On Trials

There are some add-on studies in which the combination of rTMS with antidepressants was investigated. These trials showed a greater improvement in patients receiving additional rTMS, and this effect could be observed already after the third rTMS session. Although these results are quite similar, caution is needed in the evaluation and comparison of studies. In the trial by Conca et al. [37] (n = 24), there was no sham group, and 5 different antidepressants were used with a homogenous distribution of the serotonin selective reuptake inhibitor between the groups (8 vs. 9) but with a preponderance of amitriptyline in the add-on group (4 vs. 1). In addition, rTMS parameters differed from those shown in the review by Gershon et al. [34] which are supposed to be more effective than stimulation at 8 different sites, use of a circular coil, frequency of 0.17 Hz at 1.9 T (corresponding to the maximal output of the device), 10 days of treatment, and 400 total pulses.

Garcia-Toro et al. [38] reported that in patients (n = 40) suffering from drug-resistant major depression real, but not sham, HF-rTMS was associated with a significant decrease in the HDRS scores, but only 12 patients achieved a decrease of more than 50%. They concluded that left prefrontal HF-rTMS was effectively associated with antidepressant treatment, although the size effect was small. However, the same authors found no effect of HF-rTMS compared with sham rTMS in 22 patients (6 dropped out) treated during 10 days with sertraline among a group of 28 patients (12 were initially nonmedicated and 16 failed a trial with a single antidepressant) [30]. There are differences in technical parameters that have to be considered, i.e. shorter treatment with lower total number of pulses, lower pulse intensity, and use as a sham rTMS of an active coil angulated at 90°, which has been shown to have active properties [39].

Hausmann et al. [40] compared the effects of rTMS with sham rTMS in 41 patients with major depression (3 dropped out). Group A1 (n = 12) received unilateral active stimulation consisting of HF-rTMS over the LDLPFC and subsequent sham low-frequency (LF) rTMS over the right dorsolateral prefrontal cortex (RDLPFC). Group A2 (n = 13) received simultaneous bilateral active stimulation consisting of HF-rTMS over the LDLPFC and LF-rTMS over the RDLPFC. Group C (n = 13) received bilateral sham stimulation. All patients were treated with different nontricyclic antidepressants. No significant differences were found in the outcome among the three groups, although the improvement in the rTMS groups was quantitatively superior to placebo in all assessments. Besides technical differences between Hausmann et al. [40] and the methodology suggested by Gershon et al. [34], such as the use of a lower number of pulses and a shorter treatment period, the use of four different antidepressants makes comparison with other studies problematic.

Rumi et al. [41] evaluated 46 outpatients meeting the DSM-IV [42] criteria for nonpsychotic depressive episode who were randomly assigned to receive either rTMS (n = 22) or sham rTMS (n = 24) during 4 weeks over the LDLPFC in a double-blind controlled trial. All patients were concomitantly taking amitriptyline (mean dose 110 mg/day). The rTMS group received 20 sessions (5 sessions per week) of 5-Hz rTMS (120% of MT and 1,250 pulses per session). Sham stimulation followed the same schedule, however, using a sham coil. The efficacy variables were the 17-item HDRS [43], the Montgomery-Åsberg Depression Rating Scale (MADRS) [44], a Visual Analogue Scale, and the Clinical Global Impression. Tolerability was assessed by clinical examination and a safety screening of TMS side effects. rTMS had a significantly faster response to amitriptyline. There was a significant decrease in HDRS scores, already after the first week of treatment ($p < 0.001$ compared with baseline and $p < 0.001$ compared with sham). The decrease in HDRS scores in the rTMS group was significantly superior compared with the sham group throughout the study ($p < 0.001$ at the fourth week). These contradictory findings reinforce the necessity for standardization of rTMS parameters before definitive conclusions about the efficacy of this approach can be drawn. It is important to note the absence of seizures during rTMS treatment concomitant with tricyclic antidepressants and the use of a 120% MT intensity that is one of the highest intensities used in known TMS studies.

Rossini et al. [45], in a 5-week, double-blind, randomized, sham-controlled study, recruited 99 inpatients suffering from a major depressive episode (DSM-IV criteria). The patients were randomly assigned to receive venlafaxine, sertraline, or escitalopram in combination with a 2-week period of sham or active 15-Hz rTMS on the left dorsolateral prefrontal cortex. The active rTMS group showed a significantly faster reduction in HDRS scores compared with the sham group ($p = 0.0029$). The response and remission rates were significantly greater in the active rTMS group after the stimulation period ($p = 0.002$ and $p = 0.003$, respectively), but not at the endpoint. We found no significant difference in HDRS score reduction among the 3 drugs administered, either in the active or in the sham group. These findings support the efficacy of rTMS in hastening the response to antidepressant drugs in patients with major depressive disorder. The effect of rTMS seems to be unaffected by the specific concomitantly administered drug.

However, paroxetine could not be augmented as the study by Poulet et al. [46] revealed; 19 patients with nonresistant major depression were recruited and randomly assigned to sham (coil at an angle of 45°, corresponding almost to a real stimulation) or real rTMS over the LDLPFC at 10 Hz, 80% of MT intensity for 10 days. The authors concluded that there is a similar action delay with both rTMS and antidepressant medications. Both therapeutic strategies could implicate an identical or analogous monoaminergic mechanism, and therefore, rTMS could not to be a trigger for the drug action. Further studies including a third arm with active rTMS and placebo paroxetine should help to solve this question.

A further study indicating a possible augmentation property of rTMS as an add-on strategy was published by Su et al. [47]. A total of 30 medication-resistant patients with DSM-IV major depressive disorder or bipolar disorder (most recent episode depressed) completed 10 sessions of active or sham rTMS: 10 patients at each of 2 frequencies, faster (20 Hz) or slower (5 Hz), at 100% MT, and 10 patients at sham stimulation. Patients at both stimulation frequencies demonstrated a superior reduction of depression severity compared to sham stimulation (active = 55.7% vs. sham = 16.3%). The response rate for active rTMS was 60%, in contrast to 10% for the sham treatment.

According to a congress report [48], a randomized double-blind sham-controlled multicenter trial was performed in order to investigate the efficacy of rTMS as add-on treatment in depression. One hundred and twenty-seven patients with moderate to severe depressive episodes were included in seven centers and randomly assigned to real or sham stimulation. Real stimulation parameters were 10 Hz, 110% of MT, 2,000 stimuli per day on 15 working days, above the LDLPFC. rTMS was performed as an add-on treatment to simultaneously started standardized antidepressant medication. Treatment outcome was assessed with established depression rating scales (Beck Depression Inventory, HDRS, and MADRS). In both, the real rTMS ($n = 62$) and the sham-stimulated group ($n = 65$), the intent-to-treat response rate was 31% ($p = 0.962$, confidence interval 0.5–2.2). The real/sham rTMS groups showed reductions of the mean rating scores relative to the initial scores: Beck Depression Inventory 39%/32%, HDRS 43%/38%, and MADRS 38%/39%. The differences were not significant. The presented multicenter trial does not support previous reports of smaller samples indicating an antidepressant effect of rTMS in medicated patients. Further exploration of the possible efficacy of other stimulation protocols or within selected subpopulations of patients is necessary.

Finally, considering rTMS as an add-on treatment in depression, the question still remains as to which antidepressant drugs may work well with rTMS [49].

Combination of Different rTMS Parameters as an Augmentation Strategy

As mentioned in previous sections of this chapter, studies of rTMS in depression have found antidepressant effects when HF-rTMS (≥1 Hz) is applied over the left prefrontal cortex. A few studies have also reported success with LF-rTMS to the right prefrontal cortex. Both HF-rTMS and LF-rTMS have been reported to work better in areas with cerebral hypometabolism or hypermetabolism, respectively. Based on this concept, Garcia-Toro et al. [50] studied 30 medication-resistant patients with major depression who were randomized into three groups. The first group received sham rTMS and the second group received active rTMS (20-Hz rTMS to the left prefrontal cortex and 1-Hz rTMS to the right prefrontal cortex). The third group, however, received active rTMS that was focused on different regions of the brain after examination with single photon emission computed tomography (20-Hz rTMS to an area of relatively low activity and 1-Hz rTMS to an area showing relatively high activation). This study demonstrated that combined 20- and 1-Hz rTMS was effective, but no additional advantages were obtained by focusing rTMS on areas identified by single photon emission computed tomography as showing high versus low levels of functional activity.

Another trial performed by Conca et al. [51] investigated the augmentation properties of rTMS combining low and high frequencies. Thirty-six depressed medicated inpatients were recruited and assigned to three different rTMS treatment modalities as an add-on strategy (each n = 12). In group 1, a stimulus intensity of 110% of the MT was used with a frequency of 10 Hz over the LDLPFC. The RDLPFC was stimulated in the same session with 110% MT at 1 Hz. In group 2, the patients were stimulated only over the LDLPFC with alternating trains of 110% MT at 10 Hz and trains of 110% MT at 1 Hz in the same session. In group 3, high-frequency stimulation over the LDLPFC was performed as an internal control group. None of the treatment modalities was superior but different side effects were observed. The findings observed in this trial suggest that rTMS, at varying frequencies and stimulation placements, evokes different psychoactive effects of clinical relevance. Similar results were found by Hausmann et al. [40] in a trial performed with 41 medication-free patients with major depression suggesting that rTMS as an add-on strategy, applied in a unilateral and a bilateral stimulation paradigm, does not exert an additional antidepressant effect. Regarding its efficacy, other longer trials with larger sample sizes, and with different parameters combined together are needed to evaluate this new strategy.

Besides possible advantages of combination strategies, there are also potential side effects that cannot be overlooked. Side effects of rTMS in general are seldom and weak such as cephalea and local pain. However, psychotomimetic activities of rTMS, switching into mania phenomena and, in a few cases, epileptic seizures have been reported [51–55].

Conclusion

According to all data seen to date, TMS is not ruled out as a new antidepressant treatment strategy. The contradictory findings, in some clinical trials, stress the need for standardization of rTMS parameters, before definitive conclusions about the efficacy of this approach can be drawn. Systematic and large-scale studies are needed to identify patient populations most likely to benefit, and treatment parameters most likely to produce success. Regarding augmentation studies and add-on studies, in particular, the question has been raised as to which antidepressant drugs may work well with rTMS. Studies with fixed-dose monotherapy and more homogeneity in clinical and demographic features are needed in future clinical trials. In addition to its potential clinical role, TMS promises to provide insights into the pathophysiology of depression through research designs with the ability of TMS to alter brain activity [56–61].

References

1 Lopez AD, Murray CC: The global burden of disease, 1990–2020. Nat Med 1998;4:1241–1243.

2 Elkin I, Shea MT, Watkins JT, et al: National Institute of Mental Health Treatment of Depression Collaborative Research Program. General effectiveness of treatments. Arch Gen Psychiatry 1989;46:971–982.

3 Katon W, Von Korff M, Lin E, et al: Collaborative management to achieve treatment guidelines. Impact on depression in primary care. JAMA 1995;273:1026–1031.

4 Leon AC, Olfson M, Broadhead WE, et al: Prevalence of mental disorders in primary care. Implications for screening. Arch Fam Med 1995;4:857–861.

5 Steffens DC, Krishnan KR, Helms MJ: Are SSRIs better than TCAs? Comparison of SSRIs and TCAs: a meta-analysis. Depress Anxiety 1997;6:10–18.

6 Greenberg P, Corey-Lisle PK, Birnbaum H, Marynchenko M, Claxton A: Economic implications of treatment-resistant depression among employees. Pharmacoeconomics 2004;22:363–373.

7 Segal Z, Vincent P, Levitt A: Efficacy of combined, sequential and crossover psychotherapy and pharmacotherapy in improving outcomes in depression. J Psychiatry Neurosci 2002;27:281–290.

8 Hollon SD, Jarrett RB, Nierenberg AA, Thase ME, Trivedi M, Rush AJ: Psychotherapy and medication in the treatment of adult and geriatric depression: which monotherapy or combined treatment? J Clin Psychiatry 2005;66:455–468.

9 Gaudiano BA, Beevers CG, Miller IW: Differential response to combined treatment in patients with psychotic versus nonpsychotic major depression. J Nerv Ment Dis 2005;193:625–628.

10 DeBattista C: Augmentation and combination strategies for depression. J Psychopharmacol 2006;20(suppl):11–18.

11 Lisanby SH, Morales O, Payne N, Kwon E, Fitzsimons L, Luber B, Nobler MS, Sackeim HA: New developments in electroconvulsive therapy and magnetic seizure therapy. CNS Spectr 2003;8: 529–536.
12 Bolwig TG: Putative common pathways in therapeutic brain stimulation for affective disorders. CNS Spectr 2003;8:490–495.
13 Nobler MS, Sackeim HA, Prohovnik I, Moeller JR, Mukherjee S, Schnur DB, Prudic J, Devanand DP: Regional cerebral blood flow in mood disorders. 3. Treatment and clinical response. Arch Gen Psychiatry 1994;51:884–897.
14 Sackeim HA, Prudic J, Devanand DP, Kiersky JE, Fitzsimmons L, Moody BJ, McElhinney MC, Coleman EA, Settembrino JM: Effects of stimulus intensity and electrode placement on the efficacy and cognitive effects of electroconvulsive therapy. N Engl J Med 1993;328:839–846.
15 George MS, Wassermann EM, Post RM: Transcranial magnetic stimulation: a neuropsychiatric tool for the 21st century. J Neuropsychiatry Clin Neurosci 1996;8:373–382.
16 Pascual-Leone A, Valls-Sole J, Wassermann EM, Hallett M: Responses to rapid-rate transcranial magnetic stimulation of the human motor cortex. Brain 1994;117:847–858.
17 Pascual-Leone A, Valls-Sole J, Wassermann EM, Brasil-Neto J, Cohen LG, Hallett M: Effects of focal transcranial magnetic stimulation on simple reaction time to acoustic, visual and somatosensory stimuli. Brain 1992;115:1045–1059.
18 Conca A, Hrubos W, Di Pauli J, Peschina W, König P, Hinterhuber H, Hausmann A: Transcranial magnetic stimulation and brain imagings. Nervenheilkunde 2003;22:359–364.
19 Pascual-Leone A, Hallett M: Induction of errors in a delayed response task by repetitive transcranial magnetic stimulation of the dorsolateral prefrontal cortex. Neuroreport 1994;5:2517–2520.
20 Hausmann A, Weis C, Marksteiner J, Hinterhuber H, Humpel C: Chronic repetitive transcranial magnetic stimulation enhances c-*fos* in the parietal cortex and hippocampus. Brain Res Mol Brain Res 2000;76:355–356.
21 Conca A, Peschina W, König P, Fritzsche H, Hausmann A: Effect of chronic repetitive transcranial magnetic stimulation on regional cerebral blood flow and regional cerebral glucose uptake in drug treatment-resistant depressives. A brief report. Neuropsychobiology 2002;45:27–31.
22 George MS, Ketter TA, Post RM: What functional imaging studies have revealed about the brain basis of mood and emotion; in Panksepp J (ed): Advances in Biological Psychiatry. Greenwich, JAI Press, 1996, pp 63–113.
23 Kimbrell TA, Little JT, Dunn RT, Frye MA, Greenberg BD, Wasserman EM, Repella JD, Danielson AL, Willis MW, Benson BE, Speer AM, Osuch E, George MS, Post RM: Frequency dependence of antidepressant response to left prefrontal repetitive transcranial magnetic stimulation (rTMS) as a function of baseline cerebral glucose metabolism. Biol Psychiatry 1999;46:1603–1613.
24 Pascual-Leone A, Rubio B, Pallardó F, Catalá MD: Rapid-rate transcranial magnetic stimulation of left dorsolateral prefrontal cortex in drug-resistant depression. Lancet 1996;348:233–237.
25 George MS, Wassermann EM, Kimbrell TA, Little LT, Williams WE, Danielson AL, Greenberg BD, Hallett M, Post RM: Mood improvement following daily left prefrontal repetitive transcranial magnetic stimulation in patients with depression: a placebo-controlled crossover trial. Am J Psychiatry 1997;154:1752–1756.
26 George MS, Lisanby SH, Sackeim HA: Transcranial magnetic stimulation. Arch Gen Psychiatry 1999;56:300–311.
27 Klein E, Kreinin I, Chistyakov A, Koren D, Mecz L, Marmur S, Ben-Shachar D, Feinsod M: Therapeutic efficacy of right prefrontal slow repetitive transcranial magnetic stimulation in major depression. Arch Gen Psychiatry 1999;56:315–320.
28 Padberg F, Zwanzger P, Thoma H, Kathmann N, Haag C, Greenberg BD, Hampel H, Möller HJ: Repetitive transcranial magnetic stimulation (rTMS) in pharmacotherapy-refractory major depression: comparative study of fast, slow and sham rTMS. Psychiatry Res 1999;88:163–171.
29 Berman RM, Narasimhan M, Sanacora G, Miano AP, Hoffman RE, Hu XS, Charney DS, Boutros NN: A randomized clinical trial of repetitive transcranial magnetic stimulation in the treatment of major depression. Biol Psychiatry 2000;47:332–337.
30 Garcia-Toro M, Mayol A, Arnillas H, Capllonch I, Ibarra O, Crespi M, Mico J, Lafau O, Lafuente L: Modest adjunctive benefit with transcranial magnetic stimulation in medication-resistant depression. J Affect Disord 2001;64:271–275.

31 George MS, Nahas Z, Molloy M, Speer AM, Oliver NC, Li XB, Arana GW, Risch SC, Ballenger JC: A controlled trial of daily left prefrontal cortex TMS for treating depression. Biol Psychiatry 2000;48:962–970.

32 Loo C, Mitchell P, Sachdev P, McDarmont B, Parker G, Gandevia S: Double-blind controlled investigation of transcranial magnetic stimulation for the treatment of resistant major depression. Am J Psychiatry 1999;156:946–948.

33 Manes F, Jorge R, Morcuende M, Yamada T, Paradiso S, Robinson RG: A controlled study of repetitive transcranial magnetic stimulation as a treatment of depression in the elderly. Int Psychogeriatr 2001;13:225–231.

34 Gershon AA, Dannon PN, Grunhaus L: Transcranial magnetic stimulation in the treatment of depression. Am J Psychiatry 2003;160:835–845.

35 Avery DH, Holtzheimer PE, Fawaz W, Russo J, Neumaier J, Dunner DL, Haynor DR, Claypoole KH, Wajdik C, Roy-Byrne P: A controlled study of repetitive transcranial magnetic stimulation in medication-resistant major depression. Biol Psychiatry 2006;59:187–194.

36 Herwig U, Schonfeldt-Lecuona C, Wunderlich AP, von Tiesenhausen C, Thielscher A, Walter H, Spitzer M: The navigation of transcranial magnetic stimulation. Psychiatry Res 2001;108:123–131.

37 Conca A, Koppi S, Konig P, Swoboda E, Krecke N: Transcranial magnetic stimulation: a novel antidepressive strategy? Neuropsychobiology 1996;34:204 –207.

38 Garcia-Toro M, Pascual-Leone A, Romera M, Gonzalez A, Mico J, Ibarra O, Arnillas H, Capllonch I, Mayol A, Tormos JM: Prefrontal repetitive transcranial magnetic stimulation as add on treatment in depression. J Neurol Neurosurg Psychiatry 2001;71:546–548.

39 Lisanby SH, Gutman D, Luber B, Schroeder C, Sackeim HA: Sham TMS: intracerebral measurement of the induced electrical field and the induction of motor-evoked potentials. Biol Psychiatry 2001;49:460–463.

40 Hausmann A, Kemmler G, Walpoth M, Mechtcheriakov S, Kramer-Reinstadler K, Lechner T, et al: No benefit derived from repetitive transcranial magnetic stimulation in depression: a prospective, single-centre, randomized, double-blind, sham-controlled 'add on' trial. J Neurol Neurosurg Psychiatry 2004;75:320–322.

41 Rumi DO, Gattaz WF, Rigonatti SP, Rosa M, Fregni F, Rosa MO, Mansur C, Myczkowski ML, Moreno RA, Marcolin MA: Transcranial magnetic stimulation accelerates the antidepressant effect of amitriptyline in severe depression: a double-blind placebo-controlled study. Biol Psychiatry 2005;57:162–166.

42 American Psychiatric Association: Diagnostic and Statistical Manual of Mental Disorders, ed 4. Washington, American Psychiatric Press, 1994.

43 Hamilton M: A rating scale for depression. J Neurol Neurosurg Psychiatry 1960;23:56–62.

44 Montgomery SA, Asberg M: A new depression scale designed to be sensitive to change. Br J Psychiatry 1979;134:382–389.

45 Rossini D, Magri L, Lucca A, Giordani S, Smeraldi E, Zanardi R: Does rTMS hasten the response to escitalopram, sertraline, or venlafaxine in patients with major depressive disorder? A double-blind, randomized, sham-controlled trial. J Clin Psychiatry 2005;66:1569–1575.

46 Poulet E, Brunelin J, Boeuve C, Lerond J, D'Amato T, Dalery J, Saoud M: Repetitive transcranial magnetic stimulation does not potentiate antidepressant treatment. Eur Psychiatry 2004;19: 382–383.

47 Su TP, Huang CC, Wei IH: Add-on rTMS for medication-resistant depression: a randomized, double-blind, sham-controlled trial in Chinese patients. J Clin Psychiatry 2005;66:930–937.

48 Herwig U, Fallgatter AJ, Hoeppner J, Eschweiler G, Kron M, Hajak G, Padberg F, Heiden A, Abler B, Eichhammer P, Grossheinrich N, Kammer T, Langguth B, Laske C, Plewnia C, Schulz M, Unterecker S, Spitzer M, Schönfeldt-Lecuona C: Antidepressant transcranial magnetic stimulation – First results of a multi-center trial. Biol Psychiatr 2006;59:97S.

49 George SM, Nahas Z, Lisanby SH, Schlaepfer T, Kozel FA, Greenberg BD: Transcranial magnetic stimulation. Neurosurg Clin North Am 2003;14:283–301.

50 Garcia-Toro M, Salva J, Daumal J, Andres J, Romera M, Lafau O, Echevarria M, Mestre M, Bosch C, Collado C, Ibarra O, Aguirre I: High (20-Hz) and low (1-Hz) frequency transcranial magnetic stimulation as adjuvant treatment in medication-resistant depression. Psychiatry Res 2006;146: 53–57.

51 Conca A, Di Pauli J, Beraus W, Hausmann A, Peschina W, Schneider H, König P, Hinterhuber H: Combining high and low frequencies in rTMS antidepressive treatment. Preliminary results. Hum Psychopharmacol 2002;17:353–356.

52 Conca A, König P, Hausmann A: Transcranial magnetic stimulation induces 'pseudoabsence seizure'. Acta Psychiatr Scand 2000;101:246–248.

53 Dolberg OT, Schreiber S, Grunhaus L: Transcranial magnetic stimulation-induced switch into mania: a report of two cases. Biol Psychiatry 2001;49:468–470.

54 Zwanzger P, Ella R, Keck ME, Rupprecht R, Padberg F: Occurrence of delusions during repetitive trancranial magnetic stimulation (rTMS) in major depression. Biol Psychiatry 2002;51:602–603.

55 Hausmann A, Kramer-Reinstadler K, Lechner-Schoner T, Walpoth M, Rupp CI, Hinterhuber H, Conca A: Can bilateral prefrontal repetitive transcranial magnetic stimulation (rTMS) induce mania? A case report. J Clin Psychiatry 2004;65:1575–1576.

56 Luborzewski A, Schubert F, Seifert F, Danker-Hopfe H, Brakemeier EL, Schlattmann P, Anghelescu I, Colla M, Bajbouj M: Metabolic alterations in the dorsolateral prefrontal cortex after treatment with high-frequency repetitive transcranial magnetic stimulation in patients with unipolar major depression. J Psychiatr Res 2006, E-pub ahead of print.

57 Zanardini R, Gazzoli A, Ventriglia M, Perez J, Bignotti S, Rossini PM, Gennarelli M, Bocchio-Chiavetto L: Effect of repetitive transcranial magnetic stimulation on serum brain derived neurotrophic factor in drug resistant depressed patients. J Affect Disord 2006;91:83–86.

58 Pogarell O, Koch W, Popperl G, Tatsch K, Jakob F, Zwanzger P, Mulert C, Rupprecht R, Moller HJ, Hegerl U, Padberg F: Striatal dopamine release after prefrontal repetitive transcranial magnetic stimulation in major depression: preliminary results of a dynamic [(123)I] IBZM SPECT study. J Psychiatr Res 2006;40:307–314.

59 Steele JD, Glabus MF, Shajahan PM, Ebmeier KP: Increased cortical inhibition in depression: a prolonged silent period with transcranial magnetic stimulation (TMS). Psychol Med 2000;30: 565–570.

60 Shajahan PM, Glabus MF, Gooding PA, Shah PJ, Ebmeier KP: Reduced cortical excitability in depression. Impaired post-exercise motor facilitation with transcranial magnetic stimulation. Br J Psychiatry 1999;174:449–454.

61 Padberg F, Schule C, Zwanzger P, Baghai T, Ella R, Mikhaiel P, Hampel H, Moller HJ, Rupprecht R: Relation between responses to repetitive transcranial magnetic stimulation and partial sleep deprivation in major depression. J Psychiatr Res 2002;36:131–135.

Demetrio Ortega Rumi
Dr. Ovidio Pires de Campos St., No. 785
05403–010 São Paulo City, SP (Brazil)
Tel./Fax +55 11 3069 6525, E-Mail drumi@usp.br

Marcolin MA, Padberg F (eds): Transcranial Brain Stimulation for Treatment of Psychiatric Disorders.
Adv Biol Psychiatr. Basel, Karger, 2007, vol 23, pp 97–109

Transcranial Magnetic Stimulation versus Electroconvulsive Therapy for the Treatment of More Severe Major Depression

Philip G. Janicak[a], *Sheila M. Dowd*[a], *Marco Antonio Marcolin*[b], *Moacyr Alexandro Rosa*[b]

[a]Department of Psychiatry, Rush University Medical Center, Chicago, Ill., USA;
[b]Psychiatric Institute, University of São Paulo, São Paulo, Brazil

Abstract

In those patients who are refractory to or intolerant of psychopharmacotherapy, electroconvulsive therapy (ECT) is often considered. A substantial number of depressed patients, however, cannot tolerate, do not respond to or are unwilling to accept ECT. There is a clear need to develop effective, better tolerated, better accepted, and less expensive therapies. Several preliminary studies, as well as reviews and meta-analyses of clinical trials, support a potential antidepressant effect with repetitive transcranial magnetic stimulation (rTMS). We will briefly review the concept of rTMS, the current data comparing rTMS to ECT, and discuss its potential role in the treatment of more severe depression. Based on the preliminary evidence, rTMS may be an alternative therapy for at least some depressed patients when used as an intermediate strategy between antidepressants and ECT. It may also be a viable augmentation strategy combined with medication or ECT for patients with more severe depression.

Transcranial magnetic stimulation (TMS) was initially utilized as a neurophysiological probe. In this context, it was found to produce mood elevation in some patients [1]. Subsequently, several preliminary studies, as well as reviews and meta-analyses of these clinical trials, supported a potential antidepressant effect with repetitive TMS (rTMS) [2–6]. Further, the recent completion of a large multicenter trial comparing real to sham rTMS confirms that this device-based therapy may provide a new alternative for the treatment of depression [7].

Current first-line treatments for depression include antidepressants, psychotherapy or their combination. In those patients who are refractory to or intolerant of psychopharmacotherapy, electroconvulsive therapy (ECT) is often considered. A substantial number of depressed patients, however, cannot tolerate, do not respond to or are unwilling to accept ECT [8]. Thus, there is a clear need to develop effective, better tolerated, better accepted and less expensive therapies. In this context, rTMS may be an alternate treatment strategy. We will review the concept of rTMS, the current data comparing rTMS to ECT, and discuss its potential role in the treatment of more severe depression.

Concept of Transcranial Magnetic Stimulation

TMS is based on Faraday's concept of electromagnetism. This device uses an electromagnetic coil applied to the scalp producing an intense, localized, fluctuating magnetic field that painlessly stimulates or inhibits a small area of the cortex. These fields are produced by a large electrical current passed from the stimulator through a line connected to the stimulation coil. The current is turned off and on in a rapid fashion (e.g. on for 1 ms or less, off for several milliseconds). Unlike electrical current, these electrically induced magnetic fields pass through various tissues (e.g. scalp, skull) and enter the brain unimpeded. Rapid ($\geq$1 Hz) rTMS produces neuronal depolarization and slow (<1 Hz) rTMS produces inhibition of neuronal firing in a localized area (e.g. 1–3 cm in depth, 1–2 cm in diameter) under the stimulating coil. Rapid rTMS temporarily increases metabolism and blood flow locally while also producing distal effects in areas of the brain which subserve the emotional and behavioral symptoms of depression [9, 10].

Transcranial Magnetic Stimulation Administration

There are several important stimulation parameters to consider when applying rTMS for therapeutic purposes (table 1). A typical acute treatment course in recent studies has been 2–6 weeks, or 10–30 treatment sessions, usually given 5 times per week. When used to treat depression, one of the major questions has been what constitutes an optimal set of TMS parameters. Existing data provide information on the most effective approach and these parameters have been refined over a series of trials, comparing real to sham rTMS or using rTMS to augment ongoing antidepressant drug therapy. These issues are discussed in more detail elsewhere in this book.

Table 1. TMS: critical parameters

Parameter	Comment
MT	Lowest intensity over primary motor cortex to produce contraction of the first dorsal interosseous or abductor pollicis brevis muscle; visually or electromyographically monitored
Stimulus coil location	Most common LDLPFC Less common RDLPFC Vertex
Stimulus coil configuration	Figure-eight, circular shape, crescent shape
Stimulus pulse(s) or train	
Intensity	80–120% of MT
Frequency	≤1–20 (CPS or Hz)
Duration	1 ms
Interpulse interval	50–100 ms
Stimulus train duration	3–6 s

Adapted from Janicak et al. [28].

Repetitive Transcranial Magnetic Stimulation versus Electroconvulsive Therapy for Major Depression

Human and animal studies noted a number of similar effects induced by rTMS, ECT (or electroconvulsive shock) and antidepressants on the endocrine system, sleep parameters, and in certain behavioral and biochemical measures that indicate potential antidepressant properties [9]. For example, antidepressants, electroconvulsive shock, and rTMS all prolong effort in a forced swim test. In animal models, TMS has also been reported to induce ECT-like changes in brain monoamines. Despite these similarities, there are several important differences in the treatment parameters utilized for ECT and TMS (table 2).

To our knowledge, 8 published trials have directly compared rTMS to ECT for more severely depressed patients [11–18]. These trials are summarized in table 3. Pridmore [19] has also reported that rTMS may be used in combination with ECT to achieve the same efficacy with fewer ECT sessions.

In an open study design, Grunhaus et al. [12] randomly assigned 40 patients with major depressive disorder (MDD) to either rTMS or right unilateral,

Table 2. ECT versus TMS: comparison of important treatment parameters

Parameter	ECT	rTMS
Resistance and deflection	high	negligible
Pain	yes	minimal
Site of stimulation	spread	focal
Seizure	necessary	undesired
Schedule	2–3 times a week	daily (Monday to Friday)
Depth	diencephalus	cortex
Wave form	brief or ultra-brief pulse	ultra-brief pulse
Pulse width	0.25–2.0 ms	0.2–1.0 ms
Cerebral induced current	biphasic	triphasic
Frequency	40–120 Hz	0.1–30 Hz
Current	0.5–0.9 A	1,000 A (in the coil)
Duration of stimulus	0.5–8 s	2 s to several minutes
Dosage parameter	seizure threshold	MT
Charge	up to 500 mC	up to 2 T

nondominant ECT (UL ECT). rTMS parameters were stimulation of the left dorsolateral prefrontal cortex (LDLPFC) at 90% motor threshold (MT) at 10 Hz for 2-second (n = 8) or 6-second trains (n = 12) with a total of 20 trains per session for up to 20 sessions. In the ECT group, 8 patients were switched to bilateral ECT because of insufficient response. The authors concluded that ECT was more effective than rTMS for patients with MDD and psychosis. In nonpsychotic MDD, however, the therapeutic effects of rTMS were similar to those of ECT. A potential confound that could affect the interpretation of their results was that those psychotically depressed patients receiving ECT were also receiving antidepressants and/or antipsychotics. In contrast, rTMS patients were not on similar concurrent medications. In addition, stimulus intensity (i.e., 90% of MT) was lower than those reported to be most effective by George et al. [20]. The authors also reported on a follow-up of responders in this trial. It was encouraging that relapse rates (i.e., 20%) did not differ between the ECT and rTMS groups at 3 and 6 months after an acute treatment course [21].

This same group published a second trial comparing rTMS to UL ECT for acute depression without psychosis [14]. Using similar stimulation parameters with rTMS, they reported that the two treatments were comparable in efficacy with an overall response rate of 58% (i.e., 23 out of 40 subjects responded). In the ECT group, 12 of 20 responded and in the rTMS group 11 of 20 responded.

Pridmore et al. [13] randomly assigned 32 patients with MDD who had failed to respond to at least one course of medication to either rTMS or ECT.

Table 3. Summary of rTMS versus ECT studies

Authors	Patients/design	Parameters	Comments
Grunhaus et al. [12]	40 MDD; random assignment; UL ECT or rTMS (8 patients switched to BL ECT); HDRS	LDLPFC; 10 Hz; 90% MT; 2-second trains (n = 8); 6-second trains (n = 12); ITIs not reported; 20 trains per session; up to 20 sessions	rTMS = ECT in nonpsychotic MDD; ECT plus meds > TMS in psychotic MDD (psychotic patients in ECT group were also on antipsychotics)
Pridmore et al. [13]	32 MDD; random assignment; UL ECT or rTMS; HDRS, BDI, VAS	LDLPFC; 20 Hz; 100% MT; 2-second trains; 28-second ITIs; 30–35 trains per session; 12 ± 3.4 sessions (mean ± SD)	rTMS = ECT; based on HDRS percent change and remission rates
Janicak et al. [11]	31 MDD; random assignment, with crossover option for nonresponders; rTMS or BL ECT; HDRS	LDLPFC; 10 Hz; 110% MT; 5-second trains; 30-second ITIs; 20 trains per session; 14 ± 3.4 sessions (mean ± SD)	rTMS = ECT; based on HDRS percent change and a priori definition of response
Grunhaus et al. [14]	40 nonpsychotic MDD; random assignment; rTMS or UL ECT (7 patients switched to BL ECT); HDRS, GAF	LDLPFC; 10 Hz; 90% MT; 6-second trains; 30-second ITIs; 20 trains per session; up to 20 sessions	rTMS = ECT; based on HDRS percent change and GAF ≥60
O'Connor et al. [15]	28 MDD; nonrandom assignment; UL ECT plus meds or rTMS alone; HDRS, cognitive battery	LDLPFC; 10 Hz; 90% MT; 8-second trains; 24-second ITIs; 20 trains per session; 10 sessions	ECT plus meds > rTMS alone; based on HDRS change; ECT greater cognitive adverse effects. ECT group had significantly higher HDRS scores versus TMS group at baseline

Table 3. (continued)

Authors	Patients/design	Parameters	Comments
McLoughlin et al. [16]	46 MDD; random assignment; HDRS (17-item); rTMS or BL ECT; HDRS, BDI-II (raters blinded)	LDLPFC; 10 Hz; 110% MT; 5-second trains; 55-second ITIs; 20 trains per session; up to 15 sessions	BL ECT > rTMS; based on HDRS percent change; patients continued on medications Both groups demonstrated significant improvement from baseline HDRS scores
Schulze-Rauschenbach et al. [17]	30 MDD; nonrandom assignment; UL ECT plus meds or rTMS plus meds; HDRS	LDLPFC; 10 Hz; 100% MT; 2-second trains; 5-second ITIs; 20–30 trains per session; 10.8 ± 1.4 sessions (mean ± SD)	rTMS = ECT; based on: HDRS percent change; rTMS superior to ECT for cognitive adverse effects
Rosa et al. [18]	42 nonpsychotic MDD; random assignment; UL ECT alone (2 patients switched to BL ECT) or rTMS alone; HDRS, VAS, CGI, cognitive battery	LDLPFC; 10 Hz; 100% MT; 10-second trains; 20-second ITIs; 20 trains per session; up to 20 sessions	rTMS = ECT; based on HDRS percent change; VAS; CGI; no cognitive differences

BDI-II = BDI version II; BL ECT = bilateral ECT; CGI = clinical global impression; GAF = global assessment of functioning; VAS = visual analog scale.

rTMS was applied to the left prefrontal cortex at 100% of MT, 20 Hz, 2-second trains, 30–35 trains/day separated by 28-second rest periods. The rTMS group had an average of 12 treatments (±3.4) and the UL ECT group had an average of 6.2 (±1.6) treatments. While the ECT group had a significantly greater percent improvement on the Beck Depression Inventory (BDI; 69 vs. 46%), blinded raters found that on the Hamilton Depression Rating Scale (HDRS), the rate of remission (i.e., a final score of ≤8) and percent improvement over the course of treatment were the same for subjects receiving either ECT or rTMS.

McLoughlin et al. [16] presented and published an abstract from the results of their randomized trial comparing rTMS to bilateral ECT (BL ECT) in 46 subjects with MDD. Blinded raters utilized the 17-item HDRS and the BDI as outcome measures. Treatment sessions involved administration of rTMS over the LDLPFC at 110% MT at 10 Hz for 20, 5-second trains with a 55-second intertrain interval (ITI). Subjects could receive up to 15 total sessions. Patients continued on their medication regimens during this trial. Based on change scores in the HDRS and BDI, they reported a significant reduction in baseline HDRS scores in both groups. The ECT group, however, had a significantly greater treatment response than the rTMS group ($p < 0.001$).

Recently, Rosa et al. [18] randomly assigned 42 patients with refractory, nonpsychotic MDD to either rTMS or right UL ECT. rTMS parameters were stimulation of the LDLPFC at 100% MT at 10 Hz for 10-second trains with a total of 20 trains per session for up to 20 sessions. In the ECT group, 2 patients were switched to bilateral ECT because of insufficient response. Response rates were relatively low in both groups (ECT = 40% and rTMS = 50%), possibly due to strict refractoriness criteria and severity of the disorder. Remission rates were equally low (ECT = 20% and rTMS = 10%). No significant differences were found between the two treatments.

Our results [11] (discussed later) are also consistent with these 5 studies. Thus, 5 of 6 randomized trials support a potential role for rTMS in patients who are considered suitable for ECT in clinical practice.

Two nonrandomized studies [15, 17] have also compared rTMS to UL ECT. O'Connor et al. [15] reported that ECT plus medication was more effective than rTMS alone in 28 subjects with MDD. ECT, however, carried a greater cognitive side effect burden. Schulze-Rauschenbach et al. [17] compared these two therapies also focusing on cognitive adverse effects. In a sample of 30 subjects with MDD, they reported response (≥50% reduction in baseline HDRS scores) rates of 46% in the ECT group and 44% in the rTMS group. Again, rTMS was superior to ECT in terms of cognitive adverse effects. Limitations in these trials, in addition to nonrandom assignment, were the use of concomitant medications and less aggressive trials of rTMS (e.g. shorter treatment course duration; lower stimulation intensities).

Table 4. Mean HDRS scores in the pilot study

	Baseline	Final	Percent change
rTMS (n = 17)	33 (±7.9)	15 (±11.0)	51 (±36)
ECT (n = 14)	34 (±8.7)	11 (±9.0)	67 (±27)
Total (n = 31)	33 (±8.0)	13 (±10.2)	58 (±33)

d.f. = 20; p = n.s; t = 1.56.

Table 5. Treatment responders in the rTMS versus ECT groups

	HDRS scores (≥50% decrease in baseline score or final score ≤8)		Response rate, %
	responders	nonresponders	
rTMS (n = 17)	7	10	41
ECT (n =14)	6	8	50

Fisher's exact test; p = n.s.

In a pilot trial, we compared rTMS to BL ECT in 31 subjects with MDD (unipolar or bipolar; psychotic or nonpsychotic) who were clinically appropriate for ECT [11]. Subjects were randomly assigned to rTMS or ECT with nonresponders to the initial treatment assignment having had the option to cross over to the alternate arm. rTMS parameters included:

- 110% MT;
- 10-Hz frequency;
- 5-second train duration (i.e., 50 pulses per train);
- 30-second ITI;
- 20 trains per session;
- 10–20 sessions total, given 5 days per week.

These parameters resulted in 1,000 stimulations per treatment over 10–20 sessions. Thus, subjects received a minimum of 10,000 stimulations and a maximum of 20,000 stimulations during a 2- to 4-week period. Those randomized to rTMS received stimulations with the Magstim Rapid Stimulator using a figure-eight insulated coil over the LDLPFC. Those randomized to ECT received 4–12 treatments with bitemporal electrode placement.

Table 6. Adverse effects associated with rTMS and ECT

	rTMS	ECT
Serious adverse effects	None	None
Mild adverse effects	Facial twitching	Short-term memory impairment
	Erythema at site of coil placement	Drowsiness shortly after treatment
	Anxiety before and during treatment	Postictal and anesthesia-induced confusion
	Localized to stimulation site: • Mild pain or discomfort • Feelings of warmth • Tapping sensation • Headache	

The primary outcome measure was the 24-item HDRS [22]. Patients received a minimum of 10 rTMS sessions or 4 ECT treatments and then ended the trial if they met the criteria for response (i.e., a 50% or greater decrease in baseline HDRS scores and a final score of 8 or lower). If they did not meet the criteria, they continued in the trial for another week before reassessment with the HDRS. If they still did not meet the criteria for response, they received one more week of treatment and then ended the trial. Tables 4 and 5 provide the percent change in the HDRS scores for the rTMS group, the ECT group, and the total sample, as well as the number of patients in each group who met the response criteria. While the trend favored ECT, there was no significant difference between these treatment groups. Further, the improvement in the ECT group was comparable to that seen in the Consortium for Research in ECT trials using a similarly matched group of patients [23]. Table 6 lists the adverse effects observed in both treatment arms. Of note, we found no evidence of cognitive adverse effects with rTMS [24]. The strengths of this trial included a more severely ill, depressed sample; random assignment; relatively aggressive rTMS and ECT treatment parameters, and the limited use of rescue medications (i.e., lorazepam or zolpidem as needed). All other psychotropics were stopped for 3 days before beginning treatment.

In summary, 5 of 8 published trials reported antidepressant equivalence between rTMS and ECT; 1 trial reported UL ECT to be superior to rTMS; 1 trial reported BL ECT to be superior to rTMS, and 1 trial found UL ECT plus medication superior to rTMS monotherapy in MDD with psychosis but comparable in efficacy to rTMS for MDD without psychosis. Participants were considered clinically appropriate for a course of ECT, usually due to treatment resistance or, to a lesser extent, medication intolerance. Six trials involved random assignment to either modality and 2 did not. Stimulation intensities for rTMS ranged from 90% to 110% MT and the number of sessions ranged from 10 to 20. There are several limitations to these trials, including:

- they are all *pilot studies* at single sites with small sample sizes;
- some included *heterogeneous groups* of depressed subjects (e.g. unipolar, bipolar; psychotic, nonpsychotic);
- 6 of 8 trials used *UL ECT*;
- most studies used *concomitant medications*;
- 2 trials used *nonrandom* assignment;
- most trials used *nonblinded* assessments[1].

What is now needed is a large, multisite, randomized, controlled trial to ascertain the relative benefit of rTMS in comparison to ECT in this more severely-ill depressed group. If found to be comparable, advantages of rTMS over ECT include the absence of seizure induction and therefore no need for anesthesia. Further, there is no evidence of cognitive disruption with rTMS. As a result, patients remain completely alert and independent during and immediately after the procedure. While an inadvertent seizure can occur, this is a rare event. The most common adverse effects with rTMS (e.g. local pain at the site of stimulation; posttreatment headaches) are usually mild and generally well tolerated. Presently, relative contraindications to the use of rTMS include metallic implants in the head, cardiac pacemakers, pregnancy, and a history of seizures. However, if determined to be effective, rTMS may be safer than medication or ECT in certain clinical scenarios (e.g. pregnancy). As an important social benefit, rTMS may engender less stigma than ECT.

Conclusion

We have reviewed the concept of rTMS for depression and current pilot studies comparing rTMS to ECT. In conclusion, rTMS may be an alternative therapy for at least some depressed patients when used as an intermediate strategy between antidepressants and ECT. It may also be a viable augmentation strategy combined with medication or ECT for patients with more severe depression [25, 26]. Compared with ECT, rTMS has a much better adverse effect

[1]Blinded assessments are difficult when comparing these two kinds of treatment, especially because of different cognitive side effect profiles and ethical impediments of sham ECT.

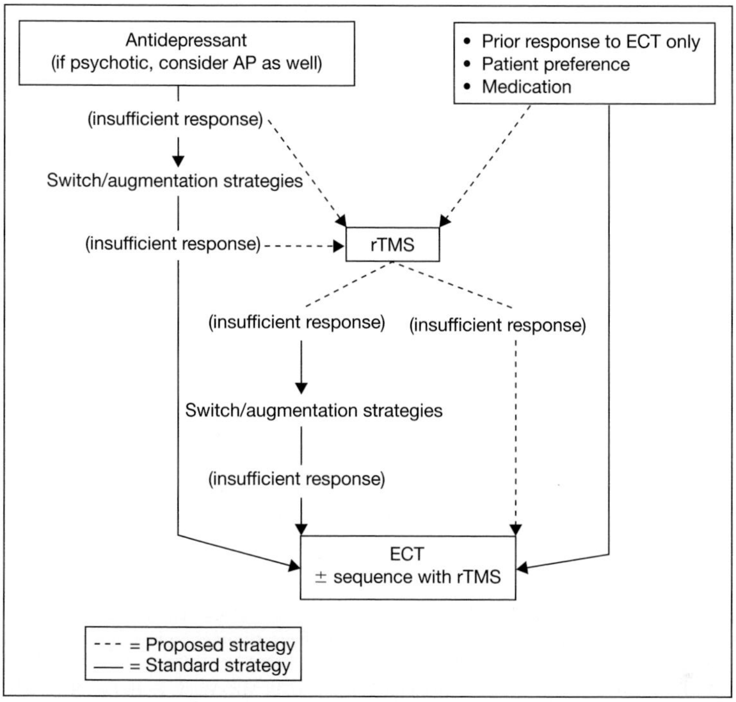

Fig. 1. The role of rTMS in a strategy for the treatment of more severe major depression (adapted from Dowd and Janicak [25]). AP = Antipsychotic.

profile including few, if any, cognitive adverse effects. It is also more efficient to administer and more cost effective (e.g. no need for anesthesia induction, seizure induction or operating room recovery monitoring). Anticipating the potential role for rTMS in the treatment of major depression, we have developed a treatment strategy that incorporates this modality (fig. 1) [25, 27, 28].

References

1 Lisanby SH, Datto CJ, Szuba MP: ECT and rTMS: past, present, and future. Depress Anxiety 2000;12:115–117.
2 McNamara B, Ray JL, Arthurs OJ, Boniface S: Transcranial magnetic stimulation for depression and other psychiatric disorders. Psychol Med 2001;31:1141–1146.
3 Holtzheimer PE, Russo J, Avery DH: A meta-analysis of repetitive transcranial magnetic stimulation in the treatment of depression. Psychopharmacology Bull 2001;35:149–169.
4 Burt T, Lisanby SH, Sackeim HA: Neuropsychiatric applications of transcranial magnetic stimulation: a meta-analysis. Int J Neuropsychopharmacol 2002;5:73–103.

5 Kozel FA, George MS: Meta-analysis of left prefrontal repetitive transcranial magnetic stimulation (rTMS) to treat depression. J Psychiatr Pract 2002;8:270–275.
6 Martin JL, Barbanoj MJ, Schlaepfer TE, Thompson E, Perez V, Kulisevesky J: Repetitive transcranial magnetic stimulation for the treatment of depression. Systematic review and meta-analysis. Br J Psychiatry 2003;182:480–491.
7 O'Reardon J, Solvason B, Janicak PG, Sampson S, Isenberg K, Nahas Z, McDonald W, Avery DH, Fitzgerald PB, Loo C, Demitrack M, George MS, Sackeim HA: Efficacy and safety of repetitive transcranial magnetic stimulation (rTMS) in the acute treatment of major depression: results of a multicenter randomized controlled trial. In preparation.
8 Fink M: Prejudice against ECT: competition with psychological philosophies as a contribution to its stigma. Convuls Ther 1997;13:253–265.
9 Post A, Keck ME: Transcranial magnetic stimulation as a therapeutic tool in psychiatry: what do we know about the neurobiological mechanisms? J Psychiatr Res 2001;35:193–215.
10 Ben-Shachar D, Belmaker RH, Grisaru N, Klein E: Transcranial magnetic stimulation induces alterations in brain monoamines. J Neural Transm 1997;104:191–197.
11 Janicak PG, Dowd SM, Martis B, Alam D, Beedle D, Krasuskai J, Strong M, Sharma R, Rosen C, Viana M: Repetitive transcranial magnetic stimulation versus electroconvulsive therapy for major depression: preliminary results of a randomized trial. Biol Psychiatry 2002;51:659–667.
12 Grunhaus L, Dannon PN, Schreiber S, Dolberg OH, Amaiz R, Lefkifker E: Repetitive transcranial magnetic stimulation is as effective as electroconvulsive therapy in the treatment of nondelusional major depressive disorder: an open study. Biol Psychiatry 2000;47:314–324.
13 Pridmore S, Bruno R, Turnier-Shea Y, Reid P, Rybak M: Comparison of unlimited numbers of rapid transcranial magnetic stimulation (rTMS) and ECT treatment sessions in major depression episode. Int J Neuropsychopharmacol 2000;3:129–134.
14 Grunhaus L, Schreiber S, Dolberg OT, Polak D, Dannon PN: A randomized controlled comparison of electroconvulsive therapy and repetitive transcranial magnetic stimulation in severe and resistant nonpsychotic major depression. Biol Psychiatry 2003;53:324–331.
15 O'Connor M, Brenninkmeyer C, Morgan A, Bloomingdale K, Thall MR, Vasile R, Pascual Leone A: Relative effects of repetitive transcranial magnetic stimulation and electroconvulsive therapy on mood and memory: a neurocognitive cost/benefit analysis. Congn Behav Neurol 2003;16:118–127.
16 McLoughlin DM, Eranti S, Mogg A, et al: A 6-month, follow-up, pragmatic randomized controlled trial of ECT and rTMS in major depression (abstract). J ECT 2005;21:59.
17 Schulze-Rauschenbach SC, Harms U, Schlaepfer TE, Maier W, Falkai P, Wagner M: Distinctive neurocognitive effects of repetitive transcranial magnetic stimulation and electroconvulsive therapy in major depression. Br J Psychiatry 2005;186:410–416.
18 Rosa MA, Gattaz WF, Pascual-Leone A, Fregni F, Rosa MO, Rumi DO, Myczkowski M, Silva MF, Mansur C, Rigonatti SP, Teixeira MJ, Marcolin MA: Comparison of repetitive transcranial magnetic stimulation and electroconvulsive therapy in unipolar non-psychotic refractory depression: a randomized single-blind study. Int J Neuropsychopharmacol 2006, E-pub ahead of print.
19 Pridmore S: Substitution of rapid transcranial magnetic stimulation treatments for electroconvulsive therapy treatments in a course of electroconvulsive therapy. Depress Anxiety 2000;12:118–123.
20 George MS, Nahas Z, Speer A, Avery D, Molloy M, Risch SC, Lorberbaum JP, Bohning DE, Post RM: How does TMS improve depression? Current hints about the role of intensity, frequency, location and dose. Biol Psychiatry 1998;43:76.
21 Dannon PN, Dolberg OT, Schreiber S, Grunhaus L: Three and six-month outcome following courses of either ECT or rTMS in a population of severely depressed individuals preliminary report. Biol Psychiatry 2002;51:687–690.
22 Hamilton M: A rating scale for depression. J Neurol Neurosurg Psychiatry 1960;23:56–62.
23 Janicak PG, Viana M, Dowd SM, Martis B, Beedle P, Alam D, Krasuski J, Strong MJ, Sharma R, Rosen C: Reply to comment on 'Repetitive transcranial magnetic stimulation versus electroconvulsive therapy for major depression: preliminary results of a randomized trial'. Biol Psychiatry 2002;52:1032–1033.
24 Martis B, Alam D, Dowd SM, Hill SK, Sharma RP, Rosen C, Pliskin N, Martin E, Carson V, Janicak P: Neurocognitive effects of repetitive transcranial magnetic stimulation in severe major depression. Clin Neurophysiol 2003;114:1125–1132.

25 Dowd SM, Janicak PG: The attraction of magnetism: how effective and safe is rTMS? Curr Psychiatry 2003;2:59–66.
26 Sackeim HA: Repetitive transcranial magnetic stimulation: what are the next steps? Biol Psychiatry 2000;48:959–961.
27 Janicak PG, Dowd SM, Strong MJ, Alam D, Beedle MD: The potential role of repetitive transcranial magnetic stimulation in treating severe depression. Psychiatr Annals 2005;35:138–145.
28 Janicak PG, Davis JM, Preskorn SH, Ayd FJ Jr, Pavuluri M, Marder S: Principles and Practice of Psychopharmacotherapy, ed 4. Philadelphia, Lippincott Williams & Wilkins, 2006, pp 317–352.

Philip G. Janicak, MD
Department of Psychiatry, Rush University Medical Center
1720 West Polk Street, Suite 107
Chicago, IL 60612 (USA)
Tel. +1 312 942 7287, Fax +1 312 942 7284, E-Mail pjanicak@rush.edu

Marcolin MA, Padberg F (eds): Transcranial Brain Stimulation for Treatment of Psychiatric Disorders.
Adv Biol Psychiatr. Basel, Karger, 2007, vol 23, pp 110–123

Transcranial Magnetic Stimulation in Schizophrenia

Marina Odebrecht Rosa[a], Paulo Belmonte-de-Abreu[b], Peter Eichhammer[c], Göran Hajak[c], Marco Antonio Marcolin[a]

[a]Psychiatric Institute, University of São Paulo, São Paulo, and [b]Departamento de Psiquiatria, Faculdade de Medicina, Universidade Federal do Rio Grande do Sul, Porto Alegre, Brazil; [c]Department of Psychiatry and Psychotherapy, University of Regensburg, Regensburg, Germany

Abstract

Repetitive transcranial magnetic stimulation (rTMS) has proven useful for the study and treatment of schizophrenic symptoms. This chapter describes the clinical studies with rTMS in schizophrenia identified by Medline search. There is evidence of an effect on positive symptoms of schizophrenia, using low-frequency (1 Hz) stimulation over the left temporoparietal cortex. There is also some evidence regarding beneficial effects on negative symptoms, mostly with high-frequency (8–20 Hz) stimulation over the prefrontal cortex, however including negative results. Overall, an effect of rTMS on positive symptoms of schizophrenia could be found, with promising but conflicting results regarding the effect on negative symptoms. There is also initial evidence of beneficial effects on other treatment-resistant symptoms, such as visual and somatic hallucinations. The results of current studies point to the importance of additional work focusing on frequency, number of stimuli applied and the length of treatment, as well as to the need of maintenance therapy.

Repetitive transcranial magnetic stimulation (rTMS) is a valuable, interesting and still intriguing tool to study and modify mood, perception and behavior in a noninvasive way, accompanied by very few side effects. It induces several effects on brain metabolism, symptoms and behaviors, described in more detail in other chapters of this book. This chapter describes major findings of therapeutic effects of rTMS in schizophrenia, and points to additional areas of research. The neurobiological effects of rTMS in men and in animals are described in previous chapters of this book.

The first part of the chapter deals with the clinical effects on brain areas and circuits involved in schizophrenia, the second investigates the effects on positive symptoms of schizophrenia, the third describes the changes of negative symptoms, and the last addresses areas where further research is needed. Clinical studies were obtained from systematic Medline review using the terms 'rTMS', 'TMS', 'repetitive transcranial magnetic stimulation' and 'schizophrenia'.

The May 2006 Pubmed search identified 20 clinical trials and among these, 12 randomized controlled trials from 1999 to 2006.

Biochemical Effects on Circuits Known to Be Altered in Schizophrenia

Neuroimaging and lesion studies linked negative symptoms to prefrontal cortex (PFC), limbic system, and basal ganglia dysfunction. The human PFC is critical for integrating emotions, cognition and autonomic nervous system regulation. Although such behaviors and symptoms have been most strongly associated with dopaminergic hypoactivity in the PFC, other neurotransmitters including norepinephrine, serotonin, and the excitatory amino acids may also play a role [1].

rTMS Studies in Humans

The early hypofrontality hypothesis in schizophrenia [2, 3] and positive rTMS findings in depression stimulated the initial studies of rTMS in schizophrenia. Overall evidence is accumulating about distributed effects of rTMS on both hemispheres and structures from the PFC, Broca's area, right and left temporoparietal cortex, basal ganglia, anterior cingulate cortex, premotor cortex, and hippocampus, with the most robust hypothesis related to local and distributed changes in excitatory and resting neurotransmitters, covering different brain circuits involved in schizophrenia.

Early Studies in Schizophrenia

Abarbanel et al. [4] used diagnostic TMS to measure parameters of cortical excitability. This study found a decreased motor threshold (MT) in line with a later study of Eichhammer and coworkers [5] indicating increased cortical excitability after motor cortex stimulation by rTMS. This finding is consistent with the theories of reduced γ-aminobutyric acid activity and increased cortical excitability in schizophrenia.

Geller et al. [6] applied low-frequency bilateral PFC rTMS (0.03 Hz, 2 T, 15 pulses on each side) and observed transient improvement in 20% of schizophrenic patients. Feinsod et al. [7] also observed improved anxiety and agitation in 70% of schizophrenic patients after 10 1-Hz right dorsolateral PFC (DLPFC) rTMS sessions over 2 weeks in an open-label design. In contrast, a double-blind controlled study by Klein et al. [8] failed to detect differences between active and inactive slow right PFC stimulation.

Rollnik et al. [9], in another double-blind controlled study, described reduced Brief Psychiatric Rating Scale (BPRS) scores after 2 weeks of left DLPFC rTMS (20 Hz) in 12 DSM-IV schizophrenic patients. A significant reduction of psychotic symptoms as indicated by reduced BPRS scores was reported, however no changes in depressive symptoms could be detected. Yu et al. [10] investigated the association of 10-Hz LPFC rTMS, P300 and prolactin levels in an open-label study of 5 medicated schizophrenic patients, and observed a partial normalization of the last-mentioned parameters.

Repetitive Transcranial Magnetic Stimulation Effect on Positive Symptoms

Increased metabolism in the left temporoparietal cortex (LTPC) and in areas of speech perception [11] was identified during visual hallucinations. LTPC 1-Hz rTMS induced changes in remote regions, presumably due to functional connections with the temporal cortex and Broca's area during speech perception. Given this, decreased auditory hallucinations secondary to LTPC stimulation could then reflect the propagation of the original stimulation through the distribution network. Hoffman et al. [12] performed a double-blind crossover design study with 3 patients with persistent auditory hallucinations (2 with schizophrenia and 1 with schizoaffective disorder) using 8-day LTPC 1-Hz rTMS, with almost total remission of hallucinations in 2 of them over 2 weeks. Later, Hoffman et al. [13] performed a crossover double-blind study with 12 medicated patients (8 with paranoid schizophrenia and 4 with schizoaffective disorder) using 4-day sham rTMS and 4-day active rTMS, with increased stimulation from 4 to 16 min. There was a significant change in hallucination scores in the active group ($p < 0.006$), with no difference in the Positive and Negative Syndrome Scale (PANSS) scores. Additionally, treatment effect was reduced in patients using anticonvulsive drugs.

In 2003, Hoffman et al. [14] published a randomized double-blind placebo-controlled study with 24 medicated drug-refractory schizophrenic/schizoaffective patients with persistent auditory hallucinations. rTMS was performed over the LTPC at the mid level between T3 and P3 of the 10–20 international EEG system during 9 days at 1 Hz (90% MT), and inactive stimulation was obtained with 45° inclinations from scalp surface. Auditory hallucinations decreased in the active group, especially voice frequency and influence over behavior. Clinical global impression (CGI) decreased, with no change on the PANSS subscales of delusions, negative symptoms or general psychopathology. There was a large variability in the duration of effects, with 52% of patients maintaining effects over at least 15 weeks. The extended sample of this study [15] with 26 additional patients (n = 50) confirmed the effects on hallucinations (p = 0.008), CGI (p = 0.0004) and frequency of hallucinations (p = 0.0014). Franck et al. [16] applied the same protocol in a schizophrenic patient that killed his mother under delusions, and observed a score reduction from 73 to 31 on the Scale for the Assessment of Positive Symptoms.

Similar results were reported by D'Alfonso et al. [17] in an open-label study of 9 schizophrenic patients with drug-resistant auditory hallucinations (7 were under clozapine and 1 under olanzapine). The protocol included 10 sessions of 20 min using 1-Hz rTMS over the temporal cortex at 80% MT. Seven out of 8 patients in the study reported a significant decrease of symptoms. Combined rTMS and clozapine appeared to be safe and efficient, deserving additional studies for further confirmation.

More recently, additional studies in Italy [18, 19], France [20, 21], Australia [22] and Korea [23] using similar methodology reported discrepant results of low-frequency rTMS for auditory hallucinations.

In detail, the randomized double-blind placebo-controlled study of Chibbaro et al. [18] in 16 medicated schizophrenics with treatment-resistant auditory hallucinations used a 45° inclination coil as control (1 Hz, 90% MT over the LTPC with 4 sessions over 4 consecutive days, 15 min each application). The scores on the Scale for the Assessment of Positive Symptoms and auditory hallucinations were significantly reduced in both groups (active and sham), but the effects persisted only in the active group (over 8 weeks).

Saba et al. [20] performed a randomized double-blind placebo-controlled study in 18 treatment-resistant medicated paranoid schizophrenics (DSM-IV) having prominent delusions and auditory hallucinations (1 Hz, 80% MT over the LTPC, 5 series of 1 min each and 60-second intervals over 10 days). Both groups had similar changes in symptoms, PANSS and CGI ($p < 0.05$), with no significant differences between the two groups ($p > 0.05$), including auditory hallucinations.

Poulet et al. [21] performed a randomized double-blind study with a crossover design in 10 patients with treatment-resistant schizophrenia (5-day sessions, 1 Hz at 90% MT, 1,000 stimuli/session, with a total of 10,000 pulses). A 56% decrease in the scores on the Hoffman Scale of Auditory Hallucination was observed with the active treatment, with the effect still present after 2-month follow-up.

In a subsequent study, Lee et al. [23] randomly allocated 39 schizophrenic patients to active or inactive rTMS over the LTPC and right temporoparietal

Table 1. Major studies of rTMS in schizophrenia: effect on positive symptoms (all 1-Hz LTPC rTMS)

Authors	Year	n	Design	Duration min	Stimuli	MT %	Duration days	Outcome
Hoffman et al. [12]	1999	3	RCT COD	4–8–12–16	2,400	80	4/4	RAH
Hoffman et al. [13]	2000	12	RCT COD	4–8–12–16	2,400	80	4/4	RAH
Hoffman et al. [14]	2003	24	RCT SC	4–8–12–16	7,920	90	9	RAH
Hoffman et al. [15]	2005	50	RCT SC	8–12–16	7,920	90	9	RAH
D'Alfonso et al. [17]	2002	9	OLS	20	12,000	80	10	RAH
Franck et al. [16]	2003	1	OLS	16	9,519	90	10	reduction in SAPS scores
Chibbaro et al. [18]	2005	16	RCT	15	3,600	90	4	reduction in SAPS scores
McIntosh et al. [24]	2004	16	RCT COD	4–8–12–16	2,400	80	4/4	no difference in PANSS scores (positive vs. general)
Saba et al. [20]	2006	16	RCT	5	3,000	80	10	no difference in PANSS scores (positive vs. negative vs. general)
Poulet et al. [21]	2005	10	RCT COD	16	10,000	90	10/10	RAH
Lee et al. [23]	2005	39	RCT	20	12,000	100	10	RAH (RTPC + LTPC)
Brunelin et al. [19]	2006	24	RCT	16	10,000	90	5	RAH
Fitzgerald et al. [22]	2005	33	RCT SC	15	9,000	90	10	RAH
Rosa et al. [25]	2006	11	RCT SC	16	9,600	90	10	

AH = Auditory hallucinations; COD = crossover design; OLS = open-label study; RAH = reduction in auditory hallucinations; RCT = randomized controlled trial; RTPC = right temporoparietal cortex; SAPS = scale for the assessment of positive symptoms; SC = sham control.

cortex (inactive: 90° coil from the skull). Thirteen patients received active LTPC, 12 active right temporoparietal cortex rTMS, and 14 received inactive treatment (7 on the right, 7 on the left side) according to the following protocol: 100% MT, 1 Hz, 20 min/day for 10 days over the LTPC (between T3/T4 and P3/P4 of the 10–20 international EEG system). Basal scores were similar among the three groups. Time effect (intrasubject comparison) revealed a significant reduction of auditory hallucinations, PANSS positive symptoms and CGI. Comparison among the groups showed a difference in PANSS positive symptoms and CGI. Post hoc analysis revealed superiority of right- and left-side rTMS compared to sham treatment, with few and transient side effects: headache (2 patients), dizziness (1 patient) and problems of concentration (1 patient). There were no significant effects of rTMS on Hoffman Scale of Hallucinations (HSH) scores, but CGI was significantly better in the active group and the mean and median PANSS scores tended to be higher in the active (right and left) rTMS group.

In a study with similar selection criteria and with a slightly different rTMS protocol (2 sessions/day), Brunelin et al. [19] observed significant improvement on auditory hallucinations after 10 sessions with 1,000 stimuli on 5 days in 14 subjects compared to sham stimulation in 10 subjects. In contrast, Fitzgerald et al. [22] and McIntosh et al. [24] both failed to detect significant changes after rTMS, although their protocols were somewhat different from each other. McIntosh et al. [24] performed a 4-day treatment, with daily duration escalating from 4 to 8, 12 and 16 min, with 15 s of rest after each minute; Fitzgerald et al. [22] applied 10 1-Hz sessions of 15 min, and both made sham stimulation with the coil placed at a 45° angle from the skull. The lack of effect could be due to the type of sham procedure they used (45° placement of the coil), or the small number of pulses in the study by McIntosh et al. [24] (table 1).

Repetitive Transcranial Magnetic Stimulation Effects on Negative Symptoms

There is now a large body of functional neuroimaging literature suggesting an association of hypofrontality in schizophrenia with negative symptoms and cognitive deficits [26]. Dolan et al. [27] showed an association of neuropsychological deficits in a group of schizophrenic patients demonstrating negative symptoms and depression with decreased DLPFC metabolism. Additionally, George and Belmaker [28] performed laterality studies during functional imaging in schizophrenia and indicated an association of LPFC hypometabolism with negative symptoms.

In line with these findings, several rTMS studies over the PFC were initiated, similar to its application in depression. One of the first studies used bilateral

PFC rTMS with 30 pulses (100% MT) [5] and evidenced a transient BPRS score reduction in 2 of 10 medicated chronically schizophrenic patients.

Cohen et al. [29] was the first to demonstrate rTMS effects on negative symptoms. They studied 6 patients with chronic schizophrenia under a stable dose of neuroleptics. The treatment procedure consisted of 2-week rTMS at 80% MT (20 Hz, 10 sessions, 2-second series over 20 min). Their major finding was a reduction of PANSS negative symptoms ($p < 0.05$). Despite a tendency to neuropsychological improvement, no change in hypofrontality was observed on repeated SPECT scans.

The use of rTMS to treat negative symptoms of schizophrenia is based, among others, on the findings of Strafella et al. [3]. This study demonstrated reduced linkage of ^{11}C-raclopride to the DLPFC and subsequent dopamine liberation in the ipsilateral caudate nucleus. Some studies demonstrated transient improvement in schizophrenia after DLPFC stimulation [30]. Despite that, this treatment did not receive a systematic investigation in treatment-resistant schizophrenia.

A further study demonstrated a partial improvement in anxiety, tension and inner restlessness in 7 of 10 schizophrenics after 10 sessions of rTMS over the right PFC (1,000 pulses) [7]. BPRS scores decreased at the endpoint, with no effect on delusions and hallucinations. A pilot study suggested improvement of negative symptoms and cognition after high-frequency (20 Hz) rTMS in the orbital PFC area (8,000 pulses) in 6 chronic schizophrenics [29]. One additional open-label study demonstrated improvement of the negative symptoms on the Scale for the Assessment of Negative Symptoms after 5 days of 10-Hz rTMS over the left DLPFC (3,500 pulses) in 10 schizophrenic patients [5]. EEG frequency bands showed hemispheric and regional changes of brain activity, decreases in the delta and beta band, increases in alpha activity in the right frontotemporal area and decreases in beta activity in the left temporal and parieto-occipital area. There was a 33% reduction of the PANSS negative scores after 1 month of 15-Hz rTMS (20 sessions, 90% MT, 35,000 pulses) in 4 patients with a stable deficit syndrome [30].

In addition, Rollnik et al. [31] documented a case report with clear improvement in BPRS scores (from 45 to 31 points) after a 20-day 2-Hz rTMS at 80% MT over the left DLPFC in a patient with treatment-resistant schizoaffective disorder. The switch to sham stimulation was followed by an increase in BPRS scores (up to 40 points). After reswitching to active stimulation, BPRS scores decreased again.

Based on the encouraging results of these case series, several randomized double-blind placebo-controlled (sham-controlled) studies were conducted. Klein et al. [8] performed the first; they applied low-frequency rTMS over the right PFC at 110% MT (1,200 pulses) in 35 schizophrenic or schizoaffective patients, without an effect on negative symptoms. Studies using high-frequency rTMS (10 Hz and 20 Hz) over the left DLPFC revealed more success. Rollnik et al. [9] performed a crossover study with active and sham rTMS treatment showing BPRS score reduction after 10 sessions of 20-Hz rTMS over the dominant PFC using 80% MT (8,000 pulses) in 12 schizophrenics. Unfortunately, the authors failed to differentiate between positive and negative symptoms. There was no difference in depressive and anxiety symptoms. In contrast, Cordes et al. [32] published a study with 10-Hz rTMS over the left DLPFC (10 sessions in 2 weeks, 110% MT, 10,000 pulses) demonstrating superiority of active over sham stimulation in PANSS negative scores. At last, Jin et al. [33] performed a randomized double-blind placebo-controlled study with a crossover design (sham control) in 27 patients with prominent negative symptoms (8- to 13-Hz rTMS over the DLPFC, 80% MT, compared to controls treated with 3- or 20-Hz rTMS and sham), with a significantly higher therapeutic effect at the peak alpha frequency of EEG.

Nahas et al. [34] described a randomized double-blind placebo-controlled study of 7 schizophrenic patients with prominent negative symptoms (20-Hz rTMS, 100% MT, 40 pulses in 2-second intervals over 20 min, total of 1,600 pulses over the left DLPFC). rTMS reduced the negatives symptoms on the Scale for the Assessment of Negative Symptoms, compared to placebo. Sachdev et al. [30] performed an open-label study in 4 schizophrenics with a stable deficit syndrome (15-Hz rTMS, 90% MT in 20 sessions over the left DLPFC), showing a significant reduction of the negative symptoms associated with functional improvement, maintained at 1-month follow-up. Jandl et al. [35] also performed an open-label study in 10 patients (10-Hz rTMS over the left DLPFC) during 15 days, with a 10% reduction of the scores on the Scale for the Assessment of Negative Symptoms (from 49 to 44 points). Holi et al. [36], on the other hand, failed to detect changes in the PANSS scores after a randomized controlled trial of 10 days with 20 trains of 5 s each and 10-Hz stimulations. Novak et al. [37] also found negative results with 20-Hz rTMS over 10 days, which indicates the need to further investigate the therapeutic effects of rTMS on negative symptoms.

Taken together, 3 of 4 randomized double-blind placebo-controlled studies using 10-Hz rTMS indicate a significant improvement of the negative symptoms [5, 32, 33]. The other studies (1 with 1-Hz [8] and 3 with 20-Hz stimulation [33, 34, 37]) failed to show this effect in schizophrenic patients. Regarding the clinical and neurobiological results, there is increasing evidence of the efficacy of 10-Hz rTMS treatment in negative symptoms, although stimulation parameters varied slightly between the reviewed studies. High-frequency rTMS (especially 10-Hz stimulation) seems to be a promising technique to improve negative symptoms in schizophrenia, although its efficacy has to be proven in randomized controlled trials with higher statistical power using larger sample sizes and improved methodology to avoid systematic bias described in previous trials.

Additionally, there is a recent study of Rosa et al. [25] in which 11 schizophrenic patients (DSM-IV) experiencing auditory hallucinations were randomly allocated to receive either 1-Hz rTMS (n = 6) or sham stimulation (n = 5) on the LTPC (with concomitant use of clozapine). All patients were required to be taking at least 350 mg of clozapine per day, for 6 months or more, and they had to have failed in at least two adequate trials with standard antipsychotic medication from two different pharmacological groups with a minimum dose of 1,000 mg of chlorpromazine equivalents. Age range was 18–50 years inclusively. A total of 160 min of rTMS (9,600 pulses) was administered over 10 days at 90% MT using a double-masked, sham-controlled, parallel design.

No differences between groups were observed in baseline psychopathology [Auditory Hallucination Rating Scale (AHRS), CGI, Visual Analog Scale, PANSS]. Treatment was well tolerated and only 1 patient in the active group complained of headache after each rTMS session (with spontaneous remission). No other adverse effects were reported.

The active group demonstrated a time effect (within-subject comparison), with a significant linear decrease in 6 of the 7 items of the AHRS, some of which persisted during follow-up: reality (week 1: $F_{1, 41} = 4.44$, $p = 0.0412$; week 2: $F_{1,41} = 9.37$, $p = 0.0039$; week 6: $F_{1,41} = 7.87$, $p = 0.0076$); attentional salience (week 1: $F_{1, 11} = 4.29$, $p = 0.0383$; week 2: $F_{1, 11} = 10.31$, $p = 0.0013$; week 6: $F_{1, 11} = 9.50$, $p = 0.0130$); frequency (week 1: $F_{1, 11} = 8.81$, $p = 0.0128$; week 2: $F_{1, 11} = 6.26$, $p = 0.0294$); length (week 1: $F_{1, 11} = 4.88$, $p = 0.0270$; week 2: $F_{1, 11} = 8.29$, $p = 0.0040$; week 6: $F_{1, 11} = 4.36$, $p = 0.0367$); number of voices (week 2: $F_{1, 11} = 14.69$, $p = 0.028$), and distress level of hallucinations (week 2: $F_{1, 11} = 19.17$, $p = 0.0011$; week 6: $F_{1, 11} = 10.51$, $p = 0.0057$).

The sham group did not show a significant decrease in reality, frequency and length, but they did reveal a significant linear decrease on the items attentional salience (week 2: $F_{1, 11} = 6.17$, $p = 0.0130$); distress level (week 2: $F_{1, 11} = 19.17$, $p = 0.0057$); number of voices (week 2: $F_{1, 11} = 17.63$, $p = 0.0015$), and loudness (week 2: $F_{1, 11} = 13.11$, $p = 0.0003$). During the follow-up (week 6), there was a significant group effect (between-subject comparison) on the items reality (fig. 1) and attentional salience (fig. 2) of the AHRS ($F_{1, 41} = 4.11$, $p = 0.0493$ and $F_{1, 11} = 4.40$, $p = 0.0360$).

Both groups showed a similar pattern of symptomatic changes on the subitems negative symptoms, general psychopathology and total score of the PANSS.

No differences across treatment modalities were observed in CGI and Visual Analog Scale at any time. Despite the high refractoriness of the sample, there was a reduction of hallucination scores in both groups that persisted during the follow-up in the active group for the items reality and attentional salience (table 2).

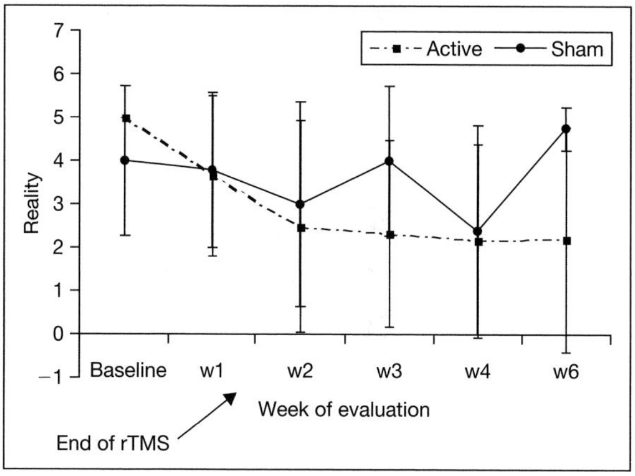

Fig. 1. AHRS mean scores (±SD) for 'reality' over time [25].

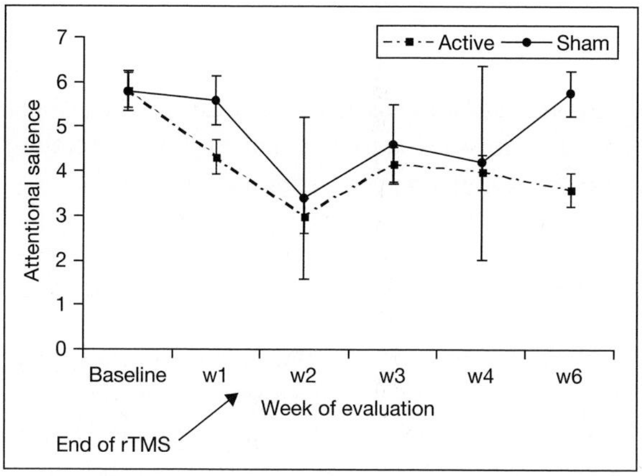

Fig. 2. AHRS mean scores (±SD) for 'attentional salience' over time [25].

Studies in Catatonia

There is only one study of rTMS in catatonia [38]. It was a case report study of a 24-year-old female patient with a history of acute psychotic episode 1 year before rTMS treatment. At baseline, she had stupor, automatic obedience, mutism, negativism and flaxy rigidity. Her psychosis remitted with haloperidol and catatonia persisted. rTMS was performed over the right PFC (80% MT, 20-Hz stimulation with a 2-second duration, 58-second intervals, 20 series/day over 10 days). Twenty-four hours after treatment, the patient woke up in the morning,

Table 2. Randomized double-blind sham-controlled studies (including crossover trials) on the treatment of negative symptoms

Authors	n	Location	Frequency, Hz	MT, %	Stimuli	p value
Klein et al. [8]	31	RPFC	1	110	1,200	n.s.
Nahas et al. [34]	8	LDLPFC	20	100	1,600	n.s.
Rollnik et al. [31]	12	DLPFC	20	80	8,000	BPRS, $p = 0.015$
Hajak et al. [5]	20	LDLPFC	10	110	10,000	PANSS NSS, $p = 0.046$
Holi et al. [36]	22	LDLPFC	10	100	10,000	n.s.
Jin et al. [33]	27	BLDLPFC	3, 10[1], 20	80	1,200, 4,000, 8,000	PANSS NSS, $p = 0.007$ at 10 Hz[1]
Cordes et al. [32]	25	LDLPFC	10	110	10,000	PANSS NSS, $p = 0.046$
Novak et al. [37]	16	LDLPFC	20	90	20,000	n.s.

BLDLPFC = Bilateral DLPFC; LDLPFC = left DLPFC; n.s. = no significant difference; NSS = negative subscale; RPFC = right PFC.

[1]Individualized alpha frequency (8–13 Hz).

walked to the bathroom and talked with other patients about her fear of aliens. Along the treatment, stupor, automatism and rigidity disappeared. The patient initiated her personal care, engaged in ward activities and begun cooperating with medical staff and family, keeping mutism over 1 additional month.

Effect on Visual Hallucinations

There is only one study of rTMS showing an effect on visual hallucinations. Merabet et al. [39] described a case report of suppression of complex visual hallucinations with 1-week 1-Hz rTMS over the occipital pole. Despite methodological limitations, the study provides initial support for further interventions in these and other dimensions of psychopathology, deserving additional studies with an improved design.

rTMS in Somatic Hallucinations

There is no report of any intervention in somatic hallucinations, despite the common occurrence of this kind of hallucinations in schizophrenia, and little is known about its anatomy and physiology. Nevertheless, due to impairment and personal suffering associated with these symptoms, there is a need for additional investigation focusing on specific patterns of somatic hallucinations (stomach, feet, hands, head, genitals); each one may be treated with a different protocol.

References

1 Goff DC, Evins AE: Negative symptoms in schizophrenia: neurobiological models and treatment response. Harv Rev Psychiatry 1998;6:59–77.
2 Weinberger D, Berman D, Zec R: Physiologic dysfunction of dorsolateral prefrontal cortex in schizophrenia. 2. Regional cerebral blood flow evidence. Arch Gen Psychiatry 1986;43: 114–124.
3 Strafella AP, Paus T, Barrett J, Dagher A: Repetitive transcranial magnetic stimulation of the human prefrontal cortex induces dopamine release in the caudate nucleus. J Neurosci 2001;21: RC157.
4 Abarbanel JM, Lemberg T, Yaroslavski U, Grisaru N, Belmaker RH: Electrophysiological responses to transcranial magnetic stimulation in depression and schizophrenia. Biol Psychiatry 1996;40:148–150.
5 Hajak G, Marienhagen J, Langguth B, Werner S, Binder H, Eichhammer P: High-frequency repetitive transcranial magnetic stimulation in schizophrenia: a combined treatment and neuroimaging study. Psychol Med 2004;34:1157–1163.
6 Geller V, Grisaru N, Abarbanel JM, Lemberg T, Belmaker RH: Slow magnetic stimulation of prefrontal cortex in depression and schizophrenia. Prog Neuropsychopharmacol Biol Psychiatry 1997;21:105–110.
7 Feinsod M, Kreinin B, Chistyakov A, Klein E: Preliminary evidence for a beneficial effect of low-frequency, repetitive transcranial magnetic stimulation in patients with major depression and schizophrenia. Depress Anxiety 1998;7:65–68.
8 Klein E, Kolsky Y, Puyerovski M, Koran D, Chistyakov A, Feinsod M: Right prefrontal slow repetitive transcranial magnetic stimulation in schizophrenia: a double-blind sham-controlled pilot study. Biol Psychiatry 1999;46:1451–1454.
9 Rollnik JD, Huber TJ, Mogk H, Siggelkow S, Kropp S, Dengler R, et al: High frequency repetitive transcranial magnetic stimulation (rTMS) of the dorsolateral prefrontal cortex in schizophrenic patients. Neuroreport 2000;11:4013–4015.
10 Yu CC, Liao KK, Chang TJ, et al: Transcranial magnetic stimulation in schizophrenia. Am J Psychiatry 2002;159:494–495.
11 Hoffman RE, Mc Glashan TH: Synaptic elimination, neurodevelopment, and the mechanism of hallucinated 'voices' in schizophrenia. Am J Psychiatry 1997;154:1683–1689.
12 Hoffman RE, Boutros NN, Berman RM, Roessler E, Belger A, Krystal JH, Charney DS: Transcranial magnetic stimulation of left temporo-parietal cortex in three patients reporting hallucinated voices. Biol Psychiatry 1999;46:130–132.
13 Hoffman RE, Boutros NN, Hu S, Berman RM, Krystal JH, Chamey DS: Transcranial magnetic stimulation and auditory hallucinations in schizophrenia. Lancet 2000;355:1073–1075.
14 Hoffman RE, Hawkins KA, Gueorguieva R, Boutros NN, Rachid F, Carrol K, Krystal JH: Transcranial magnetic stimulation of left temporo-parietal cortex and medication-resistant auditory hallucinations. Arch Gen Psychiatry 2003;60:49–56.
15 Hoffman RE, Gueorguieva R, Hawkins KA, Varanko M, Boutros NN, Wu YT, Carrol K, Krystal JH: Temporoparietal transcranial magnetic stimulation for auditory hallucinations: safety, efficacy and moderators in a fifty-patient sample. Biol Psychiatry 2005;58:97–104.
16 Franck N, Poulet E, Terra JL, Dalery J, D'Amato T: Left temporoparietal transcranial magnetic stimulation in treatment-resistant schizophrenia with verbal hallucinations. Psychiatry Res 2003;120:107–109.
17 D'Alfonso AAL, Aleman A, Kessels RP, Schouten EA, Postma A, Van Der Linden JA, Cahn W, Greene Y, de Haan EH, Kahn RS: Transcranial magnetic stimulation of left auditory cortex in patients with schizophrenia: effects on hallucinations and neurocognition. J Neuropsychiatry Clin Neurosci 2002;14:77–79.
18 Chibbaro G, Danielle M, Alagona G, DiPasquale C, Cannavo M, Rapisarda V, Bella R, Pennisi G: Repetitive transcranial magnetic stimulation in schizophrenic patients reporting auditory hallucinations. Neurosci Lett 2005;383:54–57.

19 Brunelin J, Poulet E, Bediou B, Kallel L, Dalery J, D'Amato T, Saoud M: Low frequency repetitive transcranial magnetic stimulation improves source monitoring deficit in hallucinating patients with schizophrenia. Schizophr Res 2006;81:41–45.
20 Saba G, Verdon CM, Kalalou K, Rocamora JF, Dumortier G, Benadhira R, Stamatiadis L, Vicaut E, Lipski H, Januel D: Transcranial magnetic stimulation in the treatment of schizophrenic symptoms: a double-blind sham-controlled study. J Psychiatr Res 2006;40:147–152.
21 Poulet E, Brunelin J, Bediou B, Forgeard L, Daleru J, D'Amato T, Saoud M: Slow transcranial magnetic stimulation can rapidly reduce resistant auditory hallucinations in schizophrenia. Biol Psychiatry 2005;57:188–191.
22 Fitzgerald PB, Benitez J, Dsakalakis J, Brown T, Marston NAU, de-Castella A, Kulkarni J: A double-blind sham-controlled trial of repetitive transcranial magnetic stimulation in the treatment of refractory auditory hallucinations. J Clin Psychopharmacol 2005;25:358–362.
23 Lee SH, Kim W, Chung YC, Jung KH, Bahk WM, Jun TY, Kim KS, George MS, Chae JH: A double-blind study showing that two weeks of daily repetitive TMS over the left or right temporoparietal cortex reduces symptoms in patients with schizophrenia who are having treatment-refractory auditory hallucinations. Neurosci Lett 2005;376:177–181.
24 McIntosh A, Semple D, Tasker K, Harrison L, Owens D, Johnstone EC, Ebmeier KP: Transcranial magnetic stimulation for auditory hallucinations in schizophrenia. Psychiatry Res 2004;127:9–17.
25 Rosa MO, Rosa MA, Rigonatti SP, Cabral SB, Myczodowski M, Sartorelli MC, Tavares H, Rumi DO, Marcolin MA: Effects of repetitive transcranial magnetic stimulation on auditory hallucinations refractory to clozapine. J Clin Psychiatry 2007; in press.
26 Weinberger DR, Berman KF, Chase TN: Mesocortical dopaminergic function and human cognition. Ann NY Acad Sci 1988;537:330–338.
27 Dolan RJ, Bench CJ, Liddle PF: Dorsolateral prefrontal cortex dysfunction in the major psychoses: symptoms or disease specificity? J Neurosurg Psychiary 1993;56:1290–1294.
28 George MS, Belmaker RH: Transcranial Magnetic Stimulation in Neuropsychiatry. Washington, American Psychiatric Association, 2000.
29 Cohen E, Bernardo M, Masana J, Arrufat FJ, Navarro V, Valls-Sole J, Boget T, Barrantes N, Catarineu S, Font M, Lomena FJ: Repetitive transcranial magnetic stimulation in the treatment of chronic negative schizophrenia: a pilot study. J Neurol Neurosurg Psychiatry 1999;67: 129–130.
30 Sachdew P, Loo C, Mitchell P, Malhi G: Transcranial magnetic stimulation for the deficit syndrome of schizophrenia: a pilot investigation. Pshychiatry Clin Neurosci 2005;59:354–357.
31 Rollnik JD, Seifert J, Huber TJ, Becker H, Panning B, Schneider U, Emrich HM: Repetitive transcranial magnetic stimulation and electroconvulsive therapy in a patient with treatment-resistant schizoaffective disorder. Depress Anxiety 2001;13:103–104.
32 Cordes J, Brinkmeyer J, Kotrotsios G, Arends M, Mobascher A, Agelink MW, Wölwer W: The effect of high-frequency repetitive transcranial magnetic stimulation (rTMS) on negative symptoms and electrophysiological correlates of facial affect recognition in schizophrenia. Schizophr Bull 2005;31:510.
33 Jin Y, Potkin SG, Kemp AS, Huerta ST, Alva G, Thai TM, Carreon D, Bunney WE Jr: Therapeutic effects of individualized alpha frequency transcranial magnetic stimulation (alphaTMS) on the negative symptoms of schizophrenia. Schizophr Bull 2006;32:556–561.
34 Nahas Z, Molloy M, Risch SC, George MS: TMS in schizophrenia; in George MS, Belmaker RH (eds): Transcranial Magnetic Stimulation in Neuropsychiatry. Washington, American Psychiatric Press, 2000, pp 237–252.
35 Jandl M, Bitner A, Sack E, et al: Changes in negative symptoms and EEG in schizophrenic patients after repetitive transcranial magnetic stimulation (rTMS): an open-label study. J Neural Transm 2005;112:955–967.
36 Holi MM, Eronen M, Toivonen K, Toivonen P, Marttunen M, Naukkarinen H: Left pre-frontal repetitive transcranial magnetic stimulation in schizophrenia. Schizophr Bull 2004;30:429–434.
37 Novak T, Horacek J, Mohr P, Kopecek M, Rodriguez M, Spaniel F, Dockery C, Hoschl C: The double-blind sham-controlled study of high-frequency rTMS (20 Hz) for negative symptoms in schizophrenia: a negative results. Neuro Endocrinol Lett 2006;27:209–213.

38 Grisaru N, Chudakov B, Yaroslavsky Y, Belmaker RH: Catatonia treated with transcranial magnetic stimulation. Am J Psychiatry 1998;155:1630.
39 Merabet L, Kobayashi M, Barton J, Pascual-Leone A: Suppression of complex visual hallucinatory experiences by occipital transcranial magnetic stimulation: a case report. Neurocase 2005;39:436–440.

Marco Antonio Marcolin, MD, MPH, PhD
Institute of Psychiatry
University of São Paulo
05403-010 São Paulo (Brazil)
Tel. +55 11 3069 6525, Fax +55 11 3257 11697
E-Mail marcolin@usp.br

Marcolin MA, Padberg F (eds): Transcranial Brain Stimulation for Treatment of Psychiatric Disorders.
Adv Biol Psychiatr. Basel, Karger, 2007, vol 23, pp 124–133

Repetitive Transcranial Magnetic Stimulation in the Treatment of Obsessive-Compulsive Disorder and Other Anxiety Disorders

Saxby Pridmore[a], *Marco Antonio Marcolin*[b], *Carmen Sylvia Ribeiro*[b], *Carlos Gustavo Mansur*[b]

[a]University of Tasmania, Hobart, Australia; [b]Brain Stimulation Research Center, Institute of Psychiatry, University of São Paulo, São Paulo, Brazil

Abstract

Repetitive transcranial magnetic stimulation (rTMS) is being investigated as a treatment of psychiatric disorders. This chapter reviews publications of the treatment of anxiety disorders: obsessive-compulsive disorder (OCD), posttraumatic stress disorder (PTSD) and panic disorder (PD). No definite conclusions can be reached as insufficient work has been completed. Many reports are single-case or small case studies and there have been few blind studies. There is no standardization of the site of stimulation or treatment parameters. OCD: there is some early evidence that 10-Hz stimulation of the left dorsolateral prefrontal cortex and right dorsolateral prefrontal cortex, and 1-Hz simultaneous stimulation of the left and right supplementary motor area may reduce symptoms. PTSD: one blind study suggests 10-Hz stimulation of the right dorsolateral prefrontal cortex may reduce core symptoms (reexperiencing, avoidance and hyperarousal). PD: 3 case studies have been published; 1 found that 1-Hz stimulation of the right dorsolateral prefrontal cortex reduced symptoms and response to cholecystokinin tetrapeptide challenge. Further work will clarify the role (if any) of rTMS in the treatment of these 3 disorders.

Repetitive transcranial magnetic stimulation (rTMS) is a new technology which is being investigated as a diagnostic and therapeutic option in psychiatry (and other fields of medicine) in many centers around the world. Its potential in the treatment of anxiety disorders was first reported by Greenberg et al. [1], who examined 3 patients with various symptoms. While grouped together for categorical convenience as anxiety disorders, there is little evidence that obsessive-compulsive disorder (OCD), panic disorder (PD) and posttraumatic stress disorder (PTSD) are related pathophysiologically and they are better considered as separate disorders.

Obsessive-Compulsive Disorder and Repetitive Transcranial Magnetic Stimulation

OCD is characterized by intrusive thoughts and repetitive acts aimed at reducing anxiety or distress caused by these thoughts. Significant psychosocial impairment may occur, and resistance to treatment is observed in some cases. Treatment usually includes antidepressant medication, mainly selective serotonin reuptake inhibitors. Cognitive-behavioral therapy with exposure and response prevention technique is also effective [2, 3].

Abnormal metabolism in subcortical structures and the orbitofrontal cortex can be found in OCD patients [4–7]. Some of these findings can be normalized after treatment [8–10]. Functional neuroimaging also revealed hypermetabolism in regions of the prefrontal cortex in OCD patients [11].

A paired-pulse TMS study demonstrated increased cortical excitability in OCD patients compared to controls [12]. Increased cortical excitability has been observed in Tourette's syndrome (TS) and focal dystonia, and may further support a role for the dysfunction of subcortical structures in OCD [12].

Greenberg et al. [1] studied the effect of a single session of high-frequency rTMS (20 Hz) to the left dorsolateral prefrontal cortex (LDLPFC), right dorsolateral prefrontal cortex (RDLPFC) and occipital cortex [13]. This was an open-label study, with 12 OCD patients. Compulsive urges significantly decreased for 8 h after RDLPFC stimulation. A modest, nonsignificant reduction in compulsive urges lasting 30 min followed the stimulation of the LDLPFC. There was no significant effect for obsessions. The authors identified the limitations of their study and the need for further controlled studies.

An open-label study of the effect of rTMS in 12 patients with OCD was conducted by Sachdev et al. [14]. These researchers provided 30 sessions of high-frequency (10 Hz) rTMS to either the RDLPFC or LDLPFC. Significant and sustained clinical response was observed in about one quarter of the patients, with Yale-Brown Obsessive Compulsive Scale (YBOCS) score reductions of over 40%. Both groups had a significant reduction in obsessions and compulsions, but there was no statistical difference between the groups. The researchers also observed a tendency towards continuous improvement in symptoms until the fourth week of follow-up. However, the open design left doubts about a possible placebo effect, even with this strong response in resistant patients.

Alonso et al. [15] conducted the only double-blind, placebo-controlled study for OCD treatment with rTMS reported at the time of writing. Low-frequency

(1 Hz) rTMS was applied to the RDLPFC, using a circular coil (rather than a figure-of-eight coil). Two intensities were employed: 110 and 20% motor threshold (MT). The former was considered to be an active treatment (10 patients) and the latter was considered to be sham (8 patients). Treatment was provided 3 times per week for 6 weeks. Most patients were receiving medication. No significant therapeutic effect was observed. Two patients (both checkers) in the active treatment group responded (global reduction in the YBOCS scores), as did 1 patient (sexual/religious obsessions) in the sham treatment group. The many differences between this and other studies make comparisons problematic. However, this was a double-blind trial and strongly suggests that low-frequency rTMS using a nonfocal coil to the RDLPFC will be of little benefit in OCD.

Due to the findings of deficient motor inhibition in patients with OCD and TS, and the knowledge of the connectivity of the supplementary motor area (SMA; cortical, thalamic and basal ganglia), Mantovani et al. [16] hypothesized that low-frequency (1 Hz) rTMS to the SMA may improve the symptoms and normalize the cortical activity of patients with these conditions. This was an open study involving 10 patients with OCD and/or TS who were concurrently receiving pharmacotherapy. A figure-of-eight coil was placed in the midline such that both left SMA (LSMA) and right SMA (RSMA) were stimulated simultaneously. Ten sessions of stimulation were provided on weekdays. Assessments were conducted before treatment, at the end of weeks 1 and 2, using 9 scales including the YBOCS, the Clinical Global Impression Scale (CGI) and anxiety, depression, general psychopathology and social adjustment instruments. The CGI was completed at 1 and 3 months' follow-up. As a measure of cortical activity, resting MT was conducted bilaterally at baseline and after weeks 1 and 2.

Eight patients completed the study, with no dropouts due to side effects. At the end of the second week, there was a statistically significant symptom reduction on all scales. Three of 5 'pure' OCD patients gained clinically significant improvement in OCD symptoms (YBOCS score reduction over 40%). Sixty percent of the total sample demonstrated improvement on CGI at 3 months' follow-up. The YBOCS changes were not correlated with changes in anxiety and depression and appeared to be a specific effect of rTMS on OCD and TS. In the OCD patients, at baseline, the resting MT was asymmetrical (R < L). Following treatment, the resting MT of the right side had significantly increased, such that this asymmetry disappeared. The study lacked a control group, but the authors argue that the placebo response is low in patients with OCD and TS, and that the normalization of cortical physiology and other factors point toward an actual (as opposed to a placebo) response.

An ongoing study in the Institute of Psychiatry at the University of São Paulo, Brazil, is investigating high-frequency (10 Hz) rTMS in patients with resistant OCD who are receiving pharmacotherapy [Mansur et al., unpublished data]. Thirty patients will be selected who have failed cognitive-behavioral therapy which features exposure and response prevention. All patients are evaluated prior to treatment with the YBOCS, Hamilton Anxiety and Depression Scales, and the SF-36 Quality of Life Scale. Patients are randomized to active treatment (delivered with a figure-of-eight coil) or placebo treatment (delivered with a sham coil; stimulation at 110% MT, applied to the RDLPFC). All patients receive 30 sessions of rTMS on weekdays (6 weeks). Assessments are conducted at baseline, after week 2, on completion of treatment, and at follow-up weeks 2 and 6. At the completion of treatment, those patients in the placebo group are offered active treatment in an open fashion. At the time of writing, 11 patients have completed the study, no dropouts have occurred.

No difference between the groups (4 in the active treatment group, 7 in the sham group) has been observed using any scale. However, spectacular clinical improvement was observed in 1 patient under blind active treatment, who became practically free of symptoms for at least 3 months. Three other patients showed significant clinical improvement, engaging in activities which had been long abandoned. One of these had received blind active treatment; the other 2 had failed to respond to placebo treatment, but responded to open active treatment. No sustained clinical improvement was observed in any patient receiving placebo rTMS. While statistical analysis of data collected to this point has shown no benefit from rTMS as an adjunctive treatment in resistant OCD, the mentioned individual responses suggest benefit in a subset of patients.

Table 1 summarizes the important studies to date. The situation has changed little since the authoritative reviews of Martin et al. [17] and Dell'Osso et al. [18], both of which found insufficient published data for confident conclusions. Most studies have been open using different methodologies. The blind study by Alonso et al. [15] strongly suggests that low-frequency rTMS to the RDLPFC will be of little benefit in OCD. However, these authors used a circular coil and ideally, the study could be repeated using a focused field. High-frequency studies to the DLPFC show some promise [13, 14; Mansur et al., in preparation]. The blind study of Mansur et al. [in preparation] is yet to be completed. To this point, there is no obvious advantage of active 10-Hz stimulation of the RDLPFC. However, these authors have described some remarkable individual responses, which may indicate that a subgroup of OCD patients may benefit from this approach.

The open study by Mantovani et al. [16] is of interest as a new target site is approached. This low-frequency study (1 Hz) suggests positive results (including normalization of cortical dysfunction) after simultaneous stimulation of both SMAs. Further studies are indicated.

Table 1. rTMS studies in OCD

Author	Site	Rate (Hz)	Design	Comment
Greenberg et al. [1]	LDLPFC	20	open, 12 patients, single session	some improvement
Sachdev et al. [14]	LDLPFC RDLPFC	10	open, 12 patients, 30 sessions; RDLPFC vs. LDLPFC	significant improvement with both treatments
Alonso et al. [15]	RDLPFC	1	blind, placebo-controlled, 18 patients, 3/week, 6 weeks	no significant difference
Mantovani et al. [16]	RSMA LSMA	1	open, 10 patients with OCD or TS, 10 sessions	significant improvement
Mansur et al. [in preparation]	RDLPFC	10	blind, placebo-controlled, 10 patients so far, 30 sessions (6 weeks)	no significant difference so far

Posttraumatic Stress Disorder and Repetitive Transcranial Magnetic Stimulation

PTSD is a disorder which follows a severe, usually life-threatening event in which there is reexperiencing of the event, persistent avoidance of triggers, numbing of responsiveness (feeling of engagement) and increased arousal (including insomnia and exaggerated startle response). The pathophysiology probably includes dysfunction of the hypothalamic-pituitary-adrenal axis. The neurocircuitry is yet to be fully elucidated, but decreased hippocampal volume has been described [19].

McCann et al. [20] were the first to investigate rTMS in the treatment of people with PTSD. They reported 2 case studies. Low-frequency stimulation (1 Hz) was applied to the RDLPFC for 17 days over 3 weeks in 1 case and for 30 days over 6 weeks in the other. In each case, improvement of symptoms was reported (modified PTSD symptom scale), which persisted for less than 1 month following cessation of treatment. A comparison of pre- and posttreatment PET scans suggested a reduction in cortical metabolism, preferentially on the right. However, the first PET studies were conducted months before the experimental treatment, making firm conclusions difficult.

Grisaru et al. [21] conducted an open-design single-session study of 10 patients with PTSD. Fifteen pulses of low-frequency (0.3 Hz) rTMS were delivered to each motor cortex. General improvement was observed using the CGI. There was also improvement in the core symptoms of avoidance (Impact of Event Scale), and anxiety and somatization (Symptom Check List-90). These effects lasted up to 7 days.

Rosenberg et al. [22] conducted an open study of 12 patients with PTSD and depression. Ten sessions of rTMS were applied to the LDLPFC in two groups of 6 patients, one receiving 1-Hz and the other 5-Hz stimulations. Scoring instruments were: the SCID-C, Hamilton Depression Rating Scale, Profile of Mood States, University of Southern California Repeatable Episodic Memory Test, and the Mississippi Scale of Combat Severity. The responses of the groups were not reported separately, as there were no differences. Overall, there was improvement in mood, anxiety (Tension-Anxiety and Anger-Hostility Subscales of the Profile of Mood States) and sleep, but no improvement in PTSD core symptoms (intrusive memories, avoidance, and hypervigilance). There was significant improvement on the Hamilton Depression Rating Scale, which was sustained at 2 months' follow-up. The authors concluded that 1- and 5-Hz rTMS to the LDLPFC appeared to be a useful adjunct in the treatment of refractory PTSD. Stimulation of the LDLPFC is effective in the treatment of primary depression and the associated sleep disturbance. This study provides evidence suggesting that depression associated with PTSD is also responsive. (The LDLPFC coil placement of this study was different to that used by many others. Most place the coil 5 cm anterior to the point of maximal stimulation of the thumb; Rosenberg et al. [22] placed the coil 4 cm anterior and 2 cm laterally.)

Recently, Cohen et al. [23] conducted the first double-blind, placebo-controlled trial of rTMS in the treatment of patients with PTSD. Twenty-four patients were divided into 3 groups: sham, low-frequency (1 Hz), and high-frequency (10 Hz) stimulation to the RDLPFC. Ten sessions were provided. The 10-Hz but not the 1-Hz group showed significant therapeutic effects compared to the sham group. At 2 weeks' follow-up, a significant reduction in core PTSD symptoms (reexperiencing, avoidance and hyperarousal) was observed.

Table 2 summarizes the available studies to date. Rosenberg et al. [22] have shown that 1-Hz rTMS to the LDLPFC (using their location) may be useful in treating depression associated with PTSD. Only one blind study has been conducted [23]. This suggests 10-Hz stimulation to the RDLPFC may be of use in the treatment of the core symptoms of PTSD. Replication is awaited.

Table 2. rTMS studies in PTSD

Author	Site	Rate (Hz)	Design	Comment
McCann et al. [20]	RDLPFC	1	case study, 2 patients	transient improvement in PTSD symptoms
Grisaru et al. [21]	bilateral MC	0.3	open, 12 patients	transient improvement in avoidance, anxiety and somatization
Rosenberg et al. [22]	LDLPFC*	1 5	open, 12 patients with PTSD plus depression	improved mood, anxiety and sleep, no change in intrusive memories, avoidance and hypervigilance
Cohen et al. [23]	RDLPFC	sham 1 10	blind, sham-controlled, 24 patients	10 Hz significantly superior to 1 Hz and sham in reducing reexperiencing, avoidance and hyperarousal

LDLPFC* = Atypical coil placement; MC = motor cortex.

Panic Disorder and Repetitive Transcranial Magnetic Stimulation

PD is familiar to all psychiatrists. The pathophysiology is poorly understood; noradrenalin, serotonin and GABA pathways have all been implicated. The efficacy of rTMS in the treatment of PD has not been comprehensively studied. Three case reports have been published.

Garcia-Toro et al. [24] treated 3 patients with PD using low-frequency (1 Hz) rTMS and later alternate applications of low- and high-frequency (20 Hz) rTMS, to the RDLPFC. Slight improvement in symptoms was observed, but this was not clinically significant.

Zwanzger et al. [25] reported the treatment of a patient with PD with 10 sessions of low-frequency (1 Hz) rTMS to the RDLPFC. In addition to clinical instruments, cholecystokinin tetrapeptide (CCK-4) challenge was delivered before and after treatment and plasma cortisol and ACTH were determined. After treatment, marked improvement in panic was reported. Moreover, compared to the pretreatment CCK-4 challenge, the symptomatic, as well as the cortisol and ACTH response to the posttreatment challenge was markedly reduced. Symptoms remained reduced at 4 weeks' follow-up.

Guaiana and Mortimer [26] reported the treatment of a case with a 10-year history of PD. Low-frequency (1 Hz) stimulation was applied to the right frontal area for 9 sessions, with no benefit. High-frequency (20 Hz) was then applied to the left frontal area 3 times per week for 20 sessions. Panic symptoms and agoraphobia were reportedly dramatically reduced by this second approach and improvement was sustained for 6 months.

Conclusion

No definite conclusions regarding rTMS in the treatment of anxiety disorders are possible as insufficient work has been performed. Many reports are single-case or small case studies, and few are blind. There is no standardization of the site of stimulation or treatment parameters.

While grouped together for categorical convenience, there is little evidence that OCD, PTSD and PD are related disorders and they can be considered as separate entities. Most work has been done with OCD. There is some evidence [14] that 10-Hz stimulation of the LDLPFC and RDLPFC may have beneficial effects. So far, this has not been supported by Mansur et al. [in preparation], but their work is proceeding. Mantovani et al. [16] have simultaneously stimulated both LSMA and RSMA with 1 Hz, with encouraging results, including normalization of cortical activity. This is an open study and a controlled study is now indicated.

PTSD has received some attention and a blind study by Cohen et al. [23] suggests high-frequency (10 Hz) stimulation of the RDLPFC may reduce core symptoms (reexperiencing, avoidance and hyperarousal).

PD reports include 3 case studies. These have all involved stimulation of the RDLPFC or the right frontal area. One reported negative findings. Zwanzger et al. [25] found that 1-Hz stimulation to the RDLPFC reduced symptoms and reduced the response to CCK-4 challenge.

Further work is required to clarify the role (if any) of rTMS in the treatment of these 3 disorders.

References

1 Greenberg BD, McCann UD, Benjamin J, Murphy AD: Repetitive TMS as a probe in anxiety disorders: theoretical considerations and case reports. CNS Spectr 1997;2:47–52.

2 Foa E, Steketee GS, Ozarow BJ: Behavior therapy with obsessive-compulsives: from the theory to treatment; in Mavinakalian M, Turner S, Michelson L (eds): Obsessive-Compulsive Disorder: Psychological and Pharmacological Treatment. New York, Plenum, 1985.

3 Mawson D, Romm L: Clomipramine and exposure for chronic obsessive-compulsive rituals: 2-year follow-up and further findings. Br J Psychiatry 1982;140:11–18.

4 Baxter LR Jr, Phelps ME, Mazziotta JC, Guze BH, Schwartz JM, Selin CE: Local cerebral glucose metabolic rates in obsessive-compulsive disorder. A comparison with rates in unipolar depression and in normal controls. Arch Gen Psychiatry 1987;44:211–218.

5 Swedo S, Schapiro M, Grady C, Cheslow D, Leonard H, Kumar A, Friedland R, Rapoport S, Rapoport J: Cerebral glucose metabolism in childhood-onset obsessive-compulsive disorder. Arch Gen Psychiatry 1989;46:518–523.
6 Rauch SL, Savage CR: Neuroimaging and neuropsychology of the striatum: bridging basic science and clinical practice. Psychiatr Clin North Am 1997;20:741–768.
7 Busatto GF, Buchpiguel CA, Zamignani DR, Garrido GE, Glabus MF, Rosario-Campos MC, Castro CC, Maia A, Rocha ET, Mcguire PK, Miguel EC: Regional cerebral blood flow abnormalities in early-onset obsessive-compulsive disorder: an exploratory SPECT study. J Am Acad Child Adolesc Psychiatry 2001;40:347–354.
8 Baxter LR Jr, Schwartz JM, Bergman KS, Szuba MP, Guze BH, Mazziotta JC, Alazraki A, Selin CE, Ferng HK, Munford P: Caudate glucose metabolic rate changes with both drug and behavior therapy for obsessive-compulsive disorder. Arch Gen Psychiatry 1992;49:681–689.
9 Benkelfat C, Nordahl TE, Semple WE, King AC, Murphy DL, Cohen RM: Local cerebral glucose metabolic rates in obsessive-compulsive disorder. Patients treated with clomipramine. Arch Gen Psychiatry 1990;47:840–848.
10 Schwartz JM, Stoessel PW, Baxter LR Jr, Martin KM, Phelps ME: Systematic changes in cerebral glucose metabolic rate after successful behavior modification treatment of obsessive-compulsive disorder. Arch Gen Psychiatry 1996;53:109–113.
11 Saxena S, Rauch SL: Functional neuroimaging and the neuroanatomy of obsessive-compulsive disorder. Psychiatr Clin North Am 2000;23:563–570.
12 Greenberg BD, Zieman U, Corá-Locatelli G, Harmon A, Murphy DL, Keel JC, Wassermann EM: Altered cortical excitability in obsessive-compulsive disorder. Neurology 2000;54:142.
13 Greenberg BD, George MS, Martin JD, Benjamin J, Schlaepfer TE, Altemus M, Wassermann EM, Post RM, Murphy DL: Effect of prefrontal repetitive transcranial magnetic stimulationin obsessive-compulsive disorder: a preliminary study. Am J Psychiatry 1997;154:867–869.
14 Sachdev PS, McBride R, Loo CK, Mitchell PB, Malhi GS, Croker VM: Right versus left prefrontal transcranial magnetic stimulation for obsessive-compulsive disorder: a preliminary investigation. J Clin Psychiatry 2001;62:981–984.
15 Alonso P, Pujol J, Cardoner N, Benlloch L, Merchón JM, Capdevila A, Vallejo J: Right prefrontal repetitive transcranial magnetic stimulation in obsessive-compulsive disorder: a double-blind, placebo-controlled study. Am J Psychiatry 2001;158:1143–1145.
16 Mantovani A, Lisanby S, Fulvio P, Ulivelli M, Castrogiovanni P, Rossi S: Repetitive transcranial magnetic stimulation (rTMS) in the treatment of obsessive-compulsive disorder (OCD) and Tourette's syndrome (TS). Int J Neuropsychopharmacol 2006;8:1–6.
17 Martin JL, Barbanoj MJ, Pérez V, Sacristán M: Transcranial magnetic stimulation for the treatment of obsessive-compulsive disorder (Cochrane review); in The Cochrane Library. Chichester, Wiley, 2004, issue 2.
18 Dell'osso B, Altamura CA, Allen A, Hollander E: Brain stimulation techniques in the treatment of obsessive-compulsive disorder: current and future directions. CNS Spectr 2005;10:966–997.
19 Bremner J, Vythilingam M, Vermetten E: MRI and PET study of deficits in hippocampal structure and function in women with childhood sexual abuse and posttraumatic stress disorder. Am J Psychiatry 2003;160:924–932.
20 McCann UD, Krimbell TA, Morgan CM, Anderson T, Geraci M, Benson BE, Wassermann EM, Willis MW, Post RM: Repetitive transcranial magnetic stimulation for posttraumatic stress disorder. Arch Gen Psychiatry 1998;55:276–279.
21 Grisaru N, Amir M, Cohen H, Kaplan Z: Effect of transcranial magnetic stimulation in posttraumatic stress disorder: a preliminary study. Biol Psychiatry 1998;44:52–55.
22 Rosenberg PB, Mehndiratta RB, Mehndiratta YP, Wamer A, Rosse RB, Balish M: Repetitive transcranial magnetic stimulation treatment of comorbid posttraumatic stress disorder and major depression. J Neuropsychiatry Clin Neurosci 2002;14:270–276.
23 Cohen H, Kaplan Z, Kotler M, Kouperman I, Moisa R, Grisaru N: Repetitive transcranial magnetic stimulation of the right dorsolateral prefrontal cortex in posttraumatic stress disorder: a double-bind, place-controlled study. Am J Psychiatry 2004;161:515–524.
24 Garcia-Toro M, Salva Coll J, Crespi Font M, Andres Tauler J, Aguirre Orue I, Bosch Calero C: Panic disorder and transcranial magnetic stimulation. Actas Esp Psiquiatr 2002;30:221–224.

25 Zwanzger P, Minov C, Ella R, Schüle C, Baghai T, Möller H, Rupprecht R, Padberg F: Transcranial magnetic stimulation for panic. Am J Psychiatry 2002;159:315–316.
26 Guaiana G, Mortimer A: Efficacy of transcranial magnetic stimulation in panic disorder: a case report. Aust N Z J Psychiatry 2005;39:1047.

Carlos Gustavo Mansur, MD
Brain Stimulation Research Center, University of São Paulo, Institute of Psychiatry
R. Dr. Ovidio Pires de Campos, 785
05403–010 São Paulo (Brazil)
Tel. +55 11 3069 6525, Fax +55 11 3069 6525, E-Mail cgmansur@yahoo.com

Marcolin MA, Padberg F (eds): Transcranial Brain Stimulation for Treatment of Psychiatric Disorders.
Adv Biol Psychiatr. Basel, Karger, 2007, vol 23, pp 134–154

Repetitive Transcranial Magnetic Stimulation in Non-Psychiatric Disorders: Pain, Parkinson's Disease, Stroke, Tinnitus

Jean-Pascal Lefaucheur[a], *Eman M. Khedr*[b]

[a]Service de Physiologie, Explorations Fonctionnelles, Hôpital Henri-Mondor, Créteil, France; [b]Department of Neurology, Assiut University Hospital, Assiut, Egypt

Abstract

Repetitive transcranial magnetic stimulation (rTMS) is a potent tool for modifying neural activities at the stimulated site and at a distance along functional anatomical connections. Since various neurological diseases are associated with dysfunction of neural pathways that include the cortex, therapeutic application of rTMS was considered, aiming at favourably influencing previously altered neural circuitry. This review highlights the emerging potential of rTMS to produce measurable clinical effects in chronic neuropathic pain, Parkinson's disease, motor stroke recovery, and tinnitus. In all these domains, there is growing evidence that rTMS might alleviate, at least transiently, various symptoms or impairments, depending on stimulus site or frequency. The optimization of the parameters of stimulation for each application is the key point before using rTMS as a therapeutic tool in daily neurological practice. Attempts to reach this objective benefit from functional neuroimaging or cortical excitability studies, but remain based on empirical hypotheses. Further insights into the mechanisms of action and controlled multicentre trials in large series of patients are needed to confirm the rTMS potential in neurological diseases, since the development of an alternative transcranial approach (direct current stimulation) or surgical implantation of epidural electrodes is a serious challenge to the future therapeutic application of rTMS.

Repetitive transcranial magnetic stimulation (rTMS) is a non-invasive technique that allows cortical activity to be transiently and focally modified. The electrical field, which is induced in the brain, excites or inhibits neural structures that are located under the coil or at a distance, functionally connected with the stimulated area. By reversing activity changes in disturbed or lesioned networks, rTMS has therapeutic potential for various neurological diseases.

Low-frequency rTMS (at a frequency around 1 Hz) and high-frequency rTMS (at 5 Hz or more) are thought to produce long-term synaptic depression and potentiation, respectively. Current developments of rTMS in neurological settings include chronic neuropathic pain, Parkinson's disease (PD), stroke recovery and tinnitus.

Repetitive Transcranial Magnetic Stimulation in Pain

Considering the analgesic effects provided by chronic motor cortex stimulation (MCS) with surgically implanted epidural electrodes [1], rTMS was applied in patients with chronic neuropathic pain (table 1). Pioneering studies were based on very low frequency of stimulation (0.2 Hz) [2, 3], compared to the frequencies used in implanted chronic MCS (20–55 Hz) [1]. High frequencies of stimulation (10 or 20 Hz) were subsequently used in most rTMS studies performed in patients with neuropathic pain [4–10]. Pain relief requires focal cortical stimulation (figure-of-eight coil) with a slightly different targeting between rTMS and the implanted procedure of MCS. The best target is the motor cortical area corresponding to the painful zone for epidural stimulation, but an adjacent zone for rTMS. This may result from differences in the pattern of the induced current flow between rTMS and epidural cortical stimulation and the recruited populations of fibres [11].

Mechanisms and Sites of Action

The stimulation of the motor cortex was thought to affect the sensoridiscriminative aspects of pain, as shown by improved sensory thresholds after rTMS [12] or switching 'on' the implanted epidural MCS [13]. This influence was specific for thermonociceptive signals conveyed by the spinothalamic tract, precluding a mechanism of pain relief due to the reinforcement of the lemniscal 'gate control' over the nociceptive system.

MCS may also impact on intracortical motor circuitry. We found that motor cortex rTMS restored defective intracortical inhibition assessed by a paradigm of paired TMS pulses in patients with neuropathic pain [14]. Motor cortex inhibition is associated with the existence of 20-Hz cortical oscillations that are abolished in the presence of pain [15] but could be restored by MCS.

MCS effects on pain also depend on the recruitment of fibres located within the motor cortex but projecting to remote structures, such as the thalamus, insular cortex, and brainstem [16]. All these structures could mediate the concomitant effects of MCS on spontaneous pain and innocuous thermal sensory perception. For instance, MCS might reduce pain-related hyperactivity in thalamic relays or interfere with abnormal thalamothalamic or thalamocortical

Table 1. Effects of rTMS in patients with chronic pain

Authors	Pain origin	Target; frequency; intensity of stimulation	Number and duration of trains	Percentage of pain relief; comparison with placebo condition; duration of the effects
Lefaucheur et al. [4]	Thalamic (n = 6) or brainstem (n = 6) stroke, brachial plexus lesion (n = 6)	M1; 80% RMT; 0.5 Hz /10 Hz	1 train of 20 min/20 trains of 5 s (600/1,000 pulses)	10-Hz rTMS: 20%; 0.5-Hz sham rTMS: 4–7% ($p = 0.001$ vs. sham coil; 7 responders); not determined
Lefaucheur et al. [5]	Thalamic stroke (n = 7), trigeminal nerve lesion (n = 7)	M1; 80% RMT; 10 Hz	20 trains of 5 s (1,000 pulses)	10-Hz rTMS: 30%; sham rTMS 0% ($p = 0.01$ vs. sham coil; 8 responders); around 1 week
Lefaucheur et al. [7]	Thalamic (n = 12) or brainstem (n = 12) stroke, trigeminal nerve (n = 12), brachial plexus (n = 12) or spinal cord (n = 12) lesion	M1; 80% RMT; 10 Hz	20 trains of 5 s (1,000 pulses)	10-Hz rTMS: 21%; sham rTMS: 9% ($p = 0.0002$ vs. sham coil; 39 responders); not determined
Khedr et al. [8]	Stroke (n = 24), trigeminal nerve lesion (n = 24)	M1; 80% RMT; 20 Hz	10 trains of 10 s (2,000 pulses); 5 sessions for 1 week	20-Hz rTMS: 45%; sham rTMS: 5% ($p < 0.001$ vs. angled coil; 20-Hz rTMS: 22 responders, sham rTMS: 4 responders); 2 weeks at least after the last session
Hirayama et al. [9]	Thalamic (n = 7) or brainstem (n = 5) stroke, trigeminal nerve (n = 3), brachial plexus (n = 2), or spinal cord (n = 3) lesion	M1/S1/PMC/SMA; 90% RMT; 5 Hz	10 trains of 10 s (500 pulses)	5-Hz rTMS, best cortical target (M1): 28% ($p < 0.01$ vs. angled coil; 10 responders); around 3 days

André-Obadia et al. [10]	Thalamic (n = 8) or brainstem (n = 2) stroke, trigeminal nerve (n = 1), brachial plexus (n = 1), nerve trunk (n = 1), or spinal cord (n = 1) lesion	M1; 90% RMT; 1 Hz/20 Hz	1 train of 26 min/20 trains of 4 s (1,600 pulses)	Sham/1-Hz/20-Hz rTMS: 8/–2/11% [$p > 0.05$ vs. angled coil (20 Hz); sham rTMS: 4 responders, 1-Hz rTMS: 1 responder, 20-Hz rTMS: 5 responders]; around 1 week
Lefaucheur et al. [14]	Thalamic (n = 8) or brainstem (n = 2) stroke, brachial plexus (n = 4) nerve trunk (n = 4), or spinal cord (n = 4) lesion	M1; 90% RMT; 1 Hz/10 Hz	1 train of 20 min/20 trains of 6 s (1,200 pulses)	10-Hz rTMS: 33%; sham rTMS: 11% ($p = 0.002$ vs. sham coil); not determined
Irlbacher et al. [unpublished]	Thalamic (n = 3) or brainstem (n = 7) stroke, spinal cord lesion (n = 3), phantom limb pain (n = 14)	M1; 95% RMT; 1 Hz/5 Hz	Unknown (500 pulses); 5 sessions for 1 week	Sham/1-Hz/5-Hz rTMS: 10/6/5% [$p = 0.08$ (1 Hz)/0.06 (5 Hz) vs. sham coil; 2 responders, whatever the type of rTMS]; not determined
Lefaucheur et al. [unpublished]	Thalamic stroke (n = 13), trigeminal nerve (n = 13), brachial plexus (n = 10) or spinal cord (n = 10) lesion	M1; 90% RMT; 1 Hz/10 Hz	1 train of 20 min/20 trains of 6 s (1,200 pulses)	10-Hz rTMS: 24%; 1-Hz sham rTMS: 5–10% ($p < 0.0001$ vs. sham coil); not determined
Lefaucheur et al. [unpublished]	Thalamic (n = 5) or brainstem (n = 4) stroke, trigeminal nerve (n = 14), brachial plexus (n = 4), nerve trunk (n = 4), or spinal cord (n = 5) lesion	M1; 90% RMT; 10 Hz	20 trains of 10 s (2,000 pulses)	10-Hz rTMS, best cortical target: 27/37% (face/hand pain); 11 responders/8 responders; around 1 week

Only studies performed with a figure-of-eight coil in patients with chronic neuropathic pain have been taken into consideration and case reports have been omitted. M1 = Primary motor cortex; PMC = premotor cortex; RMT = resting motor threshold; S1 = primary sensory cortex.

oscillations. The low rate of rTMS efficacy in patients with brainstem stroke or spinal cord lesion [7] could be explained by the involvement of these structures in descending modulation of nociception.

MCS could also impact on structures that participate in the motivational-affective aspect of pain, such as the cingulate/orbitofrontal cortex [16]. This was correlated to the beneficial effects of motor cortex rTMS on capsaicin-induced acute pain [17]. In addition, paired TMS pulses applied over the anterior cingulate cortex reduced the perception of painful laser stimuli found in normals [18], while rTMS applied over the right dorsolateral prefrontal cortex (DLPFC) increased the tolerance to cold-induced pain [19]. Finally, in a depressive patient suffering from drug-resistant facial pain due to teeth removal, repeated sessions of 20-Hz rTMS delivered to the left DLPFC frankly decreased pain scores, unrelated to mood changes [20].

Several rTMS cortical targets have been assessed for their ability to relieve pain, including parietal targets [21]. Stimulation over the primary motor cortex was found to produce significant analgesic effects, but maybe not on all the aspects of chronic pain. Further work is awaited to better define the optimal target of cortical stimulation according to the multifaceted presentation of neuropathic pain.

Duration of the Analgesic Effects and Predictive Factor for Implantation

Following a single motor cortex rTMS session, the maximal analgesic effect is delayed by 2–4 days and pain level can remain significantly reduced for about a week [5]. This is consistent with the delayed clinical changes observed for chronically implanted MCS at the time of programming. Therefore, synaptic plasticity (long-term potentiation or depression) and expression of secondary messengers are thought to explain this delay of action.

Following a single session, the analgesic effects are delayed, but also short-lived and thereby incompatible with a durable control of chronic pain. Repeated sessions on consecutive days are able to produce cumulative effects and to extend the effects of a single session [8]. This can be valuable for pain control during a limited period, e.g. while waiting for the surgical implantation of a cortical stimulator [6]. However, it is worth implanting electrodes to make permanent the analgesic effects that are transiently induced by rTMS.

Various studies suggested the use of TMS to predict the outcome of a subsequent chronic epidural stimulation [2, 3, 6, 10]. We experienced that pain decrease by more than 40% after a single, active rTMS session was always associated with a good surgical outcome, whereas the absence of response to rTMS did not indicate the result of the implanted procedure. Therefore, rTMS could support but not exclude the indication of MCS implantation.

The Place of rTMS in the Management of Chronic Pain

The place of rTMS as a therapeutic strategy in chronic neuropathic pain or as a selection tool for surgical implantation will depend on methodological and technical developments, e.g. changing pulse waveform or coil orientation, or conditioning rTMS session with a previous short-duration rTMS train applied at low intensity and high frequency ('theta burst') or a weak anodal or cathodal transcranial direct current stimulation [22]. At present, rTMS effects on chronic pain are quite low (from 20 to 45% relief of pain) and short-lived. To enhance the analgesic effects induced by rTMS, it is probably helpful to repeat the sessions and to increase stimulus frequency and intensity. Navigation systems dedicated to rTMS could also strengthen the reproducibility of cortical targeting, and thereby make the clinical results more reliable [9]. In the future, non-invasive transcranial cortical stimulation might be an alternative procedure to surgical MCS in order to treat chronic neuropathic pain.

Repetitive Transcranial Magnetic Stimulation in Parkinson's Disease

Various clinical results gave evidences for the therapeutic potential of cortical stimulation in PD. First in 1979, mapping the motor cortex with electrical stimulation during neurosurgical operations, Woolsey et al. [23] induced a transient improvement of rigidity and tremor in 2 PD patients. More recently, MCS applied to treat patients with chronic pain led to concomitant improvement of motor disorders, mainly tremor, related to the underlying neurological lesion at the origin of pain [24–26]. But more definitive arguments have been provided by rTMS studies in PD patients (table 2), supported at present by the first clinical results of chronically implanted cortical stimulation [27, 28].

Cortical Dysfunction in PD

Imaging studies showed that the supplementary motor area (SMA) and the DLPFC were hypoactive in PD [29]. EEG studies were also consistent with SMA hypoactivity [30–32] that could play a role in akinesia. Findings are more controversial for the primary motor cortex (M1), which was found to be hypoactive in patients with early, untreated PD, but hyperactive in advanced parkinsonism [29]. These changes correspond to primary or compensatory mechanisms related to treatment or to adaptive motor strategies.

Cortical excitability studies with single or paired TMS pulses revealed an excessive corticospinal output at rest in PD patients, concomitant to or resulting from a reduced intracortical inhibition [33]. This excessive descending

Table 2. Effects of rTMS in patients with PD

Authors	Patients	Stimulus frequency, Hz	Total pulse number	Results
Primary motor cortex stimulation				
Pascual-Leone et al. [35]	6	5	–	Movement and reaction time shortening
Siebner et al. [36]	12	5	750	Movement time shortening
Siebner et al. [37]	10	5	750	UPDRS-III improvement (reduced rigidity and bradykinesia contralateral to the stimulation)
Khedr et al. [38]	36 (19 active, 17 sham)	5	2,000/day × 10 days	UPDRS-III and walking speed improvement
Bornke et al. [39]	12	10	?	UPDRS-III improvement
Lefaucheur et al. [40]	12	10	2,000	UPDRS-III improvement (reduced rigidity and bradykinesia contralateral to the stimulation)
Lefaucheur et al. [40]	12	0.5	600	UPDRS-III improvement (reduced rigidity bilaterally)
Dias et al. [60]	20 (10 active, 10 sham)	5	2,250	Speech improvement
Khedr et al. [41]	45 (35 active, 10 sham)	25	3,000/day × 6 days	UPDRS-III, walking speed, key-tapping speed and self-assessment scale improvement
Khedr et al. [41]	20 (10 active, 10 sham)	10	3,000/day × 6 days	UPDRS-III mild improvement
Supplementary motor area stimulation				
Boylan et al. [42]	10	10	2,000	Increase in reaction time and deterioration of writing
Koch et al. [47]	10	5	2,500	No significant effect on time perception
Koch et al. [43]	8	5	900	No significant effect on dyskinesia and UPDRS-III
Koch et al. [43]	8	1	900	Reduced dyskinesia without effect on UPDRS-III

Premotor cortex stimulation				
Buhmann et al. [50]	10	1	1,200	Changes in motor cortex excitability, as assessed by a TMS paired-pulse paradigm, depending on levodopa intake
Mir et al. [51]	10	5	1,500	Normalization of motor evoked potential amplitude in on-drug patients, but no effect in off-drug patients
Dorsolateral prefrontal cortex stimulation				
Fregni et al. [45]	42 (21 active, 21 sham)	15	3,000/day × 10 days	Improvement of depression score similar to fluoxetine, with better results than fluoxetine on cognitive and motor scores
Koch et al. [47]	10	5	2,500	Time perception improvement
Boggio et al. [46]	25 (13 active, 12 sham)	15	3,000/day × 10 days	Improvement in neuropsychological testing similar to fluoxetine
Dias et al. [60]	20 (10 active, 10 sham)	15	3,000	Improvement of depression score without speech effects
Fernandez del Olmo et al. [48]	13 (8 active, 5 sham)	10	450	No significant effect on motor performance
Both motor and dorsolateral prefrontal cortex stimulation				
Lomarev et al. [61]	18	25	1,200/day × 8 days	Improvement in walking time and reduced bradykinesia for the right hand

Only studies performed with a figure-of-eight coil and based on clinical assessment (at least for primary motor cortex stimulation) have been taken into consideration. UPDRS-III = Unified PD rating scale, motor score.

corticospinal drive could be associated with rigidity. During movement preparation or execution, intracortical or thalamocortical facilitatory inputs may fail to activate correctly all the cortical areas involved in the intended movement, leading to akinesia or bradykinesia [34]. These observations support the therapeutic potential of cortical stimulation for advanced parkinsonism.

Application of rTMS in PD

The first rTMS study in PD showed improvement of reaction and movement times during M1 stimulation at high frequency (5 Hz) [35]. Moreover, improvement can last beyond the time of stimulation [36] and reach a significant level on clinical motor scores after single or repeated rTMS sessions delivered at high frequency (5–25 Hz) over M1 [37–41].

When applied over the SMA, rTMS worsened motor performance of PD patients at high frequency (10 Hz) [42], but improved apomorphine-induced dyskinesia at low frequency (1 Hz) [43]. At low frequency (0.5 Hz), DLPFC stimulation was initially found to increase motor performance concomitantly with depression relief [44]. However, subsequent studies showed that DLPFC stimulation induced antidepressant and cognitive effects, but no motor effects in PD patients [45–48]. The premotor cortex was not yet targeted in a clinical study of PD patients, although low-frequency premotor cortex stimulation was shown to enhance intracortical motor inhibitory processes more efficaciously than direct M1 stimulation in normals [49]. However, the premotor-motor interaction is absent in 'off-drug' PD patients and only partially restored by levodopa intake [50, 51].

The effects of rTMS on PD motor disturbances could be located within the motor cortex [40], or in any hypo- or hyperactive remote structures that are functionally connected with the motor cortex in corticobasal ganglia loops. In PD patients as in normals, 10-Hz rTMS over M1 or DLPFC induced a focal release of endogenous dopamine in the ipsilateral striatum (putamen, caudate nucleus), probably via corticostriatal projections [52–54]. A single TMS pulse delivered over M1 can also impact on neural activities in the subthalamic nucleus [55]. The striatum and subthalamic nucleus receive major glutamatergic inputs from various cortical areas and the degenerative process leads to a high level of oscillatory synchronization between the cortex and the basal ganglia in PD [56]. The generation of a stimulus-locked activity breaking the abnormal synchronization in corticobasal ganglia loops might contribute to the therapeutic efficacy of deep brain stimulation concomitantly with the restoration of defective cortical inhibitory processes [57–59].

Therapeutic Perspectives of Cortical Stimulation in PD

Several points argue for the value of the cortical target in PD, such as the occurrence of bilateral effects in case of unilateral stimulation, or the improvement of speech when the stimulation is centred over the mouth cortical representation [67]. In the management of PD, rTMS could be applied to select patients for epidural stimulation, as proposed in chronic pain. In addition, repeated rTMS sessions could have therapeutic potential by providing long-lasting effects [41, 61]. However, the respective value of transcranial and epidural cortical stimulation remains to be determined, compared to deep brain stimulation, in daily practice.

Repetitive Transcranial Magnetic Stimulation in Motor Stroke Recovery

Many studies have documented the changes in cortical organization that occur after motor stroke, particularly on the side of the lesion [62]. In addition, there is a balance of function between the two hemispheres that is controlled by interhemispheric inhibition. The stroke-affected hemisphere can be doubly disabled, by the stroke itself and by an imbalanced inhibition from the non-stroke hemisphere. In this model, increased activity in the affected hemisphere will promote recovery of the paretic limbs, as well as decreased inhibition from the non-stroke hemisphere.

The development of rTMS and transcranial direct current stimulation allowed the imbalance of activity between hemispheres to be modulated for enhancing stroke recovery. For instance, post-stroke motor performance improved after inhibiting the unaffected hemisphere by low-frequency rTMS [63–65] or cathodal transcranial direct current stimulation [66] or exciting the affected hemisphere by high-frequency rTMS [67, 68] or anodal transcranial direct current stimulation [66, 69]. Results provided by rTMS application are summarized in table 3. A recent study also showed that high-frequency epidural stimulation of the peri-infarct cortical region significantly promoted recovery from motor stroke in combination with rehabilitative training [70]. The authors speculate that stimulation maximized functional plasticity of the remaining connections from the damaged hemisphere.

Modulation of Neuroplasticity and Improvement of Stroke Recovery by rTMS

One concept to improve recovery from stroke is to decrease the excitability of the unaffected hemisphere and thereby to reduce its potentially detrimental inhibitory effect on the affected hemisphere [62]. In healthy subjects, a decrease in transcallosal inhibition from one hemisphere can increase the functional abilities of the other hemisphere [71]. This reasoning is supported by cases of stroke patients who improved after a subsequent disruption of the

Table 3. Effects of rTMS in motor stroke recovery

Authors	Patients	Duration after stroke	Site of stimulation	Stimulus frequency; intensity	Number and duration of trains	Results
High-frequency rTMS applied over the affected hemisphere						
Khedr et al. [67]	52 hemiplegic (26 active, 26 sham)	Less than 10 days	M1, affected hemisphere	3 Hz;120% RMT	10 trains of 10 s (300 pulses) × 10 sessions	Improvement on various disability scales for stroke
Kim et al. [68]	15 hemiparetic	6–41 months	M1, affected hemisphere	10 Hz; 80% RMT	8 trains of 2 s (160 pulses)	Enhanced movement accuracy and speed in motor task learning
Low-frequency rTMS applied over the unaffected hemisphere						
Mansur et al. [64]	10 hemiparetic	Less than 12 months	M1 or PMC, unaffected hemisphere	1 Hz; 100% RMT	1 train of 10 min (600 pulses)	Improvement in reaction time and motor performance regarding the affected hand (better for M1 than PMC stimulation)
Fregni et al. [63]	15 hemiparetic (10 active and 5 sham)	At least 1 year after stroke	M1, unaffected hemisphere	1 Hz; 100% RMT	1 train of 20 min (1,200 pulses) × 5 sessions	Improvement in reaction time and motor performance regarding the affected hand that lasted for 2 weeks
Takeuchi et al. [65]	20 hemiparetic (10 active, 10 sham)	6–54 months	M1, unaffected hemisphere	1 Hz; 90% RMT	1 train of 25 min (1,500 pulses)	Improvement in pinch acceleration of the affected hand

Only studies performed with a figure-of-eight coil have been taken into consideration and case reports have been omitted. M1 = Primary motor cortex; PMC = premotor cortex; RMT = resting motor threshold.

healthy hemisphere by another stroke [72]. Similarly, the forced use of the affected limb by immobilization of the healthy arm ('constraint-induced therapy') can enhance motor stroke recovery in association with excitability decrease in the healthy motor cortex and excitability increase in the affected motor cortex [73]. Conversely, imaging studies revealed hyperactivation in the unaffected hemisphere of patients with poor recovery [62] and TMS studies showed increased transcallosal inhibition from the unaffected to the affected hemisphere [74].

Mansur et al. [64] showed as a proof of concept that inhibition of the intact motor cortex by rTMS applied at 1 Hz in 8 patients within a year of stroke improved motor performance of the paretic hand. However, rTMS only provided short-lasting effects following a single session. As in depression [75], the magnitude and duration of the clinical effects of rTMS increased with the number of rTMS sessions in stroke studies [63, 67]. Following 5 consecutive sessions of low-frequency rTMS of the unaffected hemisphere in old stroke patients, Fregni et al. [63] found significant motor improvement of the affected hand that lasted for 2 weeks. Khedr et al. [67] showed that 10 consecutive days of high-frequency rTMS applied at 3 Hz on the affected motor area also improved durably the clinical outcome in early stroke patients.

Mechanisms of Action of rTMS in Stroke Recovery

It is well known that rTMS can affect synaptic long-term potentiation and depression by modulating neurotransmitter availability and postsynaptic receptor density in cortical layers underlying the stimulus site and among those connected to them. In theory, this could mediate neuroprotection locally and interfere with diaschisis at a distance [76].

Based on this concept, Khedr et al. [67] hypothesized that stimulating around the infarct area would increase neuronal survival rate and facilitate clinical recovery associated with physical therapy. Paus et al. [77] noted a positive correlation between the regional cerebral blood flow around the ischemic area [as measured by single photon emission computed tomography, or positron emission tomography (PET)] and the number of TMS pulse trains at the stimulation site. Lack of response to real rTMS in the patients who had the largest infarcts suggests that the success of the technique may depend at least on the existence of surviving neurons at the site of stimulation. In addition, Khedr et al. [67] employed a relatively high stimulus intensity (120% of resting motor threshold) to increase excitability of motor cortical regions adjacent to the infarct zone that may be recruited during voluntary contraction to compensate the loss of function of the damaged area. Actually, a stimulus of this intensity can induce a current in cortical layers at a distance of 2–3 cm from the stimulation site when applied in healthy subjects. Thus, improvement of motor performance may occur because of

Table 4. Effects of rTMS in patients with tinnitus

Authors	Patients	Stimulus frequency; intensity	Number and duration of trains	Results
Brief rTMS trains applied at high frequency over various sites				
Plewnia et al. [83]	14	10 Hz; 120% RMT	1 train of 3 s (30 pulses)	8 responders for left temporal/temporoparietal stimulation
Fregni et al. [84]	7	10 Hz; 120% RMT	1 train of 3 s (30 pulses)	3 responders for left temporal/temporoparietal stimulation
De Ridder et al. [85]	114	3–20 Hz; 90% RMT	1 train of 10–66 s (200 pulses)	28 good and 32 partial responders to active rTMS, 38 responders to sham rTMS; rTMS applied over the auditory cortex contralateral to tinnitus; positive correlation between tinnitus suppression and rTMS frequency
Londero et al. [86]	13	10 Hz; 120% RMT	1 train of 3 s (30 pulses)	1 responder for non-specific stimulation site
Long rTMS trains applied at low frequency over the auditory cortex located by functional neuroimaging				
Eichammer et al. [87]	3	1 Hz; 110% RMT	1 train of 33 min (2,000 pulses) × 5 days	1 responder for active but not sham-rTMS (sham coil system); 1 responder and 1 non-responder for both active and sham-rTMS
Kleinjung et al. [89]	14	1 Hz; 110% RMT	1 train of 33 min (2,000 pulses) × 5 days	8 responders for active rTMS, 5 non-responders, 1 worsened patient
Londero et al. [86]	13	1 Hz; 120% RMT	1 train of 20 min (1,200 pulses)	5 responders for the auditory cortex target stimulation (effects delayed by several days), 1 responder for the control (occipital) target stimulation

Only studies performed with a figure-of-eight coil have been taken into consideration and case reports have been omitted. RMT = Resting motor threshold.

a direct effect of the stimulus on the underlying brain tissue or because of an effect on its connections with other cortical/subcortical structures.

Recommendations for Future Studies

Many open questions remain to be settled. (1) For how long does the improvement of function persist after rTMS interventions? (2) What is the optimal time for starting the rTMS treatment after stroke? (3) Should electroencephalographic examination be performed to exclude those patients at greater risk of developing seizures? (4) Could rTMS trials for stroke recovery benefit from navigation systems dedicated to rTMS? To solve these questions, further clinical controlled trials are needed based on large series of patients with various times after stroke and long-term follow-up.

Repetitive Transcranial Magnetic Stimulation in Tinnitus

Tinnitus is a very common clinical condition, often related to a lesion of the cochlea or auditory nerve, secondary to presbyacusis, Ménière's disease, noise, barotrauma, or drug ototoxicity, among other conditions [78]. There is evidence for the contribution of peripheral auditory structures in tinnitus perception [79]. However, the fact that tinnitus may persist after total cochlear and auditory nerve removal demonstrates that tinnitus is also a central phenomenon, probably due to synaptic plastic changes within the auditory pathway resulting from the peripheral lesion [80]. In analogy to chronic pain, auditory deafferentation-induced plasticity in subcortical or cortical structures might cause or perpetuate tinnitus, associated with primary and secondary auditory cortex hyperactivation [81]. Limbic structures were also thought to play a role regarding the cognitive and affective components of tinnitus [82].

The rate of failure of classical therapies applied in tinnitus leaves some room to the development of new treatments. Taking into account tinnitus-associated auditory cortex dysfunction, auditory cortex rTMS was considered as a therapeutic application. Several studies have investigated the effects of rTMS on tinnitus, with brief trains of high-frequency rTMS or prolonged trains of low-frequency rTMS over the auditory cortex (table 4).

Clinical Effects of Low- or High-Frequency rTMS in Tinnitus

First, Plewnia et al. [83] applied brief trains of high-frequency TMS over various scalp positions in patients with tinnitus, to interrupt tinnitus by creating a 'virtual lesion' of the auditory cortex. Stimulation applied to the left temporoparietal cortex, corresponding to the secondary auditory cortical areas, significantly, but temporarily, reduced tinnitus. This result has recently been confirmed [84], even in a large sample of 114 tinnitus patients [85], but not by all authors [86].

The use of low-frequency rTMS appeared more consistent with the purpose of treating tinnitus by reducing auditory cortex hyperactivity. Eichhammer et al. [87] investigated 3 patients suffering from disabling tinnitus with 1-Hz rTMS applied over the site of maximal auditory cortex activation shown by a PET study. A neuronavigation system dedicated to rTMS targeting enabled to stimulate more reliably the PET-defined target. In 2 patients, the active rTMS session was followed by a clear improvement, which was sustained in 1 case after a prolonged treatment period over 4 weeks [88]. This short case series was followed by a sham-controlled study of 14 patients with chronic tinnitus using the same rTMS procedure. A significant improvement in tinnitus severity was found after the active rTMS sessions when compared to the placebo condition, even 6 months beyond the time of stimulation [89]. Londero et al. [86] applied rTMS in a series of 13 patients suffering from unilateral long-lasting disabling tinnitus using an fMRI-defined target contralateral to the perceived tinnitus. Low-frequency (1 Hz) stimulation of the fMRI target clearly relieved tinnitus in half of the patients with a delay of several days. All these data indicate a potential use of rTMS for tinnitus treatment. Prolonged clinical improvement should be considered on the basis of repeated rTMS sessions.

Mechanisms of Action and Shortcomings of rTMS in Tinnitus

The site of action of rTMS in tinnitus remains debatable. The deep location of Heschl's gyrus does not support a direct effect of rTMS on the primary auditory cortex. However, rTMS-induced current in the superficial lateral superior temporal gyrus could propagate to Heschl's gyrus by functional connections [90]. In addition, low-frequency rTMS over the left temporal cortex induced functional changes not only in the stimulated cortical areas, but also contralaterally to the stimulation and in both thalami [91]. One may hypothesize that rTMS could relieve tinnitus by acting on bilateral auditory corticothalamic projections, supporting the existence of thalamocortical dysrhythmia at the origin of tinnitus.

The side of the stimulation is also questionable. Some authors applied stimulation over the auditory cortex contralateral to the tinnitus [85, 86], whereas others targeted the left hemisphere, whatever tinnitus lateralization [83, 89]. The left predominance of auditory cortex hyperactivation may relate to functional asymmetry in the processing of tonal frequency between the auditory cortices [92]. Whether this interhemispheric difference in tonotopical organization plays a role for the generation of tinnitus is debated.

Various methodological points should also be considered for rTMS studies in tinnitus. First, the placebo condition must be optimal owing to the importance of the placebo effect in patients treated for tinnitus. Second, validated questionnaires should be developed to assess rTMS effects on sensoridiscriminative aspects of tinnitus severity rather than on its consequences. Finally, in spite of promising results, the optimal parameters of stimulation are not clearly defined. In particular, imaging studies can provide large areas of activation within the temporal cortex and it may be difficult to choose between several possible targets.

Conclusions

In chronic neuropathic pain, PD, motor stroke recovery, and tinnitus, there are growing evidences that rTMS might alleviate, at least transiently, various symptoms or impairments. Nevertheless, the definition of the parameters of stimulation remained rather empirical, except for stimulus frequency that depends on the intention of inhibiting or rather exciting a targeted cortical region. The optimization of the parameters of stimulation in each clinical indication is the key point before proposing rTMS as a therapeutic tool in daily neurological practice. Further insights into the mechanisms of action of rTMS with respect to the underlying disease-related cortical activity changes and well-controlled multicentre randomized trials in large series of patients are still needed to confirm the rTMS potential in neurological diseases. This is a serious challenge to future therapeutic application of rTMS, because chronic epidural cortical stimulation trials have been performed in all four conditions considered in this review. In the future, the question is not to wonder whether some neurological diseases might benefit from cortical stimulation but rather to determine the best target, parameters of stimulation and type of procedure (implanted vs. transcranial).

References

1 Nguyen JP, Lefaucheur JP, Keravel Y: Motor cortex stimulation; in Simpson BA (ed): Pain Research and Clinical Management. vol 15: Electrical Stimulation and the Relief of Pain. Amsterdam, Elsevier Science, 2003, pp 197–209.

2 Migita K, Uozumi T, Arita K, Moden S: Transcranial magnetic coil stimulation of motor cortex in patients with central pain. Neurosurgery 1995;36:1037–1040.

3 Canavero S, Bonicalzi V, Dotta M, Vighetti S, Asteggiano G: Low-rate repetitive TMS allays central pain. Neurol Res 2003;25:151–152.

4 Lefaucheur JP, Drouot X, Keravel Y, Nguyen JP: Pain relief induced by repetitive transcranial magnetic stimulation of precentral cortex. Neuroreport 2001;12:2963–2965.

5 Lefaucheur JP, Drouot X, Nguyen JP: Interventional neurophysiology for pain control: duration of pain relief following repetitive transcranial magnetic stimulation of the motor cortex. Neurophysiol Clin 2001;31:247–252.

6 Lefaucheur JP, Drouot X, Ménard-Lefaucheur I, Nguyen JP: Neuropathic pain controlled for more than a year by monthly sessions of repetitive transcranial magnetic cortical stimulation. Neurophysiol Clin 2004;34:91–95.
7 Lefaucheur JP, Drouot X, Ménard-Lefaucheur I, Zerah F, Bendib B, Cesaro P, Keravel Y, Nguyen JP: Neurogenic pain relief by repetitive transcranial magnetic cortical stimulation depends on the origin and the site of pain. J Neurol Neurosurg Psychiatry 2004;75:612–616.
8 Khedr EM, Kotb H, Kamel NF, Ahmed MA, Sadek R, Rothwell JC: Longlasting antalgic effects of daily sessions of repetitive transcranial magnetic stimulation in central and peripheral neuropathic pain. J Neurol Neurosurg Psychiatry 2005;76:833–838.
9 Hirayama A, Saitoh Y, Kishima H, Shimokawa T, Oshino S, Hirata M, Kato A, Yoshimine T: Reduction of intractable deafferentation pain by navigation-guided repetitive transcranial magnetic stimulation (rTMS) of the primary motor cortex. Pain 2006;122:22–27.
10 André-Obadia N, Peyron R, Mertens P, Mauguière F, Laurent B, Garcia-Larrea L: Transcranial magnetic stimulation for pain control double-blind study of different frequencies against placebo, and correlation with motor cortex stimulation efficacy. Clin Neurophysiol 2006;117:1536–1544.
11 Di Lazzaro V, Oliviero A, Pilato F, Saturno E, Dileone M, Meglio M, Cioni B, Papacci F, Tonali PA, Rothwell JC: Comparison of descending volleys evoked by transcranial and epidural motor cortex stimulation in a conscious patient with bulbar pain. Clin Neurophysiol 2004;115:834–838.
12 Johnson S, Summers J, Pridmore S: Changes to somatosensory detection and pain thresholds following high frequency repetitive TMS of the motor cortex in individuals suffering from chronic pain. Pain 2006;123:187–192.
13 Drouot X, Nguyen JP, Peschanski M, Lefaucheur JP: The antalgic efficacy of chronic motor cortex stimulation is related to sensory changes in the painful zone. Brain 2002;125:1660–1664.
14 Lefaucheur JP, Drouot X, Ménard-Lefaucheur I, Keravel Y, Nguyen JP: Motor cortex rTMS restores defective intracortical inhibition in chronic neuropathic pain. Neurology, in press.
15 Raij TT, Forss N, Stancak A, Hari R: Modulation of motor-cortex oscillatory activity by painful Aδ- and C-fiber stimuli. Neuroimage 2004;23:569–573.
16 Garcia-Larrea L, Peyron R, Mertens P, Gregoire MC, Lavenne F, Le Bars D, Convers P, Mauguière F, Sindou M, Laurent B: Electrical stimulation of motor cortex for pain control: a combined PET-scan and electrophysiological study. Pain 1999;83:259–273.
17 Tamura Y, Okabe S, Ohnishi T, Saito D, Arai N, Mochio S, Inoue K, Ugawa Y: Effects of 1-Hz repetitive transcranial magnetic stimulation on acute pain induced by capsaicin. Pain 2004;107: 107–115.
18 Kanda M, Mima T, Oga T, Matsuhashi M, Toma K, Hara H, Satow T, Nagamine T, Rothwell JC, Shibasaki H: Transcranial magnetic stimulation (TMS) of the sensorimotor cortex and medial frontal cortex modifies human pain perception. Clin Neurophysiol 2003;114:860–866.
19 Graff-Guerrero A, González-Olvera J, Fresán A, Gómez-Martín D, Méndez-Núñez JC, Pellicer F: Repetitive transcranial magnetic stimulation of dorsolateral prefrontal cortex increases tolerance to human experimental pain. Brain Res Cogn Brain Res 2005;25:153–160.
20 Reid P, Pridmore S: Improvement in chronic pain with transcranial magnetic stimulation. Aust NZ J Psychiatry 2001;35:252.
21 Töpper R, Foltys H, Meister IG, Sparing R, Boroojerdi B: Repetitive transcranial magnetic stimulation of the parietal cortex transiently ameliorates phantom limb pain-like syndrome. Clin Neurophysiol 2003;114:1521–1530.
22 Lefaucheur JP: New insights into the therapeutic potential of non-invasive transcranial cortical stimulation in chronic neuropathic pain. Pain 2006;122:11–13.
23 Woolsey CN, Erickson TC, Gilson WE: Localization in somatic sensory and motor areas of human cerebral cortex as determined by direct recording of evoked potentials and electrical stimulation. J Neurosurg 1979;51:476–506.
24 Nguyen JP, Pollin B, Feve A, Geny C, Cesaro P: Improvement of action tremor by chronic cortical stimulation. Mov Disord 1998;13:84–88.
25 Franzini A, Ferroli P, Servello D, Broggi G: Reversal of thalamic hand syndrome by long-term motor cortex stimulation. J Neurosurg 2000;93:873–875.
26 KatayamaY, Oshima H, Fukaya C, Kawamata T, Yamamoto T: Control of post-stroke movement disorders using chronic motor cortex stimulation. Acta Neurochir Suppl 2002;79:89–92.

27 Canavero S, Bonicalzi V, Paolotti R, Castellano G, Greco-Crasto S, Rizzo L, Davini O, Maina R: Therapeutic extradural cortical stimulation for movement disorders: a review. Neurol Res 2003;25:118–122.
28 Pagni CA, Altibrandi MG, Bentivoglio A, Caruso G, Cioni B, Fiorella C, Insola A, Lavano A, Maina R, Mazzone P, Signorelli CD, Sturiale C, Valzania F, Zeme S, Zenga F: Extradural motor cortex stimulation (EMCS) for Parkinson's disease. History and first results by the study group of the Italian neurosurgical society. Acta Neurochir Suppl 2005;93:113–119.
29 Brooks DJ: Neuroimaging in Parkinson's disease. NeuroRx 2004;1:243–254.
30 Dick JP, Rothwell JC, Day BL, Cantello R, Buruma O, Gioux M, Benecke R, Berardelli A, Thompson PD, Marsden CD: The Bereitschaftspotential is abnormal in Parkinson's disease. Brain 1989;112:233–244.
31 Pulvermuller F, Lutzenberger W, Muller V, Mohr B, Dichgans J, Birbaumer N: P3 and contingent negative variation in Parkinson's disease. Electroencephalogr Clin Neurophysiol 1996;98:456–467.
32 Rossini PM, Babiloni F, Bernardi G, Cecchi L, Johnson PB, Malentacca A, Stanzione P, Urbano A: Abnormalities of short-latency somatosensory evoked potentials in parkinsonian patients. Electroencephalogr Clin Neurophysiol 1989;74:277–289.
33 Lefaucheur JP: Motor cortex dysfunction revealed by cortical excitability studies in Parkinson's disease: influence of antiparkinsonian treatment and cortical stimulation. Clin Neurophysiol 2005;116:244–253.
34 Chen R, Kumar S, Garg RR, Lang AE: Impairment of motor cortex activation and deactivation in Parkinson's disease. Clin Neurophysiol 2001;112:600–607.
35 Pascual-Leone A, Valls-Sole J, Brasil-Neto JP, Cammarota A, Grafman J, Hallett M: Akinesia in Parkinson's disease. 2. Effects of subthreshold repetitive transcranial motor cortex stimulation. Neurology 1994;44:892–898.
36 Siebner HR, Mentschel C, Auer C, Conrad B: Repetitive transcranial magnetic stimulation has a beneficial effect on bradykinesia in Parkinson's disease. Neuroreport 1999;10:589–594.
37 Siebner HR, Rossmeier C, Mentschel C, Peinemann A, Conrad B: Short-term motor improvement after sub-threshold 5-Hz repetitive transcranial magnetic stimulation of the primary motor hand area in Parkinson's disease. J Neurol Sci 2000;178:91–94.
38 Khedr EM, Farweez HM, Islam H: Therapeutic effect of repetitive transcranial magnetic stimulation on motor function in Parkinson's disease patients. Eur J Neurol 2003;10:567–572.
39 Bornke Ch, Schulte T, Przuntek H, Muller T: Clinical effects of repetitive transcranial magnetic stimulation versus acute levodopa challenge in Parkinson's disease. J Neural Transm Suppl 2004;68:61–67.
40 Lefaucheur JP, Drouot X, Von Raison F, Ménard-Lefaucheur I, Cesaro P, Nguyen JP: Improvement of motor performance and modulation of cortical excitability by repetitive transcranial magnetic stimulation of the motor cortex in Parkinson's disease. Clin Neurophysiol 2004;115:2530–2541.
41 Khedr EM, Rothwell JC, Shawky OA, Ahmed MA, Hamdy A: Effect of daily repetitive transcranial magnetic stimulation on motor performance in Parkinson's disease. Mov Disord 2006;21: 1311–1316.
42 Boylan LS, Pullman SL, Lisanby SH, Spicknall KE, Sackeim HA: Repetitive transcranial magnetic stimulation to SMA worsens complex movements in Parkinson's disease. Clin Neurophysiol 2001;112:259–264.
43 Koch G, Brusa L, Caltagirone C, Peppe A, Oliveri M, Stanzione P, Centonze D: rTMS of supplementary motor area modulates therapy-induced dyskinesias in Parkinson disease. Neurology 2005;65:623–625.
44 Dragasevic N, Potrebic A, Damjanovic A, Stefanova E, Kostic VS: Therapeutic efficacy of bilateral prefrontal slow repetitive transcranial magnetic stimulation in depressed patients with Parkinson's disease: an open study. Mov Disord 2002;17:528–532.
45 Fregni F, Santos CM, Myczkowski ML, Rigolino R, Gallucci-Neto J, Barbosa ER, Valente KD, Pascual-Leone A, Marcolin MA: Repetitive transcranial magnetic stimulation is as effective as fluoxetine in the treatment of depression in patients with Parkinson's disease. J Neurol Neurosurg Psychiatry 2004;75:1171–1174.
46 Boggio PS, Fregni F, Bermpohl F, Mansur CG, Rosa M, Rumi DO, Barbosa ER, Odebrecht Rosa M, Pascual-Leone A, Rigonatti SP, Marcolin MA, Araujo Silva MT: Effect of repetitive TMS and

fluoxetine on cognitive function in patients with Parkinson's disease and concurrent depression. Mov Disord 2005;20:1178–1184.

47 Koch G, Oliveri M, Brusa L, Stanzione P, Torriero S, Caltagirone C: High-frequency rTMS improves time perception in Parkinson disease. Neurology 2004;63:2405–2406.

48 Fernandez del Olmo M, Bello O, Cudeiro J: Transcranial magnetic stimulation over dorsolateral prefrontal cortex in Parkinson's disease. Clin Neurophysiol, in press.

49 Bäumer T, Lange R, Liepert J, Weiller C, Siebner HR, Rothwell JC, Munchau A: Repeated premotor rTMS leads to cumulative plastic changes of motor cortex excitability in humans. Neuroimage 2003;20:550–560.

50 Buhmann C, Gorsler A, Bäumer T, Hidding U, Demiralay C, Hinkelmann K, Weiller C, Siebner HR, Munchau A: Abnormal excitability of premotor-motor connections in de novo Parkinson's disease. Brain 2004;127:2732–2746.

51 Mir P, Matsunaga K, Gilio F, Quinn NP, Siebner HR, Rothwell JC: Dopaminergic drugs restore facilitatory premotor-motor interactions in Parkinson disease. Neurology 2005;64:1906–1912.

52 Strafella AP, Paus T, Barrett J, Dagher A: Repetitive transcranial magnetic stimulation of the human prefrontal cortex induces dopamine release in the caudate nucleus. J Neurosci 2001;21:RC157.

53 Strafella AP, Paus T, Fraraccio M, Dagher A: Striatal dopamine release induced by repetitive transcranial magnetic stimulation of the human motor cortex. Brain 2003;126:2609–2615.

54 Strafella AP, Ko JH, Grant J, Fraraccio M, Monchi O: Corticostriatal functional interactions in Parkinson's disease: a rTMS/[^{11}C]raclopride PET study. Eur J Neurosci 2005;22:2946–2952.

55 Strafella AP, Vanderwerf Y, Sadikot AF: Transcranial magnetic stimulation of the human motor cortex influences the neuronal activity of subthalamic nucleus. Eur J Neurosci 2004;20: 2245–2249.

56 Williams D, Tijssen M, Van Bruggen G, Bosch A, Insola A, Di Lazzaro V, Mazzone P, Oliviero A, Quartarone A, Speelman H, Brown P: Dopamine-dependent changes in the functional connectivity between basal ganglia and cerebral cortex in humans. Brain 2002;125:1558–1569.

57 Cunic D, Roshan L, Khan FI, Lozano AM, Lang AE, Chen R: Effects of subthalamic nucleus stimulation on motor cortex excitability in Parkinson's disease. Neurology 2002;58:1665–1672.

58 Däuper J, Peschel T, Schrader C, Kohlmetz C, Joppich G, Nager W, Dengler R, Rollnik JD: Effects of subthalamic nucleus (STN) stimulation on motor cortex excitability. Neurology 2002;59: 700–706.

59 Pierantozzi M, Palmieri MG, Mazzone P, Marciani MG, Rossini PM, Stefani A, Giacomini P, Peppe A, Stanzione P: Deep brain stimulation of both subthalamic nucleus and internal globus pallidus restores intracortical inhibition in Parkinson's disease paralleling apomorphine effects: a paired magnetic stimulation study. Clin Neurophysiol 2002;113:108–113.

60 Dias AE, Barbosa ER, Coracini K, Maia F, Marcolin MA, Fregni F: Effects of repetitive transcranial magnetic stimulation on voice and speech in Parkinson's disease. Acta Neurol Scand 2006;113:92–99.

61 Lomarev MP, Kanchana S, Bara-Jimenez W, Iyer M, Wassermann EM, Hallett M: Placebo-controlled study of rTMS for the treatment of Parkinson's disease. Mov Disord 2006;21:325–331.

62 Ward NS, Cohen LG: Mechanisms underlying recovery of motor function after stroke. Arch Neurol 2004;61:1844–1848.

63 Fregni F, Boggio PS, Valle AC, Rocha RR, Duarte J, Ferreira MJL, Wagner T, Fecteau S, Rigonatti SP, Riberto M, Freedman SD, Pascual-Leone A: A sham-controlled trial of a 5-day course of repetitive transcranial magnetic stimulation of the unaffected hemisphere in stroke patients. Stroke 2006;37:2115–2122.

64 Mansur CG, Fregni F, Boggio PS, Riberto M, Gallucci-Neto J, Santos CM, Wagner T, Rigonatti SP, Marcolin MA, Pascual-Leone A: A sham stimulation-controlled trial of rTMS of the unaffected hemisphere in stroke patients. Neurology 2005;64:1802–1804.

65 Takeuchi N, Chuma T, Matsuo Y, Watanabe I, Ikoma K: Repetitive transcranial magnetic stimulation of contralesional primary motor cortex improves hand function after stroke. Stroke 2005;36: 2681–2686.

66 Fregni F, Boggio PS, Mansur CG, Wagner T, Ferreira MJ, Lima MC, Rigonatti SP, Marcolin MA, Freedman SD, Nitsche MA, Pascual-Leone A: Transcranial direct current stimulation of the unaffected hemisphere in stroke patients. Neuroreport 2005;16:1551–1555.

67 Khedr EM, Ahmed MA, Fathy N, Rothwell JC: Therapeutic trial of repetitive transcranial magnetic stimulation after acute ischemic stroke. Neurology 2005;65:466–468.

68 Kim YH, You SH, Ko MH, Park JW, Lee KH, Jang SH, Yoo WK, Hallett M: Repetitive transcranial magnetic stimulation-induced corticomotor excitability and associated motor skill acquisition in chronic stroke. Stroke 2006;37:1471–1476.

69 Hummel F, Celnik P, Giraux P, Floel A, Wu WH, Gerloff C, Cohen LG: Effects of non-invasive cortical stimulation on skilled motor function in chronic stroke. Brain 2005;128:490–499.

70 Brown JA, Lutsep HL, Weinand M, Cramer SC: Motor cortex stimulation for the enhancement of recovery from stroke: a prospective, multicenter safety study. Neurosurgery 2006;58:464–473.

71 Kobayashi M, Hutchinson S, Theoret H, Schlaug G, Pascual-Leone A: Repetitive TMS of the motor cortex improves ipsilateral sequential simple finger movements. Neurology 2004;62:91–98.

72 Vuilleumier P, Hester D, Assal G, Regli F: Unilateral spatial neglect recovery after sequential strokes. Neurology 1996;46:184–189.

73 Liepert J, Hamzei F, Weiller C: Lesion-induced and training-induced brain reorganization. Restor Neurol Neurosci 2004;22:269–277.

74 Murase N, Duque J, Mazzocchio R, Cohen LG: Influence of interhemispheric interactions on motor function in chronic stroke. Ann Neurol 2004;55:400–409.

75 Gershon AA, Dannon PN, Grunhaus L: Transcranial magnetic stimulation in the treatment of depression. Am J Psychiatry 2003;160:835–845.

76 Rossi S, Rossini PM: TMS in cognitive plasticity and the potential for rehabilitation. Trends Cogn Sci 2004;8:273–279.

77 Paus T, Jech R, Thompson CJ, Comeau R, Peters T, Evans AC: Transcranial magnetic stimulation during positron emission tomography: a new method for studying connectivity of the human cerebral cortex. Neuroscience 1997;17:3178–3184.

78 Lockwood AH, Salvi RJ, Burkard RF: Tinnitus. N Engl J Med 2002;347:904–910.

79 Nicolas-Puel C, Faulconbridge RL, Guitton M, Puel JL, Mondain M, Uziel A: Characteristics of tinnitus and etiology of associated hearing loss: a study of 123 patients. Int Tinnitus J 2002;8: 37–44.

80 Eggermont JJ, Roberts LE: The neuroscience of tinnitus. Trends Neurosci 2004;27:676–682.

81 Rauschecker JP: Auditory cortical plasticity: a comparison with other sensory systems. Trends Neurosci 1999;22:74–80.

82 Holgers KM, Zoger S, Svedlund K: Predictive factors for development of severe tinnitus suffering – Further characterisation. Int J Audiol 2005;44:584–592.

83 Plewnia C, Bartels M, Gerloff C: Transient suppression of tinnitus by transcranial magnetic stimulation. Ann Neurol 2003;53:263–266.

84 Fregni F, Marcondes R, Boggio P, Marcolin MA, Rigonatti SP, Sanchez TG, Nitsche M, Pascual-Leone A: Transient tinnitus suppression induced by repetitive transcranial magnetic stimulation and transcranial direct current stimulation. Eur J Neurol 2006;13:996–1001.

85 De Ridder D, Verstraeten E, Van der Kelen K, De Mulder G, Sunaert S, Verlooy J, Van de Heyning P, Moller A: Transcranial magnetic stimulation of tinnitus: influence of tinnitus duration on stimulation parameter choice and maximal suppression. Otol Neurotol 2005;26:616–619.

86 Londero A, Lefaucheur JP, Malinvaud D, Brugieres P, Peignard P, Nguyen JP, Avan P, Bonfils P: Stimulation magnétique du cortex auditif dans les acouphènes invalidants. Résultats préliminaires. Presse Med 2006;35:200–206.

87 Eichhammer P, Langguth B, Marienhagen J, Kleinjung T, Hajak G: Neuronavigated repetitive transcranial magnetic stimulation in patients with tinnitus: a short case series. Biol Psychiatry 2003;54:862–865.

88 Langguth B, Eichhammer P, Wiegand R, Marienhegen J, Maenner P, Jacob P, Hajak G: Neuronavigated rTMS in a patient with chronic tinnitus. Effects of 4 weeks treatment. Neuroreport 2003;14:977–980.

89 Kleinjung T, Eichhammer P, Langguth B, Jacob P, Marienhagen J, Hajak G, Wolf SR, Strutz J: Long-term effects of repetitive transcranial magnetic stimulation (rTMS) in patients with chronic tinnitus. Otolaryngol Head Neck Surg 2005;132:566–569.

90 Brugge JF, Volkov IO, Garell PC, Reale RA, Howard MA: Functional connections between auditory cortex on Heschl's gyrus and on the lateral superior temporal gyrus in humans. J Neurophysiol 2003;90:3750–3763.

91 May A, Hajak G, Ganssbauer S, Steffens T, Langguth B, Kleinjung T, Eichhammer P: Structural brain alterations following 5 days of intervention: dynamic aspects of neuroplasticity. Cereb Cortex, in press.
92 Liegeois-Chauvel C, Giraud K, Badier JM, Marquis P, Chauvel P: Intracerebral evoked potentials in pitch perception reveal a functional asymmetry of the human auditory cortex. Ann NY Acad Sci 2001;930:117–132.

Prof. Jean-Pascal Lefaucheur
Service de Physiologie, Explorations Fonctionnelles, Hôpital Henri-Mondor
51, avenue de Lattre-de-Tassigny
FR–94010 Créteil (France)
Tel. +33 1 4981 2694, Fax +33 1 4981 4660, E-Mail jean-pascal.lefaucheur@hmn.aphp.fr

Marcolin MA, Padberg F (eds): Transcranial Brain Stimulation for Treatment of Psychiatric Disorders. Adv Biol Psychiatr. Basel, Karger, 2007, vol 23, pp 155–171

Magnetic Seizure Therapy for the Treatment of Depression

Sarah H. Lisanby, Angel V. Peterchev

Brain Stimulation and Therapeutic Modulation Division, Department of Psychiatry, Columbia University College of Physicians and Surgeons, New York State Psychiatric Institute, New York, N.Y., USA

Abstract

Cognitive side effects limit the clinical utility of electroconvulsive therapy (ECT), the most effective and rapidly acting treatment for severe depression. Studies suggest that prefrontal cortical involvement may be important to preserving the efficacy of ECT, while seizure spread to the medial temporal lobes may be related to its amnestic side effects. However, the scalp and skull shunt the flow of electricity, limiting control over current spread with ECT. Magnetic fields enter the brain unimpeded, allowing enhanced control over the site of stimulation and seizure initiation compared to ECT. Magnetic seizure therapy (MST) involves the induction of a seizure under general anesthesia using high-frequency repetitive transcranial magnetic stimulation. MST was developed to reduce the cognitive side effect burden of convulsive therapy through focal seizure induction in the prefrontal cortex. Work to date supports the feasibility of MST in the nonhuman primate and in patients with depression. Preliminary results indicate that seizures induced with MST are more focal, result in less involvement of hippocampal and deep brain structures, and have a better acute side effect profile than those induced with ECT. Future directions for the clinical development of MST technology are discussed.

Electroconvulsive therapy (ECT) retains an important position in treatment algorithms for major depressive disorder and bipolar disorder because it remains the most effective and rapidly acting treatment available for treatment-resistant depression (TRD) [1]. Despite advances in psychotherapeutic and psychopharmacological interventions for major depression, a disturbingly large proportion of depressed patients are not adequately treated with presently available strategies. The results of the Sequenced Treatment Alternatives to Relieve Depression trial bring the magnitude of the problem presented by TRD into sharp focus. Nearly 80% of the 2,876 Sequenced Treatment Alternatives to

Relieve Depression trial participants had chronic or recurrent major depression at study entry, and 72% of the sample failed to remit following a standardized trial of citalopram [2]. Even more alarming, approximately 75% failed to remit with a second antidepressant trial [3]. ECT could be an effective treatment for such patients with TRD who fail to respond to second-line and third-line pharmacotherapy. Given the prevalence of depression worldwide, why is there an apparent mismatch between the number of patients who could benefit from ECT and those who receive it?

The well-documented and recognized cognitive side effects of ECT remain an impediment to its widespread use. Concerns regarding the memory loss associated with ECT among clinicians and patients alike frequently effectively restrict its use in many cases to a last resort treatment, or prevent its use entirely. Withholding ECT from patients who could benefit from it is unfortunate considering its unmatched efficacy, even in highly severe and treatment-resistant cases. If there were an available form of convulsive therapy with a more favorable risk/benefit ratio, it would likely be used earlier in the course of illness and could bring effective treatment to those suffering with the considerable morbidity and disability associated with TRD.

Advances in the methodologies for focal brain stimulation using electromagnetic fields present new avenues for the study and potentially for the treatment of mood disorders. These novel technologies include repetitive transcranial magnetic stimulation (rTMS), magnetic seizure therapy (MST), deep brain stimulation, vagus nerve stimulation, transcranial direct current stimulation and modifications of ECT. While none of these technologies appear remotely close to completely replacing ECT, they represent alternative strategies that may expand the spectrum of available treatment options, and they are likely to add important information regarding the pathophysiology of depression and the mechanisms of action of effective treatments.

This chapter reviews the current status of MST to improve the risk/benefit ratio of convulsive therapy in the treatment of severe depression. By coupling the therapeutic power of seizures with the focality of magnetic fields, MST holds the promise of retaining the efficacy of ECT, but with fewer cognitive side effects. This chapter critically reviews how close MST is to fulfilling that promise, and presents a research agenda for further study with this novel intervention.

Definitions and Comparison with Repetitive Transcranial Magnetic Stimulation

MST refers to the use of rTMS to induce a therapeutic seizure from a focal region of the cerebral cortex [4–6]. Both MST and rTMS utilize rapidly alternating magnetic fields applied to the scalp. In the case of rTMS, the level of stimulation is selected to be subconvulsive and administered to an alert, unanesthetized subject. In the case of MST, the level of stimulation is designed to intentionally induce a seizure in an anesthetized subject. Coupling the superior spatial precision of magnetic fields with the unparalleled antidepressant action of seizures, MST was designed to be a more tolerable form of convulsive therapy than ECT.

Since MST is more invasive than subconvulsive stimulation with rTMS, MST is under development for those patients in whom subconvulsive rTMS is inadequate to effectively treat their depression. As reviewed elsewhere in this book, work with subconvulsive rTMS in depression has been promising [7, 8]. While rTMS has compared favorably with ECT in some head-to-head comparisons, those comparisons are necessarily limited by the lack of blinding of the patients [9–11]. One recent study found ECT to be superior to rTMS in the nonpsychotic subtype [12]. Further, most studies agree that ECT has a faster speed of response and remains more effective than rTMS in the psychotic subtype of depression. The need for continued parallel development of both subconvulsive and convulsive methods to treat depression is supported by the substantial heterogeneity in depression subtypes, severity and response profiles.

Role of Convulsive Therapy in Current Psychiatric Practice

ECT has remained in continuous clinical use since its inception approximately 70 years ago due to its as yet unsurpassed efficacy in treating severe acute depression. Today, ECT continues to play an important role in the treatment of severe depression, catatonia, both the depressed and manic phases of bipolar disorder, and resistant schizophrenia, especially for patients who cannot tolerate or who have not responded to psychotropic medications [1]. Vagus nerve stimulation was approved by the US FDA for the long-term adjunctive management of TRD, but ECT remains the only somatic treatment with proven efficacy in the acute management of TRD [13]. It is estimated that 1–2 million individuals receive ECT each year worldwide, with utilization increasing. ECT is uniquely suited for the treatment of the most severely ill depressed and psychotic patients because of its fast onset of action, exceptionally high response rate (especially in psychotic depression), and profound acute beneficial effect on suicidality, a major source of morbidity and mortality from depression [14, 16]. Were there a treatment modality that carried the efficacy of ECT without its cognitive side effects, its usage could become much higher than the estimated

100,000 patients/year who receive ECT in the USA and might more closely match the percentage of patients estimated to suffer from TRD.

Despite the indisputable therapeutic advantages of ECT, its amnestic side effects substantially reduce its tolerability and clinical utility. Retrograde amnesia is the most persistent adverse effect of ECT [15–18]. Most patients have gaps in memory for events that occurred close in time to ECT, but retrograde amnesia may extend several months or years. Memories of an autobiographical nature are spared to a greater degree than memories of an impersonal nature [15]. Nevertheless, loss of memory for one's life is frequently cited among the reasons patients offer when they reject a trial (or retrial) of ECT. While retrograde amnesia frequently improves during the months following ECT, recovery may be incomplete, with prolonged amnesia for events that occurred close to the time of treatment [19]. Moreover, ECT possesses a high relapse rate with some patients showing a return to illness within a few weeks after completing acute treatment, highlighting the need for effective maintenance strategies [20].

Rationale for Focal Seizure Induction as a Means of Reducing Amnestic Effects of Convulsive Therapy

The literature suggests that focal seizure induction may be a strategy to reduce the side effects of ECT while retaining its efficacy. If successful, focal seizure induction could bring the most effective intervention yet available to more patients earlier in the course of treatment. The rationale for focal seizure induction with MST is built upon the finding that the efficacy and side effects of ECT are largely determined by the site of seizure initiation and by the patterns of seizure spread. Variations in the ECT technique (e.g. electrode placement, pulse width, and electrical dosage) can lower its side effects substantially [21–23]. Patterns of functional change in prefrontal regions are reported to be associated with the antidepressant action, while functional changes in the medial temporal lobe have been associated with the amnestic effects of ECT. Specifically, ECT is associated with mossy fiber sprouting (MFS), the growth of a new synaptic connection in the dentate gyrus (i.e. within the hippocampus) [24–26]. Apparently not necessary for antidepressant action since MFS is not observed with antidepressant medications, MFS seen in response to seizures is thought to disrupt the normal functioning of the hippocampus in animal seizure models [27]. Our data suggest that focal seizure induction from prefrontal structures, avoiding temporal structures, is not associated with marked anatomical changes in the hippocampus and thus may be a means of reducing the cognitive side effects of ECT [28–30].

Electrical versus Magnetic Means of Focal Seizure Induction

The relative advantages of using magnetic fields to induce focal seizures rather than the direct application of electricity to the scalp derived from the physics of brain stimulation. The scalp and skull impede the flow of electricity applied directly to the scalp, resulting in broadly distributed fields that are difficult to focus and control [4, 31]. Individual differences in scalp and skull anatomy will confound these factors, making standardization across individuals difficult and perhaps in part contributing to the high degree of variability seen across individuals in ECT seizure threshold [32]. Changing electrode placement is clearly beneficial, as in the switch from bilateral to unilateral electrode placement, but the resultant seizures are still bilaterally generalized. Novel electrode configurations and pulse characteristics are under development, yet focal seizure initiation will likely remain difficult to achieve reliably.

In contrast, MST has theoretical advantages relative to electrical approaches because magnetic fields pass through tissue (including the scalp and skull) without impedance and can be more precisely targeted [33]. Magnetic fields delivered with TMS and MST penetrate only about 2–4 cm deep from the scalp (depending upon coil configuration), which can be an advantage since it avoids direct stimulation of deeper structures (like the hippocampus). In vivo measurements in non-human primates support the hypothesis that MST-induced current and the resulting seizures are more focal than typically seen with ECT [34]. This enhanced control represents a means to focus the treatment to the cortical structures thought to mediate antidepressant effects and to reduce seizure spread to medial temporal structures implicated in the amnestic side effects of ECT.

Magnetic Seizure Therapy Device Development

MST is delivered with rTMS devices that have been custom modified to permit reliable seizure induction in anesthetized subjects (fig. 1). The anticonvulsant action of anesthesia has posed the greatest challenge to MST device design, and can be reduced through proper selection of anesthetic agents with less impact on seizure threshold and the action of rTMS (discussed below) [35]. Some of the factors to be taken into account in the design of MST devices include the coil configuration, range of output parameters, heat tolerance, power requirements for the device, and pulse characteristics.

Coil Selection

As a result of their differing magnetic field distributions, different coil types and scalp placements result in dramatically different effects on the topographical

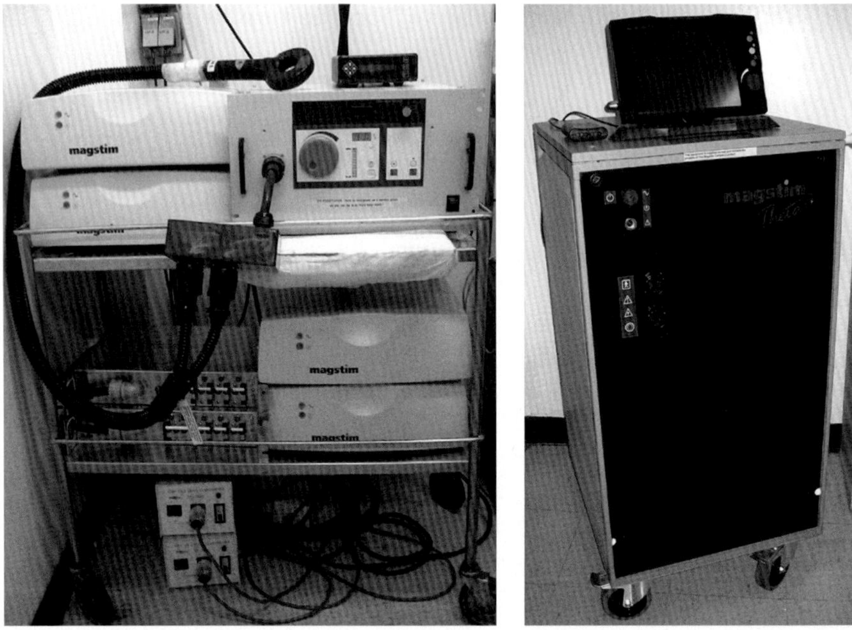

a *b*

Fig. 1. Current MST devices. ***a*** Prototype MST device powered by four capacitor chargers, in use for nonhuman primate studies. ***b*** Integrated MST device, in use for human MST (Magstim Theta®).

spread of the resultant seizure. The relatively nonfocal round coil [both flat (fig. 2a) and curved (fig. 2b) configurations] has been more efficient in inducing seizures than the more focal double-cone (fig. 2c) and figure-of-eight (fig. 2d) coil configurations [30, 36]. In addition to resulting in different seizure thresholds, coils differ in the topography of the seizures that they induce. The nonfocal round coil produces greater seizure activity across a wider region, whereas the more focal double-cone coil produces more localized seizure activity on the dorsal and frontal surfaces of the brain with its peak underlying the intersection of the coil windings. This control of seizure onset and spread enables the empirical testing of the relations among individual seizure characteristics and clinical outcome. Such work should shed light on the mechanisms of action of ECT and guide the development of novel interventions for depression.

Novel coil designs are under development to extend the depth of penetration and enable seizure induction from structures that may be deeper than the outer surface of the cortex [37, 38]. Altering the rate of drop-off of field

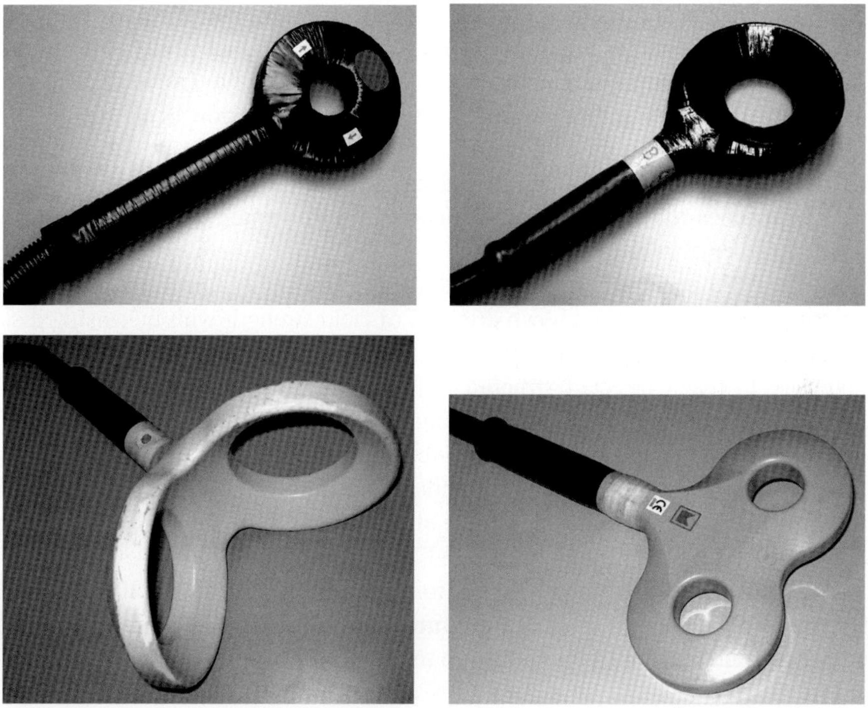

Fig. 2. Representative MST coils: flat round (***a***), curved round (***b***), double-cone (***c***), figure-of-eight (***d***). The most efficient coils for MST have been the round coil (flat and curved) and double-cone configurations.

strength as a function of distance through changes in coil design may be helpful and should be explored, but it is considered theoretically impossible to focus stimulation with rTMS at depth without any stimulation of overlying brain structures [39, 40]. Other coil modifications include the use of metal cores to intensify field strength and permit device operation at lower power requirements [41].

Parameters of Stimulation

Work with rTMS had already shown that rTMS can induce seizures inadvertently if given at sufficiently intense parameters of stimulation [42, 43]. Seizure risk with rTMS can be increased by increasing intensity above motor threshold, increasing frequency, lengthening train duration, or by shortening the intertrain interval [44]. The relative efficiency of these parameter modifications in increasing seizure risk has not been systematically examined, but the ECT literature suggests that lower levels of stimulus packing (which refers to the number of pulses per unit time) are more efficient [45]. This literature would argue in favor of the ability to sustain long trains of stimulation in preference to excessively high frequencies given for short durations. These considerations led to the current MST device design that can sustain peak output for up to 10 s, which matches the longest trains of stimulation commonly delivered by the modern generation of ECT devices.

The TMS literature suggests that intensity is a highly important parameter of stimulation, due to the known drop-off of field strength with increasing distance from the coil [39]. Thus with MST it is important to provide sufficient intensity to reach targeted structures at levels sufficient to induce neuronal depolarization despite the anticonvulsant effects of anesthesia. All of the work to date with MST has operated the device at maximal stimulator output, which is approximately double the typical motor threshold, to ensure that intensities were sufficient to overcome anesthetic effects.

The first monkey and human MST cases were treated at 40–50 Hz, compared with 1–20 Hz typically used for subconvulsive rTMS [30, 36, 46]. Current MST devices (fig. 1) deliver stimulation at 100 Hz, 100% intensity (2 T at the coil surface) for trains lasting up to 10 s.

Heating

Increasing output parameters will increase heating of the coil and device components. Large and nonfocal coils experience less heating than smaller focal coils. Proper material selection, precooling, and active cooling systems can minimize these constraints. The magnetic pulse shape also affects coil heating. Briefer pulses use less energy to produce neuronal depolarization, and result in less coil heating [47, 48].

It is not just the coils that heat up with high levels of rTMS, it is also the EEG electrodes. Nonmetallic EEG electrodes are now available for use in the fMRI environment that reduce the risk of scalp burns with MST.

Power Requirements

The higher output of the MST device introduces larger electrical supply demands than standard rTMS devices, but design improvements have made the present model more compact and feasible to implement in clinical settings. For example, while the early MST devices required 8–16 separate 20-A rated circuits, the current model operates on only two 3-phase power sources. Further reduction of power consumption could be possible by optimizing the coil design and pulse shape [41, 47, 49].

Pulse Characteristics

All MST devices generate biphasic sinusoidal magnetic pulses like those used in conventional rapid-rate rTMS stimulators. Conventional biphasic pulses induce electrical currents with similar magnitudes in both polarities, in contrast to monophasic pulses that induce current with one preferential polarity. The reason for the use of biphasic pulses is technical. Presently, biphasic devices have substantially higher power efficiency and less coil heating than monophasic devices [50].

An increasing number of studies have examined the relative effectiveness of different pulse characteristics with rTMS [51–53]. A review of 1-Hz rTMS studies in healthy subjects concluded that the stimulation site, duration, and current direction play an important role in outcome, and that the pulse configuration likely contributes as well [54]. Thus, pulse parameters could potentially be optimized to enhance neuromodulatory effects. Similar considerations might be expected to apply to MST as well.

Anesthesia for Magnetic Seizure Therapy

Since MST involves intentional seizure induction with the potential of generalization to the motor cortex, the procedure is performed under anesthesia with the medical and physiological monitoring procedures performed during standard ECT (EKG, pulse oximetry, end-tidal CO_2, blood pressure, EEG, and motor manifestations using the 'cuff technique'). Anesthesia and the associated physiological monitoring are not utilized with subconvulsive rTMS, where the risk of seizure is low when safety guidelines are followed [43, 55]. The reason for employing anesthesia during convulsive therapy (ECT and MST) is to protect the body from musculoskeletal injury during motor convulsion through succinylcholine-induced muscular paralysis. Ultimately, if truly focal seizure induction may be achieved such that motor generalization reliably does not occur, then muscular paralysis may not be necessary. However, procedures for preventing motor generalization are not yet defined so the routine use of anesthesia is recommended for MST at present.

Anesthetic regimens differ in their impact upon MST. These considerations are presented in depth in White et al. [35]. Briefly, it has been recognized that certain anesthetic medications, such as thiopental and propofol, increase seizure threshold and shorten seizure duration with ECT. The same is true with MST, but with MST the impact is more critical with the use of devices that are already close to seizure threshold. Methohexital is widely considered an anesthetic of choice for ECT [1], and has also been used successfully with MST [30, 36, 56]. Etomidate has even less effect on seizure threshold than methohexital and has been useful in lengthening seizures with ECT. We have had good success with etomidate during

MST [57], but also note that etomidate-induced myoclonus must be carefully distinguished from the MST-induced seizure. Monitoring motor manifestations alone may be inadequate to distinguish myoclonus from seizure. EEG monitoring is essential for this differentiation and for accurate seizure detection with MST.

Finally, the appropriate timing of the duration of muscular relaxation during MST is an important consideration. With MST, as with ECT, it is optimal for the muscular relaxation to last throughout the induced seizures, but to recover prior to the point when the patient regains consciousness. In the case of ECT, it may take upwards of 30 min to an hour or more for the patient to regain orientation. In the case of MST, orientation recovery is much faster [36]. Indeed, orientation recovery can be so fast that it precedes recovery from succinylcholine, which can result in patients becoming alert while still experiencing some degree of muscular weakness. This risk can be minimized by reducing succinylcholine dosage to the minimum necessary, and through the use of a peripheral nerve stimulator to accurately time the MST delivery to coincide with the peak action of succinylcholine. We found that because MST-induced seizures were generally less robust than ECT-induced seizures in their intensity of motoric expression, patients had lower succinylcholine dosage requirements to achieve adequately modified seizures [35].

Animal Studies on the Physiological, Anatomical, and Cognitive Effects of Magnetic Seizure Therapy

We performed the first MST procedure on a rhesus monkey because seizure induction in smaller animals was prohibited by the technical considerations of coil heating (discussed above) and the coil-to-brain size ratio that constrains the intensity of the electric field induced in the brain with TMS [5]. While working with other species would have the advantage of a greater number of readily available behavioral models of depression and antidepressant action, the monkey provides the best homology to the human, and the broadest and most sophisticated models of cognitive function with which to test the hypothesis that MST will induce less amnesia than ECT.

We have now completed a study of 24 rhesus monkeys randomly assigned to receive treatment with electroconvulsive shock (ECS; at 2.5 times seizure threshold), MST (with a round coil positioned on the vertex at 2.5 times seizure threshold), or anesthesia-alone sham. We are also midway through a new study of similar design examining the effects of MST at 6 times seizure threshold. Our work in nonhuman primates to date has provided support for the safety of MST and ECS (using neuroanatomical, neuropathological, and stereological measures) [58–60], showed that MST and ECS differed in neurophysiological [34] and neuroanatomical [6, 61] measures that may relate to their differing cognitive profiles, and provided new data on hippocampal plasticity in response to convulsive interventions.

The electric field induced in the brain by MST is less intense and more confined to the superficial cortex than ECS, according to our intracerebral recordings in rhesus monkeys [34]. We found MST-induced seizures to show less robust ictal expression, less postictal suppression, less generalization to the hippocampus and deeper brain structures, and result in a less robust serum prolactin surge [62] and less immediate post-stimulus bradycardia. These physiological and neuroendocrine differences are consistent with MST having less of an impact than ECS on temporal lobe and diencephalic structures. These results are also consistent with MST exerting less of an impact on parasympathetic outflow that should, in turn, be associated with a lower risk of cardiac complications. This latter point could be especially relevant to older patients with comorbid medical conditions.

We found no neuropathological changes associated with MST or ECS upon careful and systematic neuropathological examination of the brains of rhesus monkeys following chronic treatment [58]. Stereological cell counts of 3 regions of the prefrontal cortex and 2 regions of the dentate gyrus revealed no treatment-related reductions in neuron or glial cell counts [63].

However, differences between MST and ECS in their effects on neuroplasticity were apparent. Specifically, ECS, but not MST, robustly increased MFS [61] in the dentate gyrus of rhesus monkeys [26]. A relative lack of physiological and structural changes in the hippocampus with MST may relate to its superior cognitive profile. Consistent with this hypothesis, our nonhuman primate model of the amnestic side effects of ECT revealed better outcomes with MST than with ECS [56, 60].

Clinical Studies of Magnetic Seizure Therapy

Altogether 45 patients have received MST worldwide since the first patient was treated in 2000 [30, 36, 46, 57]. In general, MST has been well tolerated with no significant adverse events or unanticipated side effects.

Initial case studies demonstrated the feasibility of performing MST in humans. The first depressed patient to receive MST experienced a 50% drop in Hamilton Depression Rating Scale ($HDRS_{24}$) scores following 4 MST sessions. MST at 40 Hz, 100% of maximal stimulator output, administered for 4 s was well tolerated with no significant side effects [30]. A second patient with medication-resistant depression received 12 MST sessions at 50 Hz, for 8 s, at maximal output and experienced remission (with an 82% drop in $HDRS_{24}$ scores and a final $HDRS_{24}$ score of 6) [46].

The first trial of MST in the USA contrasted MST and ECT in their acute cognitive side effects [36]. This double-masked, randomized, within-subject trial contrasted the acute cognitive side effects of MST with ultrabrief-pulse right unilateral ECT (selected for its exceptionally low cognitive side effect burden). We found MST to be well tolerated with fewer side effects than ECT and faster recovery of orientation, a predictor of the magnitude of long-term retrograde amnesia [17, 36]. Masked neuropsychological assessments revealed advantages of MST relative to ECT. As expected, MST and ECT did not differ on tasks more heavily dependent on prefrontal lobe function (i.e. memory for temporal order, verbal fluency), but MST showed clear advantages over ECT in cognitive domains subserved at least partly by temporal lobe structures (i.e. memory for recent events, new list learning, category fluency).

Although both ECT and MST seizures were generalized and resulted in motor convulsion, marked differences in the nature of the seizures induced by MST and ECT were seen [36]. Compared to ECT, MST seizures were shorter and showed lower ictal EEG amplitudes and less postictal suppression. While these EEG characteristics have been thought to relate to the antidepressant activity of ECT, new evidence suggests that the relations with efficacy are unclear when applied to novel forms of stimulation. For example, lower ictal EEG amplitude and less postictal suppression are also seen with ultrabrief-pulse right unilateral ECT, which has demonstrated equal antidepressant efficacy with bilateral ECT [64].

Differences were also seen between MST- and ECT-induced seizures in their degree of generalization to deeper brain structures, as indexed indirectly by the seizure-induced surge in serum prolactin and vagally mediated post-stimulation bradycardia [62]. Less intense ictal expression also has the added benefit of requiring lower doses of succinylcholine to protect the body from the motor convulsion [35].

Next, we conducted a randomized, double-masked, 2-center (New York State Psychiatric Institute and University of Texas Southwestern Medical Center) study comparing two forms of MST in their antidepressant properties and side effects [57]. This study established the feasibility and tolerability of MST in the clinical setting, and provided the first controlled data on the antidepressant efficacy of MST.

While the published reports with MST to date utilized a device that was capped at 400 pulses, the newly available 100-Hz device now permits stimulation with up to 1,000 pulses. This device has undergone testing in the rhesus monkey, and preliminary evidence suggests that even higher dosages of MST retain advantages in terms of amnestic side effects [65]. Initial human testing with this device has already demonstrated the feasibility of seizure induction from the prefrontal cortex with MST.

Future studies will be needed to characterize the long-term side effect profile and antidepressant efficacy of MST relative to ECT. These early studies are promising and are being followed up with another multicenter trial.

Future Directions for Magnetic Seizure Therapy Development

The field of MST remains young. Results of ongoing preclinical and clinical studies will undoubtedly inform the next generation of MST device. Unanswered questions remain regarding optimal dosing strategies, coil type and position, and patient selection.

Since dosage relative to seizure threshold is such an important predictor of efficacy and side effects with ECT, this may also apply to MST, though these relationships have not yet been established for MST. Studies will need to contrast different dosing strategies in their efficacy and side effects. Currently available devices now offer an expanded range of dosing options to facilitate that dose-ranging work. While rTMS technology has extended beyond typical monofrequency trains to examine the value of frequency combinations (such as priming and theta burst) [66, 67], compound frequencies have yet to be explored for MST.

Given that focality of seizure initiation and limitation of spread are goals of MST, the development of new coil designs (both winding patterns and material selections) could facilitate these goals. In particular, novel strategies to increase depth of penetration without excessively broadening the region of superficial cortex affected may also be useful.

Another aspect of dosing of MST that remains to be studied is the number of treatments per week. Presently, MST is conducted 3 times a week because that is the standard in the USA for ECT; however, there are no empirical data to guide the frequency of treatments. Given its more benign side effect profile, more frequent treatments could be feasible and tolerable.

Once optimal dosing for an acute course is established, posttreatment maintenance strategies will be needed – e.g. combination pharmacotherapy and/or maintenance MST. The potential role of maintenance MST following an acute course of ECT (or MST) has yet to be explored.

Concluding Remarks

Convulsive therapy retains an important role in psychiatry today as the most effective treatment for the acute management of severe TRD and other conditions.

Theories regarding the mechanisms of action of ECT have guided the development of newer, more focal treatments such as MST to improve the risk/benefit ratio of convulsive therapy and to expand its clinical utility. MST combines the focality of magnetic fields with the unmatched therapeutic efficacy of seizures. Work to date supports the feasibility and safety of MST. These results need to be replicated in larger samples to test the generalizability of the findings. Studies are under way to define its optimal dosing paradigm and determine its efficacy in relation to ECT. MST provides a new tool with which to further define the mechanisms of action of ECT, since MST can be used to deliver focal stimulation at specific brain sites and test hypothesized relations among the site of initiation and the spectrum of clinical effects. The results of ongoing and future studies will be helpful in determining the ultimate role of MST relative to other existing treatment strategies in treatment algorithms for TRD and other conditions.

Acknowledgements

This study was supported by NIH MH60884, Stanley Medical Research Foundation, NARSAD, and an American Federation for Aging Research Beeson Scholar Award. S.H.L. has received research support from Magstim Company, Neuronetics, and Cyberonics.

References

1 American Psychiatric Association Task Force on Electroconvulsive Therapy: The Practice of Electroconvulsive Therapy: Recommendations for Treatment, Training, and Privileging. Washington, American Psychiatric Association, 2001.
2 Trivedi MH, Rush AJ, Wisniewski SR, Nierenberg AA, Warden D, Ritz L, Norquist G, Howland RH, Lebowitz B, McGrath PJ, Shores-Wilson K, Biggs MM, Balasubramani GK, Fava M: Evaluation of outcomes with citalopram for depression using measurement-based care in STAR*D: implications for clinical practice. Am J Psychiatry 2006;163:28–40.
3 Rush AJ, Trivedi MH, Wisniewski SR, Stewart JW, Nierenberg AA, Thase ME, Ritz L, Biggs MM, Warden D, Luther JF, Shores-Wilson K, Niederehe G, Fava M: Bupropion-SR, sertraline, or venlafaxine-XR after failure of SSRIs for depression. N Engl J Med 2006;354:1231–1242.
4 Sackeim H: Magnetic stimulation therapy and ECT. Convuls Ther 1994;10:255–258.
5 Lisanby SH, Luber B, Finck AD, Schroeder C, Sackeim HA: Deliberate seizure induction with repetitive transcranial magnetic stimulation in nonhuman primates. Arch Gen Psychiatry 2001;58: 199–200 (erratum 515).
6 Lisanby SH: Magnetic seizure therapy: development of a novel convulsive technique; in Lisanby SH (ed): Brain Stimulation in Psychiatric Treatment. Arlington, American Psychiatric Publishing, Inc, 2004, vol 23, chapter 4, pp 77–116.
7 Gershon AA, Dannon PN, Grunhaus L: Transcranial magnetic stimulation in the treatment of depression. Am J Psychiatry 2003;160:835–845.
8 Burt T, Lisanby SH, Sackeim HA: Neuropsychiatric applications of transcranial magnetic stimulation: a meta analysis. Int J Neuropsychopharmacol 2002;5:73–103.
9 Grunhaus L, Dannon PN, Schreiber S, Dolberg OH, Amiaz R, Ziv R, Lefkifker E: Repetitive transcranial magnetic stimulation is as effective as electroconvulsive therapy in the treatment of nondelusional major depressive disorder: an open study. Biol Psychiatry 2000;47:314–324.

10 Grunhaus L, Schreiber S, Dolberg OT, Polak D, Dannon PN: A randomized controlled comparison of electroconvulsive therapy and repetitive transcranial magnetic stimulation in severe and resistant nonpsychotic major depression. Biol Psychiatry 2003;53:324–331.
11 Janicak PG, Dowd SM, Martis B, Alam D, Beedle D, Krasuski J, Strong MJ, Sharma R, Rosen C, Viana M: Repetitive transcranial magnetic stimulation versus electroconvulsive therapy for major depression: preliminary results of a randomized trial. Biol Psychiatry 2002;51:659–667.
12 McLoughlin D, Eranti SV, Mogg A, Pluck G, Purvis R, Edwards D: A 6-month, follow-up, pragmatic randomised controlled trial of ECT and rTMS in major depression. J ECT 2005;21:59.
13 Group UER: Efficacy and safety of electroconvulsive therapy in depressive disorders: a systematic review and meta-analysis. Lancet 2003;361:799–808.
14 Prudic J, Sackeim H: Electroconvulsive therapy and suicide risk. J Clin Psychiatry 1999;60(suppl 2): 104–110.
15 Lisanby SH, Maddox JH, Prudic J, Devanand DP, Sackeim HA: The effects of electroconvulsive therapy on memory of autobiographical and public events. Arch Gen Psychiatry 2000;57: 581–590.
16 Weiner RD: Retrograde amnesia with electroconvulsive therapy: characteristics and implications. Arch Gen Psychiatry 2000;57:591–592.
17 Sobin C, Sackeim HA, Prudic J, Devanand DP, Moody BJ, McElhiney MC: Predictors of retrograde amnesia following ECT. Am J Psychiatry 1995;152:995–1001.
18 Squire LR, Slater PC, Miller PL: Retrograde amnesia and bilateral electroconvulsive therapy. Long-term follow-up. Arch Gen Psychiatry 1981;38:89–95.
19 Donahue AB: Electroconvulsive therapy and memory loss: a personal journey. J ECT 2000;16: 133–143.
20 Sackeim HA, Haskett RF, Mulsant BH, Thase ME, Mann JJ, Pettinati HM, Greenberg RM, Crowe RR, Cooper TB, Prudic J: Continuation pharmacotherapy in the prevention of relapse following electroconvulsive therapy: a randomized controlled trial. JAMA 2001;285:1299–1307.
21 Sackeim HA, Prudic J, Devanand DP, Nobler MS, Lisanby SH, Peyser S, Fitzsimons L, Moody BJ, Clark J: A prospective, randomized, double-blind comparison of bilateral and right unilateral electroconvulsive therapy at different stimulus intensities. Arch Gen Psychiatry 2000;57:425–434.
22 Sackeim HA, Prudic J, Devanand DP, Kiersky JE, Fitzsimons L, Moody BJ, McElhiney MC, Coleman EA, Settembrino JM: Effects of stimulus intensity and electrode placement on the efficacy and cognitive effects of electroconvulsive therapy. N Engl J Med 1993;328:839–846.
23 Sackeim HA, Portnoy S, Neeley P, Steif BL, Decina P, Malitz S: Cognitive consequences of low-dosage electroconvulsive therapy. Ann NY Acad Sci 1986;462:326–340.
24 Chen AC, Shin KH, Duman RS, Sanacora G: ECS-induced mossy fiber sprouting and BDNF expression are attenuated by ketamine pretreatment. J ECT 2001;17:27–32.
25 Gombos Z, Spiller A, Cottrell GA, Racine RJ, McIntyre Burnham W: Mossy fiber sprouting induced by repeated electroconvulsive shock seizures. Brain Res 1999;844:28–33.
26 Lisanby S, Sackeim H, Dwork AJ, Underwood M, Wang X, Kassir SA, Luber B, Arango V: Effects of electroconvulsive shock and magnetic seizure therapy on mossy fiber sprouting and cellular proliferation in the primate hippocampus. Biol Psychiatry 2003;53:173S.
27 Lipp HP, Schwegler H, Heimrich B, Driscoll P: Infrapyramidal mossy fibers and two-way avoidance learning: developmental modification of hippocampal circuitry and adult behavior of rats and mice. J Neurosci 1988;8:1905–1921.
28 Lisanby SH: Update on magnetic seizure therapy: a novel form of convulsive therapy. J ECT 2002;18:182–188.
29 Lisanby SH, Morales O, Payne N, Kwon E, Fitzsimons L, Luber B, Nobler MS, Sackeim HA: New developments in electroconvulsive therapy and magnetic seizure therapy. CNS Spectr 2003;8: 529–536.
30 Lisanby SH, Schlaepfer TE, Fisch HU, Sackeim HA: Magnetic seizure therapy of major depression. Arch Gen Psychiatry 2001;58:303–305.
31 Sackeim HA, Long J, Luber B, Moeller JR, Prohovnik I, Devanand DP, Nobler MS: Physical properties and quantification of the ECT stimulus. 1. Basic principles. Convuls Ther 1994;10:93–123.
32 Lisanby SH, Devanand DP, Nobler MS, Prudic J, Mullen L, Sackeim HA: Exceptionally high seizure threshold: ECT device limitations. Convuls Ther 1996;12:156–164.

33 Barker AT, Jalinous R, Freeston IL: Non-invasive magnetic stimulation of human motor cortex. Lancet 1985;i:1106–1107.

34 Lisanby SH, Moscrip T, Morales O, Luber B, Schroeder C, Sackeim HA: Neurophysiological characterization of magnetic seizure therapy (MST) in non-human primates. Suppl Clin Neurophysiol 2003;56:81–99.

35 White PF, Amos Q, Zhang Y, Stool L, Husain MM, Thornton L, Downing M, McClintock S, Lisanby SH: Anesthetic considerations for magnetic seizure therapy: a novel therapy for severe depression. Anesth Analg 2006;103:76–80.

36 Lisanby SH, Luber B, Schlaepfer TE, Sackeim HA: Safety and feasibility of magnetic seizure therapy (MST) in major depression: randomized within-subject comparison with electroconvulsive therapy. Neuropsychopharmacology 2003;28:1852–1865.

37 Zangen A, Roth Y, Voller B, Hallett M: Transcranial magnetic stimulation of deep brain regions: evidence for efficacy of the H-coil. Clin Neurophysiol 2005;116:775–779.

38 Roth Y, Zangen A, Hallett M: A coil design for transcranial magnetic stimulation of deep brain regions. J Clin Neurophysiol 2002;19:361–370.

39 Bohning DE, Pecheny AP, Epstein CM, Speer AM, Vincent DJ, Dannels W, George MS: Mapping transcranial magnetic stimulation (TMS) fields in vivo with MRI. Neuroreport 1997;8: 2535–2538.

40 Heller L, van Hulsteyn DB: Brain stimulation using electromagnetic sources: theoretical aspects. Biophys J 1992;63:129–138.

41 Epstein CM, Davey KR: Iron-core coils for transcranial magnetic stimulation. J Clin Neurophysiol 2002;19:376–381.

42 Wassermann EM, Cohen LG, Flitman SS, Chen R, Hallett M: Seizures in healthy people with repeated 'safe' trains of transcranial magnetic stimuli. Lancet 1996;347:825–826.

43 Pascual-Leone A, Houser CM, Reese K, Shotland LI, Grafman J, Sato S, Valls-Sole J, Brasil-Neto JP, Wassermann EM, Cohen LG: Safety of rapid-rate transcranial magnetic stimulation in normal volunteers. Electroencephalogr Clin Neurophysiol 1993;89:120–130.

44 Wassermann EM: Risk and safety of repetitive transcranial magnetic stimulation: report and suggested guidelines from the International Workshop on the Safety of Repetitive Transcranial Magnetic Stimulation, June 5–7, 1996. Electroencephalogr Clin Neurophysiol 1998;108:1–16.

45 Devanand DP, Lisanby SH, Nobler MS, Sackeim HA: The relative efficiency of altering pulse frequency or train duration when determining seizure threshold. J ECT 1998;14:227–235.

46 Kosel M, Frick C, Lisanby SH, Fisch HU, Schlaepfer TE: Magnetic seizure therapy improves mood in refractory major depression. Neuropsychopharmacology 2003;28:2045–2048.

47 Davey K, Epstein CM: Magnetic stimulation coil and circuit design. IEEE Trans Biomed Eng 2000;47:1493–1499.

48 Barker AT, Garnham CW, Freeston IL: Magnetic nerve stimulation: the effect of waveform on efficiency, determination of neural membrane time constants and the measurement of stimulator output. Electroencephalogr Clin Neurophysiol Suppl 1991;43:227–237.

49 Peterchev A, Spellman T, Lisanby SH: cTMS: a novel TMS device inducing near rectangular pulses with controllable pulse width. ACNP Annu Meet Abstr, in press.

50 Jalinous R: Principles of magnetic stimulator design; in Pascual-Leone A, Davey NJ, Rothwell J, Wassermann EM, Puri BK (eds): Handbook of Transcranial Magnetic Stimulation. London, Arnold, 2002, pp 30–38.

51 Sommer M, Alfaro A, Rummel M, Speck S, Lang N, Tings T, Paulus W: Half sine, monophasic and biphasic transcranial magnetic stimulation of the human motor cortex. Clin Neurophysiol 2006;117:838–844.

52 Tings T, Lang N, Tergau F, Paulus W, Sommer M: Orientation-specific fast rTMS maximizes corticospinal inhibition and facilitation. Exp Brain Res 2005;164:323–333.

53 Taylor JL, Loo CK: Stimulus waveform influences the efficacy of repetitive transcranial magnetic stimulation. J Affect Disord, in press.

54 Sommer M, Paulus W: Pulse configuration and rTMS efficacy: a review of clinical studies. Suppl Clin Neurophysiol 2003;56:33–41.

55 Belmaker B, Fitzgerald P, George MS, Lisanby SH, Pascual-Leone A, Schlaepfer TE, Wassermann E: Managing the risks of repetitive transcranial stimulation. CNS Spectr 2003;8:489.

56 Moscrip TD, Terrace HS, Sackeim HA, Lisanby SH: Randomized controlled trial of the cognitive side-effects of magnetic seizure therapy (MST) and electroconvulsive shock (ECS). Int J Neuropsychopharmacol 2006;9:1–11.
57 Lisanby S, Husain M, Morales O, Thornton WL, White PF, Payne N, Rush AJ, Sackeim H: Controlled clinical trial of the antidepressant efficacy of magnetic seizure therapy in the treatment of major depression. ACNP Annu Meet Abstr 2003;166.
58 Dwork AJ, Arango V, Underwood M, Ilievski B, Rosoklija G, Sackeim H, Lisanby S: Absence of histological lesions in primate models of electroconvulsive therapy (ECT) and magnetic seizure therapy (MST). Am J Psychiatry 2004;161:576–578.
59 Moscrip T, Terrace H, Sackeim H, Lisanby SH: A primate model of the anterograde and retrograde amnesia produced by convulsive treatment. J ECT 2004;20:26–36.
60 Moscrip T, Terrace H, Sackeim H, Lisanby S: A primate model of the cognitive and electrophysiological effects of electroconvulsive shock (ECS) and magnetic seizure therapy (MST). J ECT 2004;20:64.
61 Scalia J, Lisanby S, Underwood M, Sackeim H, Dwork AJ, Morales O, Fung E, Arango V: The spatial distribution of mossy fiber sprouting in a non-human primate model for electroconvulsive therapy and magnetic seizure therapy. Biol Psychiatry 2004;55:207S.
62 Morales O, Luber B, Kwon E, Ellsasser R, Sackeim HA, Lisanby SH: Prolactin response to convulsive therapy: magnetic seizure therapy (MST) versus electroconvulsive shock (ECS) in nonhuman primates. J ECT 2003;19:58A.
63 Lisanby SH, Pakkenberg B, Dwork AJ, Christensen JR, Larsen KB, Scalia J, Underwood M, Sackeim HA, Arango V: Stereological and neuropathological examination of the safety of electroconvulsive shock (ECS) and magnetic seizure therapy (MST) in nonhuman primates. Biol Psychiatry 2005;57:147S.
64 Perera TD, Luber B, Nobler MS, Prudic J, Anderson C, Sackeim HA: Seizure expression during electroconvulsive therapy: relationships with clinical outcome and cognitive side effects. Neuropsychopharmacology 2004;29:813–825.
65 Lisanby S, Moscrip T, Luber B, Truesdale M, Reyes N, Trottmann L, Terrace HS: Randomized controlled trial of the cognitive side effects of magnetic seizure therapy and electroconvulsive shock. ACNP Annu Meet Abstr 2005;30:178S.
66 Iyer MB, Schleper N, Wassermann EM: Priming stimulation enhances the depressant effect of low-frequency repetitive transcranial magnetic stimulation. J Neurosci 2003;23:10867–10872.
67 Huang YZ, Edwards MJ, Rounis E, Bhatia KP, Rothwell JC: Theta burst stimulation of the human motor cortex. Neuron 2005;45:201–206.

Sarah H. Lisanby, MD
1051 Riverside Drive, Unit 21
Brain Stimulation and Therapeutic Modulation Division Department of Psychiatry
Columbia University College of Physicians and Surgeons
New York State Psychiatric Institute, New York, NY 10032 (USA)
Tel. +1 212 543 5558, Fax +1 212 543 6056, E-Mail slisanby@columbia.edu

Marcolin MA, Padberg F (eds): Transcranial Brain Stimulation for Treatment of Psychiatric Disorders.
Adv Biol Psychiatr. Basel, Karger, 2007, vol 23, pp 172–186

Induction and Modulation of Neuroplasticity by Transcranial Direct Current Stimulation

M.A. Nitsche, A. Antal, D. Liebetanz, N. Lang, F. Tergau, W. Paulus

Department of Clinical Neurophysiology, Georg August University, Göttingen, Germany

Abstract

Brain stimulation with weak direct current has recently been reintroduced as a method to elicit and modulate neuroplasticity of the human cerebral cortex. Transcranial direct current stimulation (tDCS) generates modulations of excitability during as well as up to an hour after the end of stimulation, depending on the duration of stimulation. While anodal stimulation increases excitability, cathodal stimulation reduces it. The primary mechanism is a subthreshold modification of the neuronal resting membrane potential; however, the after-effects are controlled by shifts in NMDA receptor strength. tDCS has been demonstrated to modify perceptual and cognitive functions reversibly in healthy subjects. Moreover, the results of first clinical pilot studies support its efficacy as a treatment in neurological and psychiatric diseases that are accompanied by pathological shifts in cortical activity. It is shown here that tDCS improves motor functions after stroke and reduces symptoms in tinnitus and depressed patients.

An important focus of current activities in brain research is the exploration of the properties and foundations of neuroplasticity [1, 2]. Newly developed tools such as functional imaging, sophisticated electroencephalographic and transcranial stimulation techniques enable researchers to study neuroplasticity not only in animal and slice models, but also in humans. In this context, brain stimulation with weak direct current has been awakening renewed interest as a potentially valuable tool for inducing and modulating neuroplasticity.

Some 40 years ago, the application of weak direct current was already shown to result in neuroplastic modifications. In anesthetized rats, weak direct current, delivered by intracerebral or epidural electrodes, induced activity and excitability diminutions or enhancements of the sensorimotor cortex which were stable for hours after the end of stimulation [3]. Subsequent studies revealed that these effects were dependent on protein synthesis [4] and accompanied by modifications of intracellular cAMP and calcium levels [5, 6]. Thus, they share some features with the nowadays more commonly known neuroplastic phenomena in animal experiments, namely long-term potentiation and long-term depression. Furthermore, it was demonstrated that *transcranial* application of weak direct current also induces an intracerebral current flow sufficiently large to achieve the intended effects. In monkeys, approximately 50% of the transcranially applied currents enter the brain through the skull [7] – and these results have been replicated in humans [8]. In healthy subjects, it was found that direct current stimulation changed EEG patterns and evoked potentials at the cortical level [9]. Moreover, anodal stimulation of the motor cortex was reported to optimize performance in a choice reaction time task [10, 11]. Although these early experiments in humans included some cortical stimulation, most probably the position of the electrodes used in most of the respective experiments primarily resulted in brain stem stimulation.

In the intervening years, non-invasive stimulation of the human brain via transcranial application of weak direct current was nearly forgotten. This might have been due to the lack of methods available to probe its effects on a non-phenomenological level. In the last few decades, transcranial electric and magnetic stimulation (TES, TMS), as well as functional imaging methods such as functional magnetic resonance tomography and positron emission tomography, have evolved as suitable tools to monitor changes of brain activity and excitability. Direct current stimulation has been re-evaluated and developed into a method that reliably induces and modulates neuroplasticity in the human cerebral cortex non-invasively, transcranially and painlessly in order to induce focal, prolonged – but yet reversible – shifts of cortical excitability [12–14]. This review offers an overview of the basic and functional effects of weak direct current stimulation in healthy subjects and patients suffering from neuropsychiatric disorders.

Modes of Action of Transcranial Direct Current Stimulation

Basic Features

It has now been shown in a multitude of studies that tDCS of the cerebral cortex in humans produces polarity-dependent excitability shifts during and after stimulation. Anodal tDCS enhances excitability, while cathodal stimulation diminishes it [12–14]. The efficacy of stimulation to induce the effects depends on stimulation duration, the current strength applied in relation to electrode size (and thus current density), and the orientation of the current flow

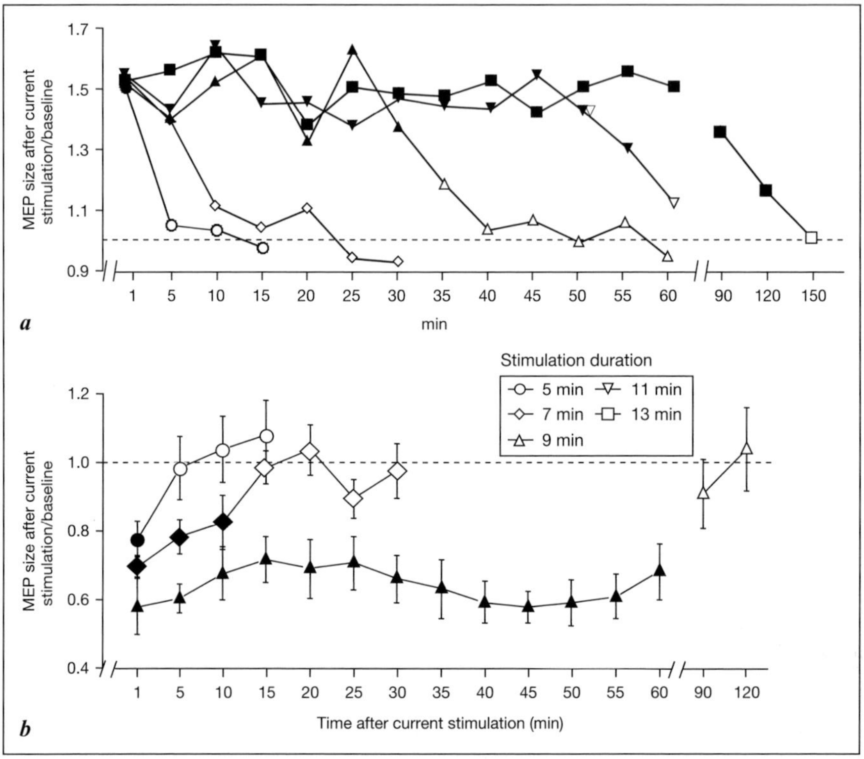

Fig. 1. tDCS of the human motor cortex modulates TMS-elicited MEP amplitudes after stimulation for up to an hour, depending on stimulation duration. Anodal stimulation (***a***) enhances, while cathodal stimulation (***b***) diminishes cortical excitability. Note that 5–7 min of stimulation results in short-lasting after-effects, while prolonged tDCS increases the duration of the after-effects overproportionally [13, 14]. Filled symbols indicate significant deviations of the MEP amplitudes relative to baseline. (With permission of *Neurology* and *Clinical Neurophysiology*).

relative to the stimulated neurons: at a current strength of 1 mA (and an electrode size of 35 cm^2), at least 3 min of tDCS are needed to induce after-effects. Conversely, if stimulated for 5 min, the minimum current strength required to induce after-effects is 0.6 mA. Prolongation of stimulation duration or increase in current strength augment the duration and strength of the after-effects [12], which can outlast the stimulation by about 1 h in healthy subjects [13, 14] (fig. 1). Moreover, as shown for the human motor cortex and for the rat hippocampus, only specific electrode positions effectively induce direct current-related shifts of excitability. Current flow along the longitudinal axis of a neuron is needed to achieve a relevant effect [12, 15].

Mechanisms of Action, as Revealed by Pharmacological and Neurophysiological Studies

The primary mechanism of tDCS for inducing cortical excitability shifts is a subthreshold modulation of the neuronal resting membrane potential. This was first shown directly in animal experiments. Here, anodal stimulation results in a subthreshold depolarization, while cathodal stimulation hyperpolarizes neuronal membranes [16, 17]. Pharmacological studies support the existence of a similar effect in humans, since here ion channel block with the voltage-dependent sodium channel blocker carbamazepine or the calcium channel antagonist flunarizine reduced the excitability-enhancing effects of anodal tDCS during stimulation, but did not influence the cathodal tDCS-generated excitability stimulation. During a short tDCS, which elicits no after-effects (stimulation duration of about 4 s), synaptic mechanisms are not involved, as shown by the absent effect of NMDA receptor antagonists, the GABA agonist lorazepam and the monoamine reuptake blocker amphetamine on the tDCS-induced excitability changes under these conditions [18–20]. Furthermore, the after-effects are not due to reverberating electrical circuits or other purely electrical phenomena, as shown in early animal experiments [4]. They depend on modifications of NMDA receptor efficacy, since these are blocked by the NMDA receptor antagonist dextromethorphan, but prolonged by the partial NMDA receptor agonist D-cycloserine [18, 21]. This tDCS polarity-dependent shift of NMDA receptor function seems to be initiated by the respective membrane potential shift and probably by the accompanying cortical activity modification, because it is prevented by the sodium channel blocker carbamazepine. Intraneuronal calcium concentration also contributes, since antagonism of calcium channels does eliminate the excitability-enhancing after-effects of anodal tDCS [18]. Similar to results obtained in animal experiments with regard to the effects of neuromodulators on neuroplasticity, the monoaminergic enhancer amphetamine consolidates the tDCS-driven excitability enhancement, probably due to β-adrenergic effects [20]. Conversely, dopaminergic (predominantly D_2) agonists seem to consolidate cathodal tDCS-generated excitability diminutions [22]. The GABAergic system is able to modulate the tDCS-induced after-effects on excitability, since at least the anodal tDCS-induced intracortical enhancement of facilitation and reduction of inhibition is abolished by lorazepam [19].

Some efforts have been made – beyond the use of pharmacology – to characterize the neuronal populations affected by tDCS. These studies have so far largely focused on motor cortical function. By comparing the size of motor-evoked potentials (MEPs) elicited by TMS with those evoked by TES, intracortical modifications can be separated from direct effects on pyramidal tract neurons. Responses to TES are dominated by direct stimulation of corticospinal axons whereas those evoked by TMS are dominated by transsynaptic activation of corticospinal neurons [23]. For the after-effects of tDCS, it has been demonstrated that TES does not modify MEPs when applied at moderate intensity – in contrast to the effect on the TMS-generated MEP amplitudes [12–14]. Thus, a predominantly intracortical effect of tDCS seems plausible. However, in another study, an impact on the TES-evoked MEP was reported for the after-effects of cathodal tDCS [24]. Since low-intensity TES, as applied in this experiment, is thought to influence the proximal aspect of pyramidal tract axons, this might be an indication for an additional membrane effect of tDCS on corticospinal neurons. Active and resting motor thresholds (MT) and input/output curves (I/O curves) resemble global measures of corticospinal excitability [25, 26]. Because within the MT paradigm TMS intensity is at threshold level by definition, the excitability of a central core region in the cortical muscle representation field is monitored here. The I/O curve serves as an index of the excitability of larger neuronal populations. Here, the slope of MEP amplitudes resulting from increased TMS intensity reflects the recruitment of neuronal populations. Active and passive MTs were not modified during anodal and cathodal tDCS or for the after-effects in one study [27]. However, they were found to be increased for the after-effects of cathodal tDCS in another study [24], probably caused by a higher current density applied in this study. For the I/O curve, anodal and cathodal tDCS influence the recruitment of neurons by TMS applied during direct current stimulation as well as during the after-effects: anodal tDCS enhances, while cathodal stimulation diminishes recruitment [27]. Thus, these results essentially confirm those obtained with single-pulse TMS. The selective effect of tDCS on the I/O curve is most probably caused by the greater population of neurons tested by this technique. The sensitivity of the I/O curve in detecting cortical excitability changes may be superior as compared to MT changes, especially because the tDCS electrodes cover a relatively large cortical area. For exploring the intracortical effects of tDCS, motor cortical inhibition and facilitation were studied [27] by a double-stimulation paradigm [28]. It was found that during tDCS intracortical facilitation is diminished by cathodal tDCS. For the after-effects of tDCS, cathodal tDCS additionally enhances inhibition, while anodal stimulation results in reversed effects [27]. However, in another study, no effect of long-lasting after-effects of tDCS on intracortical inhibition/facilitation was described [29]. It is difficult to compare the results of the two studies, since TMS test pulse amplitude, which is important for the amount of inhibition and facilitation achieved [30, 31], was not adjusted in the latter experiment, and a higher intensity of the conditioning pulse applied in that study may have led to ceiling or bottom effects. Indirect waves (I-waves) are corticospinal waves generated by motor cortex stimulation, which evolve after the first or direct corticospinal volley (direct or D-wave) and are likely under control of intracortical neuronal circuits [32].

I-wave facilitation was not influenced during short-lasting tDCS. For the after-effects, the first I-wave peak was enhanced by anodal and cathodal tDCS, while peak 4 was facilitated solely by anodal direct current stimulation [27]. The lack of a tDCS effect on I-wave facilitation by tDCS protocols which do not elicit after-effects (intra-tDCS condition) fits well with the assumption that the excitability modulation generated by tDCS in this case depends primarily on membrane polarization, while I-wave facilitation depends on synaptic mechanisms. The facilitatory effect of anodal *and* cathodal tDCS on the first I-wave within the long-lasting after-effects is surprising. Anodal stimulation may have caused an enhanced I-wave peak amplitude by increasing cortical facilitation. For the cathodal tDCS condition, this result could have been caused by a deactivating effect from inhibitory interneurons controlling the first I-wave peak, as was suggested as an explanation for the reduction of transcallosal inhibition by cathodal tDCS [33]. Alternatively, it cannot currently be ruled out that cathodal tDCS increases the excitability of subpopulations of excitatory interneurons, which influence the MEP amplitude within the first I-wave.

Taken together, the results suggest that the net corticospinal excitability modulation induced *during* tDCS, which elicits no after-effects, critically depends on membrane polarization. This is demonstrated by the results of the pharmacological studies and by the trend towards an increased slope of the I/O curve achieved by anodal tDCS and the reduced slope brought about by cathodal tDCS – but also by the little or no effect of tDCS on intracortical inhibition, facilitation and I-wave facilitation. For the *after-effects* of tDCS, the shift of the latter parameters suggests a prominent involvement of intracortical synaptic mechanisms in the resulting excitability modulations. Here, anodal tDCS increased not only the slope of the I/O curve, but also increased intracortical facilitation, diminished intracortical inhibition and increased I-wave peaks, whereas cathodal tDCS resulted in the reverse effects, with the exception of I-wave facilitation. These effects are most likely explained by tDCS-generated modifications of NMDA receptor efficacy. I/O curve, intracortical inhibition and facilitation, as well as I-wave facilitation are thought to be at least partly controlled by these receptors.

Safety Aspects

For the safety of tDCS, only limited knowledge is available so far. In general, the combination of strength of current, size of stimulated area and stimulation duration are the relevant parameters that determine the efficacy of electrical brain stimulation [34]. A formula representing these parameters is total charge [current strength (A)/area (cm^2) $\times$ stimulation duration (s)] [35]. This formula was originally developed for suprathreshold electrical stimulation, but it seems to also be appropriate for weak subthreshold direct current stimulation, because different current intensities per area will result in different amounts of neuronal de- or hyperpolarization, and it has been shown that different stimulation durations result in different time courses of the induced excitability shifts [3, 12]. Preliminary limits for a safe total charge of stimulation have been given [35]. Currently applied tDCS protocols are well below this threshold. These protocols (current strength typically 1–2 mA, electrode size between 25 and 35 cm^2, stimulation up to 20 min) should be regarded as safe, as shown by behavioural measures, EEG, serum neuron-specific enolase concentration, and diffusion-weighted and contrast-enhanced MRI measures [13, 14, 36, 37]. However, electrode positions above cranial foramina and fissures should be avoided because these could increase effective current density, and thus safety of stimulation may no longer be guaranteed.

Functional Effects of Transcranial Direct Current Stimulation

Impact of tDCS on Perception and Elementary Behaviour

In the occipital lobe, tDCS is known to be able to induce bidirectional excitability shifts of the primary visual cortex (V1). Visual cortex excitability can be monitored by determination of phosphene thresholds. Phosphenes are subjective light sensations, which are elicited by single- or double-pulse TMS of the visual cortex [38]. The phosphene threshold is the lowest TMS intensity which reliably induces phosphenes. Anodal tDCS was shown to decrease the threshold for phosphenes, while cathodal stimulation resulted in effects in the opposite direction [39]. Thus, like in the motor cortex, anodal tDCS enhances V1 excitability, while cathodal stimulation diminishes it. Likewise, it has been shown that cathodal tDCS of V1 increases contrast perception threshold [40]. In this study, anodal tDCS failed to have any effect on contrast perception, most probably due to a ceiling effect caused by the already optimum perceptual performance of the subjects without stimulation.

For the somatosensory cortex, anodal tDCS, when applied over the motor cortex representational area of the hand motor area, increases the amplitudes of somatosensory-evoked potentials (P25/N33, N33/P40) for at least 60 min after the end of stimulation [41]. Cathodal tDCS was without effect in this protocol. However, cathodal tDCS delivered over C4 – and thus perhaps more directly over the somatosensory cortex – impaired the tactile discrimination threshold [42].

With regard to elementary motor cortex function, it was demonstrated that anodal stimulation improves performance in choice reaction time tasks [10, 11, 43]. Moreover, tDCS with both polarities reduced training-induced changes of motor cortical excitability patterns and re-established the pre-use dominant pattern [44]. The most parsimonious explanation for the latter result is a deactivation of transiently, use-dependently activated networks by cathodal tDCS and a reactivation of transiently use-dependently inhibited networks by anodal tDCS. Thus, both tDCS conditions would shift the focus of excitability back to the pre-use dominant one. Furthermore, these results imply that the functional effects of tDCS may depend on task characteristics.

tDCS Affects Cognitive Performance

Since learning requires functional changes in the cortical architecture that involve excitability modulations, the induction of neuroplastic changes by weak direct current stimulation is an interesting potential tool to modulate these processes. Indeed, it was shown in some early experiments that learning processes are influenced by direct current stimulation: in monkeys, anodal stimulation of the dorsolateral prefrontal cortex improved performance in a delayed reaction time task, while cathodal stimulation of the same region worsened it [45]. The same pattern of results was found by Albert [46] and Morrell and Naitoh [47] for a conditioned avoidance task in the rabbit. Thus, an externally induced increase in cortical excitability seems to be beneficial to learning processes, while decreasing it results in a more negative outcome. This is in accordance with current opinions that long-term potentiation, which could be enhanced by an excitability elevation and diminished by a respective reduction of excitability, is the crucial mechanism for the formation of memory traces [48].

For humans, it has been shown that specifically anodal stimulation of the primary motor cortex improves implicit motor sequence learning in its acquisition phase, while stimulation of other areas, like premotor and prefrontal cortices, was without effect [43]. Likewise, anodal stimulation of the left V5, a motion-sensitive cortical area, improved learning in a visuomotor coordination task. Interestingly, cathodal tDCS of the same region improved performance of the same task in an overlearned state [49, 50]. It was speculated that different effects of tDCS on different learning phases might be due to phase specificity of neuroplastic modifications: while during learning an excitability enhancement should increase the strengthening of task-relevant synaptic connections, the benefit of suppressing task-irrelevant or distractive neuronal connections may be superior during performance of an overlearned task by shaping the task-relevant activation pattern. For implicit semantic memory processing, left frontopolar tDCS was examined. Here, anodal stimulation improved performance in a probabilistic classification learning task [51], while cathodal stimulation tended to worsen it [52].

Declarative memory can also be improved by tDCS: repetitive bilateral anodal tDCS of the dorsolateral prefrontal cortex over 30 min of total stimulation duration with a stimulation pattern of alternating 15 s on and off, applied via small electrodes with a relatively high current density, improved verbal declarative memory performance, when applied during slow-wave sleep [53]. Similarly, a significant increase in word fluency was reported after 20 min of anodal tDCS of the left dorsolateral prefrontal cortex, while cathodal stimulation decreased it mildly [36]. This effect was apparent only with a current strength of 2 mA, but not with 1 mA, which argues for a stimulation intensity-dependent effect of tDCS on the dorsolateral prefrontal cortex, in addition to that already demonstrated for the primary motor cortex [12].

Working memory is also influenced by tDCS. Fregni et al. [54] report improved performance in a three-back sequential-letter working memory task during anodal stimulation of the left dorsolateral prefrontal cortex. However, bilateral repetitive anodal and cathodal tDCS of the dorsolateral prefrontal cortex resulted in deficits of response selection and preparation in the Sternberg working memory paradigm [55]. These opposing results might be due to task characteristics, since the Sternberg paradigm demands more complex information processing than the three-back letter task, but might also be caused by the different stimulation protocols used in both studies.

Taken together, the studies undertaken so far show perceptive and behavioural effects of tDCS in relatively simple, but also complex cognitive paradigms. Although in most paradigms tested, anodal tDCS seems to improve performance, the effects depend critically on stimulation parameters (e.g. electrode position, electrode size, stimulation intensity), but also on task characteristics like complexity and learning phase. Altogether, tDCS has evolved as a useful tool to explore task-related information processing in the human cerebral cortex.

Clinical Applications

For the clinical application of tDCS, at least two main fields of interest can be identified: (a) the exploration of pathological alterations of neuroplasticity in neurological and psychiatric diseases, and (b) the evaluation of a possible clinical benefit of tDCS in these diseases. Both lines of research are still in their early days.

Pathological alterations of neuroplasticity can be studied by testing the inducibility of prolonged excitability shifts by cathodal or anodal tDCS. Moreover, combining tDCS and repetitive TMS (rTMS) might furthermore deliver information about the pathology of metaplasticity in certain neurological and psychiatric diseases. Pathology of metaplasticity was explored in patients with focal hand dystonia. In this disease, the excitability of inhibitory circuits is reduced at multiple levels of the sensorimotor system, including the hand area of the primary motor cortex. This might be caused or accompanied by a deficient function of homeostatic mechanisms, which keep cortical excitability within a normal physiological range. This hypothesis was tested by application of the homeostatic plasticity protocol introduced by Siebner et al. [29] in the respective group of patients. Here, 10 min of anodal or cathodal tDCS of the primary motor cortex are followed by 1-Hz rTMS (intensity 85% of resting MT) of the same area. In healthy subjects, anodal tDCS enhances, while cathodal tDCS reduces excitability, and this effect is reversed by subsequent rTMS. In the patients with focal hand dystonia, however, 1-Hz rTMS failed to convert the excitability enhancement induced by anodal tDCS into a clear inhibition. Moreover, cathodal tDCS did not result in a significant inhibition, nor did it modify the effect of 1-Hz rTMS on excitability [56]. Thus, homeostatic mechanisms reducing high-level cortical activity might be deficient in focal hand dystonia. The failure of cathodal tDCS alone to induce clear inhibition in this patient group might be taken as evidence for an additional, generally reduced, ability to establish inhibitory neuroplasticity.

For the evaluation of clinical benefits from tDCS-induced neuroplasticity for patients with neurological and psychiatric diseases, a limited number of pilot studies have been performed. In chronic stroke patients with paresis, motor rehabilitation can be hampered by a kind of maladaptive plasticity called 'learned non-use' [57]. Prolonged inactivity of the paretic extremity reduces its motor cortical representation and excitability, and thus compromises motor function. This may partly be caused by a contralateral motor cortex hyperactivity, which increases transcallosal inhibition of the lesioned hemisphere. Thus, enhancing excitability of the lesioned motor cortex by anodal tDCS, as well as reducing excitability of the non-lesioned contralateral one by cathodal stimulation, might improve motor function of the paretic extremity after stroke. Indeed, it was shown in chronic stroke patients with paresis of the upper limb that 20 min of anodal stimulation of the hand area in the primary motor cortex of the lesioned hemisphere improved performance with regard to fine motor skills, as evaluated by the Jebsen Taylor test [58]. In another study, it was demonstrated that 20 min of cathodal stimulation of the hand area situated within the non-leisoned cortex is equally effective [59]. The impact of short-lasting tDCS on tinnitus was tested by applying 3-min anodal, cathodal or sham stimulation to the left temporoparietal area [60]. In the motor cortex, this stimulation duration results in after-effects lasting for about 1 min after stimulation. Similar to high-frequency rTMS, anodal tDCS decreased tinnitus immediately after stimulation.

In psychiatric patients, some studies were conducted in the 1960s with a bilateral frontopolar electrode montage, and the reference electrode positioned at the knee. It was speculated that this stimulation protocol primarily stimulates the brain stem. Using this stimulation protocol, it was found that excitability-enhancing anodal stimulation diminished depressive symptoms [61], while excitability-reducing cathodal stimulation reduced manic symptoms [62].

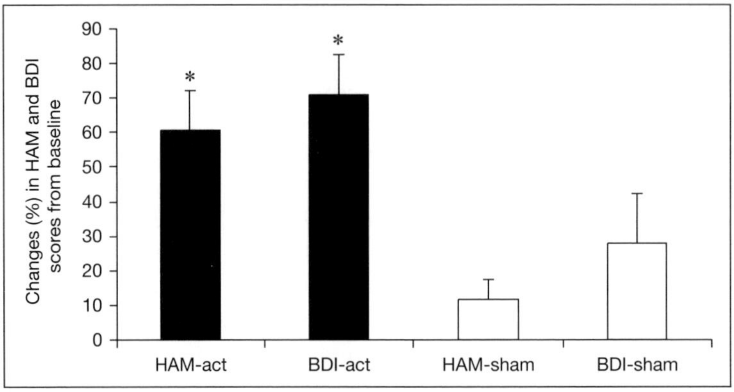

Fig. 2. Mean score changes (%) after treatment, according to the HAM and the BDI, in depressive patients treated with active tDCS (black column) and sham tDCS (white column). There was a significant improvement in depression scores measured by the HAM and the BDI after treatment only in the active tDCS group. Error bars are standard errors. Significance level (*) was assessed by the paired Student t test (comparison between the HAM and BDI scores at baseline and after treatment for both groups). Statistical significance refers to a two-tailed p value <0.05 (with permission by Fregni et al. [67]). BDI = Beck depression inventory; HAM = Hamilton depression rating scale.

Unfortunately, these results could not be replicated in all follow-up studies, possibly because of different patient subgroups, measures of changes or other factors that were not controlled for systematically (for an overview, see Lolas [63]). In schizophrenic patients, this stimulation protocol did not produce clear effects in the only study conducted [64]. In recent years, it has become increasingly clear with functional imaging methods that in depressed patients the left dorsolateral prefrontal cortex is hypoactive, while activity of the right prefrontal cortex might be increased [65]. Consequently, non-invasive stimulation techniques were applied to determine whether a normalization of prefrontal activity could diminish clinical symptoms. Indeed, activity-enhancing rTMS of the left prefrontal cortex was found to improve the clinical status of depressed patients [66]. The ability of tDCS to produce similar effects has recently been tested in a double-blind, sham-controlled pilot study [67]. Excitability-enhancing anodal tDCS of the left dorsolateral prefrontal cortex, combined with cathodal stimulation of the right frontopolar cortex, was applied for 5 alternate days in a group of patients suffering from major depression. Compared to baseline values and the sham tDCS control group, depression scores, as recorded by the Beck Depression Inventory and the Hamilton Depression Rating Scale, were significantly reduced in the treatment group (fig. 2). In view of this, tDCS could evolve as a promising new complementary method to treat depression in the future.

Although research activities with regard to clinical applications of tDCS are still in their infancy, the results obtained so far show (a) that tDCS, e.g. in combination with TMS or rTMS, could evolve as a valuable technique to study neuroplasticity as well as metaplasticity in neurological and psychiatric diseases, and (b) the possibility of using tDCS to treat diseases of the central nervous system which are accompanied by pathological alterations of cerebral excitability can be derived from the results of the aforementioned studies. However, these studies were performed mainly to prove the principle that tDCS can reduce symptoms. Thus, the stimulation durations in most cases were relatively short, stimulation intensities weak, and the effects were – perhaps with the exception of the depression study – mostly subclinical. Future studies need to show if prolonged, repetitive or stronger stimulation protocols, for which safety has to be assured, could evolve into clinically relevant improvements.

References

1 Bennett MR: The concept of long-term potentiation of transmission at synapses. Prog Neurobiol 2000;60:109–137.

2 Malenka RC, Bear MF: LTP and LTD: an embarrassment of riches. Neuron 2004;44:5–21.

3 Bindman LJ, Lippold OCJ, Redfearn JWT: The action of brief polarizing currents on the cerebral cortex of the rat (1) during current flow and (2) in the production of long-lasting after-effects. J Physiol 1964;172:369–382.

4 Gartside IB: Mechanisms of sustained increases of firing rate of neurones in the rat cerebral cortex after polarization: role of protein synthesis. Nature 1968;220:383–384.

5 Hattori Y, Moriwaki A, Hori Y: Biphasic effects of polarizing current on adenosine-sensitive generation of cyclic AMP in rat cerebral cortex. Neurosci Lett 1990;116:320–324.

6 Islam N, Aftabuddin M, Moriwaki A, Hattori Y, Hori Y: Increase in the calcium level following anodal polarization in the rat brain. Brain Res 1995;684:206–208.

7 Rush S, Driscoll DA: Current distribution in the brain from surface electrodes. Anaest Analg 1968;47:717–723.

8 Dymond AM, Coger RW, Serafetinides EA: Intracerebral current levels in man during electrosleep therapy. Biol Psychiatry 1975;10:101–104.

9 Pfurtscheller G: Changes in the evoked and spontaneous brain activity of man during extracranial polarization. Z Gesamte Exp Med 1970;152:284–293.

10 Elbert T, Lutzenberger W, Rockstroh B, Birbaumer N: The influence of low-level transcortical DC-currents on response speed in humans. Int J Neurosci 1981;14:101–114.

11 Jaeger D, Elbert T, Lutzenberger W, Birbaumer N: The effects of externally applied transcephalic weak direct currents on lateralization in choice reaction tasks. J Psychophysiol 1987;1:127–133.

12 Nitsche MA, Paulus W: Excitability changes induced in the human motor cortex by weak transcranial direct current stimulation. J Physiol 2000;527:633–639.

13 Nitsche MA, Paulus W: Sustained excitability elevations induced by transcranial DC motor cortex stimulation in humans. Neurology 2001;57:1899–1901.

14 Nitsche MA, Nitsche MS, Klein CC, Tergau F, Rothwell JC, Paulus W: Level of action of cathodal DC polarisation induced inhibition of the human motor cortex. Clin Neurophysiol 2003;114:600–604.

15 Lian J, Bikson M, Sciortino C, Stacey WC, Durand DM: Local suppression of epileptiform activity by electrical stimulation in rat hippocampus in vitro. J Physiol 2003;547:427–434.

16 Purpura DP, McMurtry JG: Intracellular activities and evoked potential changes during polarization of motor cortex. J Neurophysiol 1965;28:166–185.
17 Scholfield CN: Properties of K-currents in unmyelinated presynaptic axons of brain revealed by extracellular polarisation. Brain Res 1990;507:121–128.
18 Nitsche MA, Fricke K, Henschke U, Schlitterlau A, Liebetanz D, Lang N, Henning S, Tergau F, Paulus W: Pharmacological modulation of cortical excitability shifts induced by transcranial DC stimulation. J Physiol 2003;553:293–301.
19 Nitsche MA, Liebetanz D, Schlitterlau A, Henschke U, Fricke K, Lang N, Henning S, Frommann K, Paulus W, Tergau F: GABAergic modulation of DC-stimulation-induced motor cortex excitability shifts in the human. Eur J Neurosci 2004;19:2720–2726.
20 Nitsche MA, Grundey J, Liebetanz D, Lang N, Tergau F, Paulus W: Catecholaminergic consolidation of motor cortex plasticity in humans. Cereb Cortex 2004;14:1240–1245.
21 Nitsche MA, Jaussi W, Liebetanz D, Lang N, Tergau F, Paulus W: Consolidation of externally induced human motor cortical neuroplasticity by D-cycloserine. Neuropsychopharmacology 2004;29:1573–1578.
22 Nitsche MA, Lampe C, Antal A, Liebetanz D, Lang N, Tergau F, Paulus W: Dopaminergic modulation of DC-induced neuroplasticity in the human motor cortex. Eur J Neurosci 2006;23:1651–1657.
23 Edgley SA, Eyre JA, Lemon RN, Miller S: Comparison of activation of corticospinal neurons and spinal motor neurons by magnetic and electrical transcranial stimulation in the lumbosacral cord of the anaesthetized monkey. Brain 1997;120:839–853.
24 Ardolino G, Bossi B, Barbieri S, Priori A: Non-synaptic mechanisms underlie the after-effects of cathodal transcutaneous direct current stimulation of the human brain. J Physiol 2005;568: 553–563.
25 Abbruzzese G, Trompetto C: Clinical and research methods for evaluating cortical excitability. J Clin Neurophysiol 2002;19:307–321.
26 Chen R: Studies of human motor physiology with transcranial magnetic stimulation. Muscle Nerve Suppl 2000;9:S26–S32.
27 Nitsche MA, Seeber A, Frommann K, Klein CC, Nitsche MS, Rochford C, Liebetanz D, Lang N, Antal A, Paulus W, Tergau F: Modulating parameters of excitability during and after transcranial direct current stimulation of the human motor cortex. J Physiol 2005;568:291–303.
28 Kujirai T, Caramia MD, Day BL, Thompson PD, Ferbert A, Wroe S, Asselman P, Marsden CD: Corticocortical inhibition in human motor cortex. J Physiol 1993;471:501–519.
29 Siebner HR, Lang N, Rizzo V, Nitsche MA, Paulus W, Lemon RN, Rothwell JC: Preconditioning of low-frequency repetitive transcranial magnetic stimulation with transcranial direct current stimulation: evidence for homeostatic plasticity in the human motor cortex. J Neurosci 2004;24: 3379–3385.
30 Chen R: Interactions between inhibitory and excitatory circuits in the human motor cortex. Exp Brain Res 2004;154:1–10.
31 Stefan K, Kunesch E, Benecke R, Cohen LG, Classen J: Mechanisms of enhancement of human motor cortex excitability induced by interventional paired associative stimulation. J Physiol 2002;543:699–708.
32 Ziemann U, Rothwell JC: I-waves in motor cortex. J Clin Neurophysiol 2000;17:397–405.
33 Lang N, Nitsche MA, Paulus W, Rothwell JC, Lemon R: Effects of transcranial DC stimulation over the human motor cortex on corticospinal and transcallosal excitability. Exp Brain Res 2004;156:439–443.
34 Agnew WF, McCreery DB: Considerations for safety in the use of extracranial stimulation for motor evoked potentials. Neurosurgery 1987;20:143–147.
35 Yuen TGH, Agnew WF, Bullara LA, Jacques S, McCreery DB: Histological evaluation of neural damage from electrical stimulation: considerations for the selection of parameters for clinical application. Neurosurgery 1991;9:292–298.
36 Iyer MB, Mattu U, Grafman J, Lomarev M, Sato S, Wassermann EM: Safety and cognitive effect of frontal DC brain polarization in healthy individuals. Neurology 2005;64:872–875.
37 Nitsche MA, Niehaus L, Hoffmann KT, Hengst S, Liebetanz D, Paulus W, Meyer B-U: MRI study of human brain exposed to weak direct current stimulation of the frontal cortex. Clin Neurophysiol 2004;115:2419–2423.

38 Meyer BU, Diehl R, Steinmetz H, Britton TC, Benecke R: Magnetic stimuli applied over motor and visual cortex: influence of coil position and field polarity on motor responses, phosphenes, and eye movements. Electroencephalogr Clin Neurophysiol Suppl 1991;43:121–123.
39 Antal A, Kincses TZ, Nitsche MA, Paulus W: Manipulation of phosphene thresholds by transcranial direct current stimulation in man. Exp Brain Res 2003;150:375–378.
40 Antal A, Nitsche MA, Paulus W: External modulation of visual perception in humans. Neuroreport 2001;12:3553–3555.
41 Matsunaga K, Nitsche MA, Tsuji S, Rothwell J: Effect of trenscranial DC sensorimotor cortex stimulation on somatosensory evoked potentials in humans. Clin Neurophysiol 2004;115:456–460.
42 Rogalewski A, Breitenstein C, Nitsche MA, Paulus W, Knecht S: Transcranial direct current stimulation disrupts tactile perception. Eur J Neurosci 2004;20:313–316.
43 Nitsche MA, Schauenburg A, Lang N, Liebetanz D, Exner C, Paulus W, Tergau F: Facilitation of implicit motor learning by weak transcranial direct current stimulation of the primary motor cortex in the human. J Cogn Neurosci 2003;15:619–626.
44 Rosenkranz K, Nitsche MA, Tergau F, Paulus W: Diminution of transient motor cortex plasticity by weak transcranial direct current stimulation in the human. Neurosci Lett 2000;296:61–63.
45 Rosen SC, Stamm JS: Transcortical polarization: facilitation of delayed response performance by monkeys. Exp Neurol 1972;35:282–289.
46 Albert DJ: The effects of polarizing currents on the consolidation of learning. Neuropsychologia 1966;4:65–77.
47 Morrell F, Naitoh P: Effect of polarization on a conditioned avoidance response. Exp Neurol 1962;6:507–523.
48 Rioult-Pedotti MS, Friedman D, Donoghue JP: Learning-induced LTP in neocortex. Science 2000;290:533–536.
49 Antal A, Nitsche MA, Kincses TZ, Kruse W, Hoffmann K-P, Paulus W: Facilitation of visuo-motor learning by transcranial direct current stimulation of the motor and extrastriate visual areas in humans. Eur J Neurosci 2004;19:2888–2892.
50 Antal A, Nitsche MA, Kruse W, Hoffmann K-P, Paulus W: Visuomotor coordination is improved by transcranial direct current stimulation of the human visual cortex. J Cogn Neurosci 2004;16: 521–527.
51 Knowlton BJ, Mangels JA, Squire LR: A neostriatal habit learning system in humans. Science 1996;273:1399–1340.
52 Kincses TZ, Antal A, Nitsche MA, Bártfai O, Paulus W: Facilitation of probabilistic classification learning by transcranial direct current stimulation of the prefrontal cortex in the human. Neuropsychologia 2003;42:113–117.
53 Marshall L, Molle M, Hallschmid M, Born J: Transcranial direct current stimulation during sleep improves declarative memory. J Neurosci 2004;24:9985–9992.
54 Fregni F, Boggio PS, Nitsche M, Bermpohl F, Antal A, Feredoes E, Marcolin MA, Rigonatti SP, Silva MTA, Paulus W, Pascual-Leone A: Anodal transcranial direct current stimulation of prefrontal cortex enhances working memory. Exp Brain Res 2005;166:23–30.
55 Marshall L, Molle M, Siebner HR, Born J: Bifrontal transcranial direct current stimulation slows reaction time in a working memory task. BMC Neurosci 2005;6:23.
56 Quartarone A, Rizzo V, Bagnato S, Morgante F, Sant'Angelo A, Romano M, Crupi D, Girlanda P, Rothwell JC, Siebner HR: Homeostatic-like plasticity of the primary motor hand area is impaired in focal hand dystonia. Brain 2005;128:1943–1950.
57 Liepert J, Miltner WH, Bauder H, Sommer M, Dettmers C, Taub E, Weiller C: Motor cortex plasticity during constraint-induced movement therapy in stroke patients. Neurosci Lett 1998;250:5–8.
58 Hummel F, Celnik P, Giraux P, Floel A, Wu WH, Gerloff C, Cohen LG: Effects of non-invasive cortical stimulation on skilled motor function in chronic stroke. Brain 2005;128:490–499.
59 Fregni F, Boggio PS, Mansur CG, Wagner T, Ferreira MJL, Lima M, Rigonatti SP, Marcolin MA, Freedman SD, Nitsche MA, Pascual-Leone A: Transcranial direct current stimulation of the unaffected hemisphere in stroke patients. Neuroreport 2005;16:1551–1555.
60 Fregni F, Marcondes R, Boggio P, Marcolin MA, Rigonatti SP, Sanchez TG, Nitsche MA, Pascual-Leone A: Transient tinnitus suppression induced by repetitive transcranial magnetic stimulation and transcranial direct current stimulation. J Neurol 2006;13:996–1001.

61 Costain R, Redfearn JW, Lippold OC: A controlled trial of the therapeutic effect of polarization of the brain in depressive illness. Br J Psychiatry 1964;110:786–799.
62 Carney MW: Negative polarisation of the brain in the treatment of manic states. Ir J Med Sci 1969;8:133–135.
63 Lolas F: Brain polarization: behavioral and therapeutic effects. Biol Psychiatry 1977;12:37–47.
64 Lifshitz K, Harper P: A trial of transcranial polarization in chronic schizophrenics. Br J Psychiatry 1968;114:635–637.
65 Schutter DJ, van Honk J: A framework for targeting alternative brain regions with repetitive transcranial magnetic stimulation in the treatment of depression. J Psychiatry Neurosci 2005;30:91–97.
66 Loo CK, Mitchell PB: A review of the efficacy of transcranial magnetic stimulation (TMS) treatment for depression, and current and future strategies to optimize efficacy. J Affect Disord 2005;88:255–267.
67 Fregni F, Boggio PS, Nitsche MA, Marcolin MA, Rigonatti SP, Pascual-Leone A: Treatment of major depression with transcranial direct current stimulation. Bipolar Disord 2006;8:203–204.

M.A. Nitsche
Robert-Koch-Strasse 40
DE–37099 Göttingen (Germany)
Tel. +49 551 399571, Fax +49 551 398126, E-Mail mnitsch1@gwdg.de

Marcolin MA, Padberg F (eds): Transcranial Brain Stimulation for Treatment of Psychiatric Disorders.
Adv Biol Psychiatr. Basel, Karger, 2007, vol 23, pp 187–203

Theta Burst Stimulation

Ying-Zu Huang[a], *John C. Rothwell*[b]

[a]Department of Neurology, Chang Gung Memorial Hospital and Chang Gung University College of Medicine, Taipei, Taiwan, ROC; [b]Sobell Department of Motor Neuroscience and Movement Disorders, Institute of Neurology, University College London, London, UK

Abstract

It has proved possible in experimental animals to manipulate synaptic efficiency using direct electrical stimulation. The introduction of transcranial methods of non-invasively stimulating the human brain raised hopes that similar effects could be produced in humans, with the potential for eventual therapeutic application in disease states. However, human subjects often require lengthy conditioning with traditional repetitive transcranial magnetic stimulation (rTMS), and even then effects are often weak, variable and have only mild benefits in a therapeutic setting. To address some of these concerns, we developed novel rTMS paradigms, which can swiftly produce relatively strong and controllable long-term changes in the excitability of cortical circuits after only a few minutes of conditioning. They are based on theta burst stimulation (TBS) patterns of neuronal firing occurring in the hippocampus of animals and use low-intensity (80% of active motor threshold) stimulation to produce long-term depression-like and long-term potentiation-like effects on the motor system of conscious humans. These can be measured at an electrophysiological and behavioural level as effects that outlast the period of stimulation by over an hour. In particular, we have found that the pattern of delivery of TBS (continuous versus intermittent) is crucial in determining the direction of change in synaptic efficiency.

The nervous system has a remarkably flexible organisation that allows it to analyse, store, and react to changes inside or outside the body in an efficient and appropriate manner throughout life. This kind of complex adaptation, termed (neural) plasticity, seems to be present to a greater or lesser extent from the embryo to late life [1]. It is widely accepted that long-lasting changes in the efficiency of synaptic transmission, including long-term potentiation (LTP) and long-term depression (LTD), form the basis of neural plasticity. In the past, attention focussed on the role of plasticity in development but more recently interest has focussed on the possible role of neural plasticity in reacting to and compensating for chronic injury or neurological disease.

There are many ways of inducing plasticity naturally or artificially in animal preparations. Among them, repetitive electrical stimulation of neural pathways first introduced by Lømo, Bliss and others in the late 1960s to early 1970s is the most efficient way of achieving plasticity, and is still the most commonly used protocol. One of the most effective patterns of stimulation for producing LTP is the 'theta burst' paradigm [2], which was developed to mimic the normal pattern of neural firing in the hippocampus of rats during exploratory behaviour [3]. It consists of very short bursts of high-frequency stimulation at 100–200 Hz which are repeated at 5 Hz (the theta range of frequencies in EEG terminology) for a period of around 2 s. For example, theta burst stimulation (TBS) of Schaffer/commissural projections to the CA1 field of the rat induced LTP lasting more than 1 h in the hippocampus. LTD, in contrast, is often induced by slow-frequency (<10 Hz) stimulation [4], although in some systems continuous high-frequency stimulation may have a similar effect if the membrane potential of the postsynaptic neurone is changed, for example by concurrent synaptic activity or by artificial polarisation of the membrane [5].

The development of repetitive transcranial magnetic stimulation (rTMS), as a technique for non-invasive and painless stimulation of the human brain, led to the expectation that effects similar to those observed in animal models could be produced in conscious humans. If this were possible, it was reasoned that rTMS might have potential therapeutic applications by offering a non-invasive method of inducing plasticity in conscious humans that could be used to treat brain diseases due to hyper- or hypoexcitability in the brain.

However, the results of traditional paradigms of rTMS have been disappointing, and often weak and inconsistent. There are several possible reasons for the previous disappointing results. First, even in animal experiments, it has been difficult to demonstrate LTP/LTD in the cortex of awake and freely moving animals without the use of extended or repeated sessions of stimulation [6]. Second, concerns over safety have limited many studies on humans to the use of relatively low frequencies of stimulation of 25 Hz or (usually) below. This type of stimulation can certainly produce effects on neural systems in humans that outlast the period of stimulation, and which have some characteristics that are similar to those seen in animal studies [7]. However, conditioning with low frequencies of stimulation is slow, and in human studies the ratio of the time taken to apply the stimulation to the duration of the after-effect is only about 1:1, which is clearly not practical for a therapeutic application. In addition, the effect observed after rTMS in humans is subject to notable interindividual variability [8], and behavioural effects have been elusive [9] without the use of complex experimental paradigms [10]. Third, only protocols with regular frequency have been tried in rTMS, while successful paradigms in animal studies often use patterned stimulation, for example, theta burst stimulation (TBS). In addition, TMS in humans is relatively non-focal, and therefore cannot be used to target spatially specific neural connections. In response to these problems, we developed TMS paradigms based on TBS patterns: i.e. patterned, high-frequency stimulation using relatively low intensities.

The Effect of a Short Burst

As a preparatory investigation prior to the introduction of TBS in humans, we explored the effect of applying a single short burst of high-frequency rTMS to the human motor cortex in order to document its effects on corticospinal excitability. The safety guidelines for rTMS [11] do not extend to frequencies above 25 Hz, so we were deliberately conservative in the intensities that we applied at 50 Hz. Due to safety concerns and the availability of the equipment, we decided to use intensities of up to 80% of active motor threshold (AMT) given at 50 Hz with up to 15 pulses per burst.

We first tested the effect of burst length and intensity. In this part, we examined the changes in amplitude of motor-evoked potential (MEP) and short-interval intracortical inhibition (SICI) that occurred 20 ms after bursts at 50 Hz with different lengths and different stimulus intensities. The paradigms that test SICI in humans are thought to monitor excitability in local intracortical circuits involving $GABA_A$ergic connections [12, 13]. We delivered a short burst at three different stimulus intensities: 50, 70 and 80% of AMT. Both 5- and 15-pulse bursts were given at each stimulus intensity. Figure 1 shows the effect on MEP amplitude and SICI. At the intensities we used, both 5- and 15-pulse bursts had the same effect on MEP and SICI. Post hoc comparison of the combined data from the 5- and 15-pulse bursts with the control MEP amplitude showed that bursts at 70 and 80% AMT increased the amplitude of MEPs by approximately 38 and 48% [14], respectively, whereas they decreased the amount of SICI from 58 to 78% control and from 62 to 85% control [14], respectively. There was no effect on MEP and SICI with stimulation at 50% AMT. In addition, we also showed that H-reflex in the contralateral flexor carpi radialis was not affected by a 5-pulse burst at 80% AMT [14].

Interpreting the reduced percent SICI at 20 ms after a burst of 5 pulses is difficult because the MEP was also facilitated at that time. Although SICI is usually more prominent the larger the MEP [15], facilitation of the response might also increase the effective amplitude of the conditioning stimulus. Given that there is a 'U'-shaped dependence of SICI on conditioning intensity [13], it

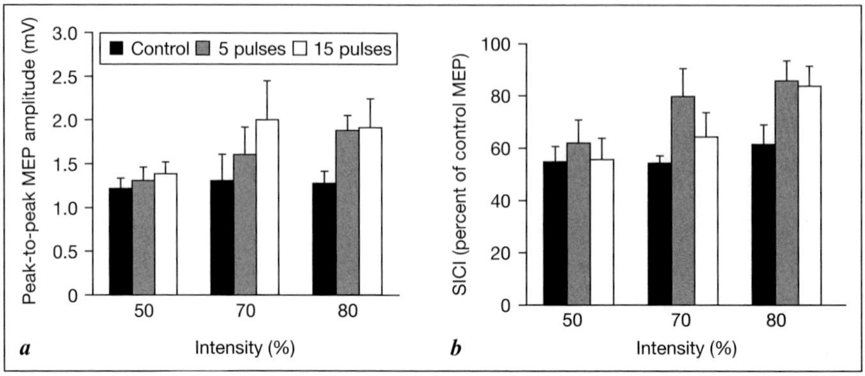

Fig. 1. The effect of bursts at 50 Hz on MEP amplitude (***a***) and SICI (***b***). SICI is expressed as a percentage of the unconditioned MEP in each subject. This figure represents group data. Error bars refer to the standard error of the measurements [14].

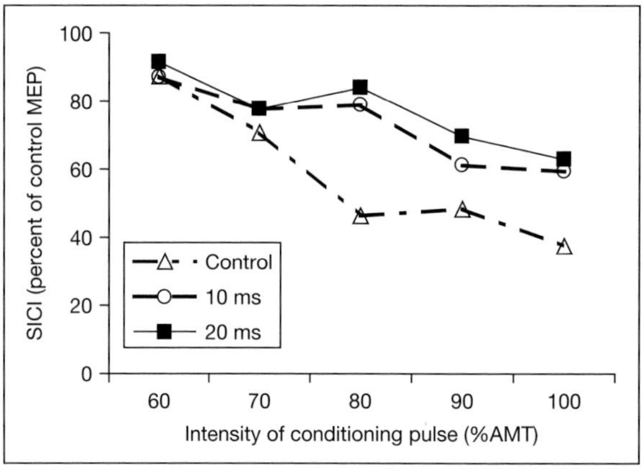

Fig. 2. The effect of a 5-pulse burst at 50 Hz and 80% AMT on the amount of SICI using different intensities of the conditioning pulse (x-axis). SICI is expressed as a percentage of the unconditioned MEP in each subject [14].

is possible that increasing the effectiveness of the conditioning stimulus would decrease SICI. In order to overcome this problem, we investigated whether the threshold for producing SICI was changed by a conditioning burst of 5 pulses at 80% AMT. SICI was tested at both 10 and 20 ms after the end of the burst, and 5 different intensities of the conditioning stimulus were used to evoke inhibition: 60, 70, 80, 90, and 100% AMT. The results (fig. 2) at 10 and 20 ms did not differ from each other but each differed from the control data in which no burst

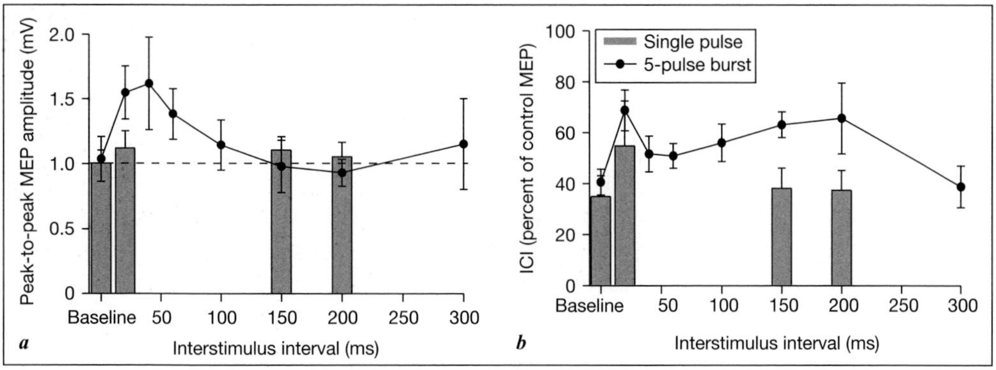

Fig. 3. Comparison of the effect of a single-pulse (bars) and a 5-pulse burst at 50 Hz (symbols and lines) both at an intensity of 80% AMT. ***a*** The time course of the effect on the MEP amplitude. ***b*** The time course of the effect on SICI presented as a percentage of unconditioned MEP. The x-axis represents the interval between the single pulse or the last pulse in the conditioning train and the time of the test MEP [14].

had been given in advance. There was significantly more inhibition in the control data at all intensities of stimulation [14].

We also checked the influence of a 5-pulse burst on the resting motor threshold (RMT) or AMT at 20 ms after the end of the burst. The RMT was significantly reduced from 53 ± 19% to 46 ± 15% by a burst of 5 pulses at 80% AMT, whereas the AMT was not significantly changed [14].

In a second stage, we looked in more detail at the effects of 5-pulse bursts delivered at 50 Hz and 80% AMT on MEP amplitude and SICI at a wider range of intervals between 20 and 300 ms after the end of each burst. We found that 5-pulse bursts at 50 Hz could produce short-lasting after-effects that were larger and longer in duration than those seen after application of a single conditioning stimulus of the same intensity (fig. 3) [14]. A single conditioning stimulus at 80% AMT had no effect on the amplitude of subsequent test MEPs at intervals of ≥20 ms. However, a burst of 5 pulses increased test MEPs at 20 and 40 ms after the end of the burst. As noted above, the low intensity of the stimuli in the burst is unlikely to have produced any descending activity in the corticospinal tract and therefore this increase in excitability is likely to be cortical in origin. The mechanism is unclear, although it is interesting to note that Valls-Sole et al. [16] also saw facilitation of test MEPs at about 50 ms after a single, larger, conditioning stimulus. One possibility is that the stimuli in the burst were at around the threshold intensity for intracortical facilitation (ICF) [17]. In this case, the first stimulus of the burst might have produced a subthreshold period of ICF which was still present when the second pulse of the burst was applied 20 ms (i.e. 50 Hz) later. This could continue for the remaining 3 pulses of the burst and result in a period of cortical facilitation resembling that seen after a single larger conditioning stimulus.

As with the MEP, a burst of 5 pulses had a stronger effect on SICI than a single pulse of the same intensity. However, the time course of the effect on SICI was longer than that on the MEP, suggesting that (at least at intervals of 150 and 200 ms) they were mediated by two separate mechanisms. There have been two previous studies of the effects of a single conditioning stimulus on SICI in the motor cortex, but the intensity of the stimulus and the interval at which SICI was tested were different to those used here. Sanger et al. [18] found that SICI was decreased 100 ms after a suprathreshold stimulus; Bestmann et al. [19] found that a stimulus which produced no SICI when given alone could increase SICI at intervals of 4 ms or less. The present data appear to show that a single stimulus of 80% AMT had no significant effect on SICI when tested 20–200 ms later.

The increase in the effect on SICI of a 5-pulse burst is not unexpected and implies some form of facilitation of the effects of each single pulse when given at a frequency of 50 Hz. However, the interpretation of the effect on SICI is complicated by the fact that the burst also increases the amplitude of MEPs. There are two possible confounding factors. First, the amplitude of the test MEP in the SICI paradigm is increased by rTMS. However, this is usually associated with a small increase in the amount of SICI [15] rather than the reduction we saw in the present experiments. In addition, we still observed a significant decrease in SICI in 3 subjects in whom we adjusted the test intensity to maintain the amplitude of the test MEP following a burst at 1 mV [14]. The second confounding factor is that previous work has shown that SICI is maximal at particular conditioning intensities (about 80–100% AMT at an SICI interval of 3 ms), and is smaller at intensities above and below that value. The 50-Hz burst, by analogy with its effect on the MEP, could have increased the effectiveness of the conditioning pulse and hence decreased SICI. This seems unlikely to have happened since we found that the 50-Hz burst increased the threshold for producing SICI and reduced the amount of inhibition at all intensities of conditioning stimulus. Finally, it should be noted that the threshold for SICI was expressed relative to AMT, and that control experiments confirmed that this was not affected by rTMS. We therefore conclude that the 50-Hz burst effect on SICI was not secondary to an effect on the excitability of the test or conditioning pulse used to measure SICI.

The 5-pulse burst of 50 Hz reduced SICI for about 200 ms. It is possible that the reduced SICI at long intervals (e.g. 150 and 200 ms) is linked to the observations of Sanger et al. [18] of a similar reduction at the same intervals after a single suprathreshold pulse. Perhaps 5 pulses of low intensity at 50 Hz can summate leading to this same mechanism. Sanger et al. [18] explained their effect as being due to an interaction between long-interval intracortical inhibition and SICI. If the 50-Hz burst were inducing this effect, it might be a useful method of invoking long-interval intracortical inhibition without the preceding MEP evoked by a single large conditioning stimulus.

The results of the short-burst study confirm that it is safe and possible to condition the human motor cortex with short bursts of 50-Hz rTMS using very low intensity pulses. We therefore felt confident to apply longer-lasting theta burst conditioning to the human cortex to study long-term after-effects at cortical synapses in a similar way as it has been so successfully applied in animal experiments.

Theta Burst Stimulation

The basic TBS pattern of rTMS is a burst containing 3 pulses of 50-Hz magnetic stimulation at 80% AMT given every 200 ms (i.e. at 5 Hz). We have investigated the effects of two different stimulation paradigms (fig. 4a). The first paradigm, which we have called intermittent theta burst stimulation (iTBS), mimics the TBS stimulation that has long been used for producing LTP in animal preparations [2, 20]. We gave the basic pattern in a short train lasting 2 s (i.e. 10 bursts), repeated every 10 s for 20 cycles (a total of 600 pulses). The second paradigm, which we have called continuous theta burst stimulation (cTBS), delivers the basic pattern in a continuous train lasting 40 s (cTBS600; i.e., 200 bursts and a total of 600 pulses) or 20 s (cTBS300; i.e., 100 bursts and a total 300 pulses). We assessed the consequences of these different stimulation paradigms by assessing the time course of changes in MEP size elicited from the contralateral first dorsal interosseous muscle by a single pulse of TMS delivered at a set intensity (the intensity required to produce an MEP of 1 mV) before and after conditioning. RMT and AMT were also measured before and at 10 min after the end of cTBS300.

We have not observed, and subjects have not reported any serious adverse effects in any of the TBS experiments so far. There was also no problem with overheating of the stimulation coil with this low intensity of stimulation. When the stimuli were given in the iTBS pattern, MEPs were facilitated after 190 s of stimulation for about 19 min (fig. 4b) [21]. This parallels the LTP phenomenon induced by TBS in animal preparations. However, when we gave all the bursts continuously without a pause, i.e. cTBS, to enhance the facilitatory effect, we surprisingly saw totally opposite results. MEPs were dramatically suppressed for about 60 min after cTBS600 (fig. 5b), even though the protocol uses the same number of stimuli as iTBS. When the cTBS was shortened from 40 to

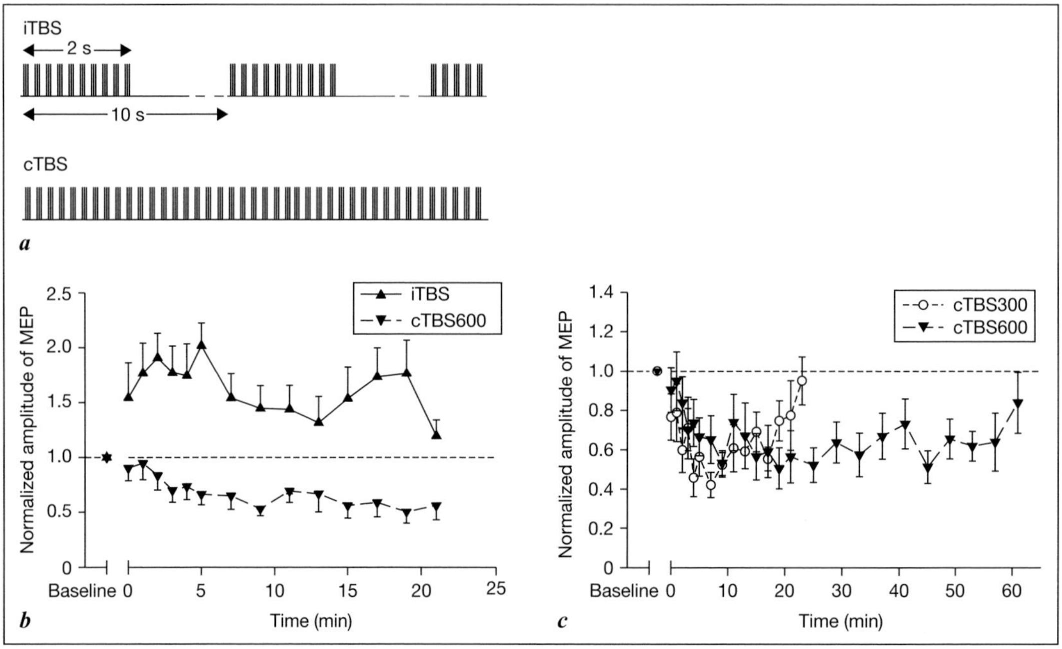

Fig. 4. Paradigms of TBS and their effects on MEPs. ***a*** Graphical illustration of the two stimulation paradigms of TBS. Each paradigm uses a TBS pattern in which 3 pulses of stimulation are given at 50 Hz, repeated every 200 ms. In the iTBS pattern, a 2-second train of TBS is repeated every 10 s for a total of 190 s (600 pulses). In the cTBS paradigm, a 20-second or 40-second train of uninterrupted TBS is given (300 or 600 pulses). ***b*** The time course of changes following conditioning with iTBS (d) or cTBS600 (f). There was a significant facilitation of MEP size following iTBS lasting for about 15 min, and a significant reduction of MEP size following cTBS lasting for nearly 60 min. ***c*** Comparison of the effects of cTBS given for 20 s [300 pulses; cTBS300 (y)] with the same paradigm given for 40 s [600 pulses; cTBS600 (f)]. There was a significant effect of duration of cTBS conditioning on the time course of the effect [significant TIME × DURATION interaction ($F_{14, 112} = 2.24$, $p < 0.05$)] with the effect of cTBS300 lasting about 20 min compared to the effect of cTBS600 which lasted about 60 min (modified from Huang et al. [21]).

20 s, i.e. cTBS300, the suppression lasted for more than 20 min (fig. 4c) [21]. Our different TBS paradigms have large effect sizes and acceptable interindividual variability compared with traditional rTMS paradigms. Thus, the mean percentage change of the MEP size in the period where the maximum effect occurred (i.e. 7–14 min after cTBS300, 15–40 min after cTBS600, 1–10 min after iTBS) was −45.0% (SD = 8.9%), −42.2% (SD = 24.0%) and 75.7% (SD = 40.9%), respectively. These effect sizes and variability compare well with traditional rTMS paradigms, such as those explored by Maeda et al. [8],

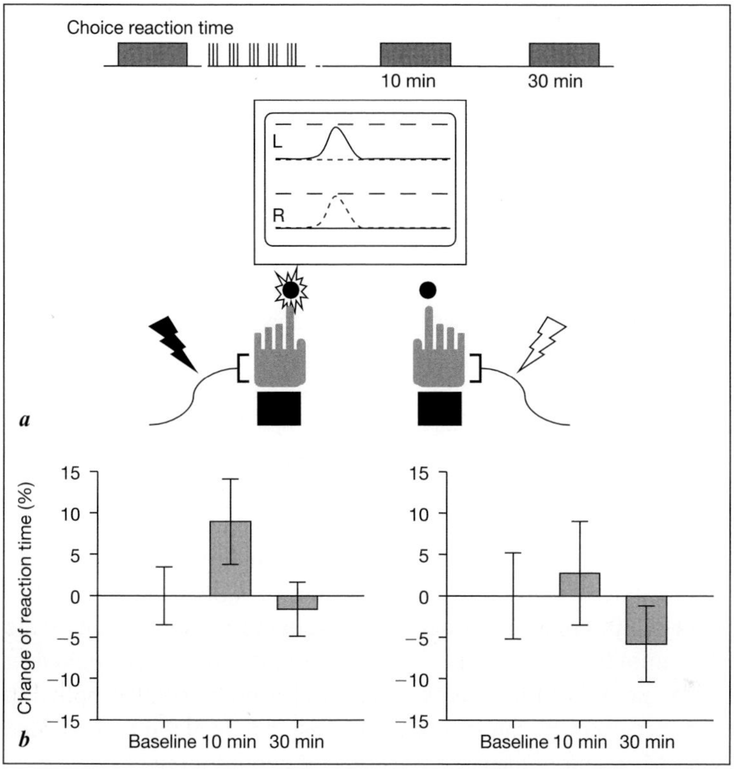

Fig. 5. The changes in choice reaction time following cTBS. ***a*** A graphical illustration of the choice reaction time task. Electrodes were attached to the ulnar side of the hands. Electrical stimuli were delivered through these electrodes in a random sequence. Subjects were instructed to press the button with the index finger of the hand stimulated as quickly as possible, when they felt a stimulus. In addition, they were asked to press the button with a certain force. Visual feedback as to the accuracy of the force with which they pressed the button was given on a screen in front of the subject. ***b*** There was a significant lengthening of reaction time in the conditioned hand 10 min after cTBS [$F(2, 16) = 4.30$, $p < 0.05$], and a significant shortening of reaction time in the unconditioned hand 30 min after cTBS [$F(2, 16) = 7.82$, $p < 0.005$]. Modified from Huang et al. [21].

where a much larger number of rTMS pulses (1,600) produced mean effects of −34.03% (SD = 37.87%) after 1 Hz and 37.87% (SD = 53.59%) after 10 Hz. In addition, we found that cTBS300 increased the RMT from 49.0 ± 8.9% to 51.0 ± 9.7% of maximum output of the magnetic stimulator, while AMT stayed unchanged [21].

Given the very low intensity of the individual pulses (80% AMT), it is highly unlikely that TBS produced any activity in descending corticospinal fibres, and therefore that there were any direct effects of TBS on the excitability of circuits in the spinal cord. However, as a further test of this, we compared the effect of cTBS300 on MEPs evoked in forearm flexor muscles with that on the spinal H-reflex evoked in the same muscles. MEPs were suppressed to 76.5% of control size in these muscles following cTBS300, but the H-reflex was not significantly affected [21].

We have therefore demonstrated that stimulation over the motor hand area in healthy subjects using frequencies of rTMS based on theta burst patterns can produce rapid changes in the function of the motor system that outlast the period of stimulation by over 60 min. These long-lasting, consistent and significant effects were produced despite very short periods of conditioning (20–192 s) and very low stimulus intensities (80% of AMT). This is in contrast to many previous paradigms of rTMS in humans, which have required much longer periods of conditioning at higher stimulus intensities to have an effect of similar duration [7].

The data show that the effects on the motor system depend on the pattern of stimulation and state of the motor system when the TBS is applied. Thus, cTBS for 20 s (cTBS300) reduces corticospinal excitability, as indicated by the decline in MEP amplitudes, whereas the same number of pulses applied at 15 Hz for the same period of time has no effect [21]. However, TBS applied in an intermittent pattern (iTBS) can increase corticospinal excitability, indicated by the increase in MEP amplitudes after this type of conditioning.

Furthermore, cTBS300 produced clear changes in a two-choice reaction task in which subjects had to press buttons with the left or right hand in response to an electrical stimulation [21]. This is the first time that a behavioural effect on such a simple task has been shown with methods of conditioning the motor cortex. In this experiment, cTBS was applied to the left hemisphere and reaction times were measured in the right (conditioned) and left (unconditioned) hands to electrical stimuli applied randomly to each hand (fig. 5a). The reaction time of the conditioned hand was slowed by cTBS by around 10% for at least 10 min, while the reaction time of the unconditioned hand remained unchanged. In addition, a decrease in reaction times 30 min after cTBS300 was noticed (fig. 5b) [21]. The finding of a significant slowing of reaction time following just 20 s of cTBS is notable, as a clear behavioural effect on such a simple task has been difficult to produce previously with other kinds of rTMS [9]. It seems likely that the significant shortening of reaction time that was observed in the unconditioned hand 30 min after conditioning is a learning effect. A similar effect was not observed in the conditioned hand, perhaps indicating that conditioning with cTBS not only affected reaction time, but also motor learning. It is also possible that the hypofunction of the left hemisphere caused by TBS produced a reciprocal hyperfunction of the right hemisphere, facilitating motor responses in the unconditioned hand via a similar mechanism to that observed in human subjects following unilateral stroke [22]. However, further experiments are needed to address these possibilities directly.

Mechanisms of Theta Burst Stimulation

MEPs evoked in the forearm flexor muscles by a standard pulse of TMS were smaller after cTBS, whereas spinal H-reflexes in the same muscle were unaffected. The simplest explanation for this is that spinal motoneurones and the synaptic input from the H-reflex are unaffected by cTBS, and that changes in MEP are due to changes in the excitability of circuits in the cortex. Since MEPs evoked in hand and forearm muscles by TMS pulses are produced by transsynaptic excitation of corticospinal projection neurones [23], this would imply either an increase in the effectiveness of that synaptic input or an increase in the baseline excitability of the corticospinal neurones that receive it. A lack of effect of TBS on spinal circuits would also be consistent with the very low intensity (80% AMT) of the pulses we employed for TBS: well below the threshold for evoking any direct corticospinal effects. However, it is possible that the population of spinal motoneurones tested by the H-reflex is different from that activated by the MEP, so that a small spinal component to the MEP change may exist.

As further evidence that TBS has an effect on the excitability of intrinsic cortical circuits, we measured SICI and ICF before and after iTBS and cTBS300 using a standard paired-pulse paradigm. We assessed SICI at interstimulus intervals of 2 and 3 ms using a conditioning intensity of 80% AMT, and ICF at interstimulus intervals of 10 and 15 ms with a conditioning intensity of 90% AMT. Because cTBS increased the RMT but keeps AMT the same, we adjusted the intensity of the test stimuli while assessing SICI and ICF after TBS to maintain the amplitude of test MEPs at approximately 1 mV. We found that SICI was significantly increased following iTBS, while ICF remained the same. In contrast, cTBS reduced the amount of SICI and ICF (fig. 6) [21].

The paradigms that test SICI and ICF in humans are thought to monitor excitability in local intracortical circuits, some of which involve $GABA_A$ergic connections [12, 13]. This makes it highly likely that a change in SICI and ICF is due to an effect on the excitability of connections in these circuits. It is interesting to note that, like the MEP data, effects of TBS depend on the pattern of stimulation. Thus, both SICI and ICF are suppressed following cTBS. The effects of iTBS are less pronounced, with the only significant effect being an

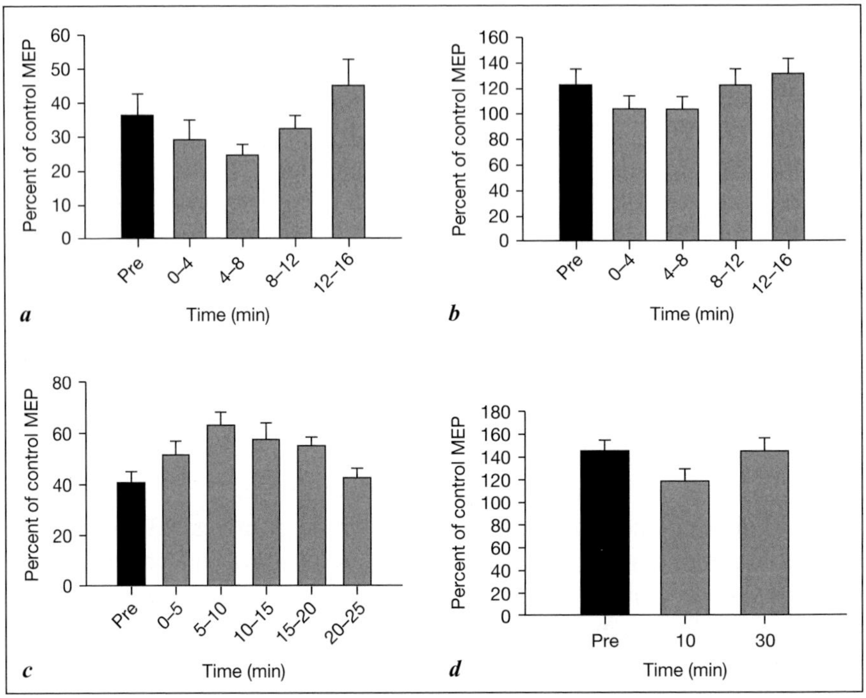

Fig. 6. The effect of iTBS and cTBS on SICI and ICF. SICI was significantly increased following iTBS [F(4, 24) = 5.01, $p < 0.005$] (***a***), but was reduced following cTBS [F(5, 30) = 3.75, $p < 0.01$] (***c***). ICF was not significantly altered following iTBS (***b***), but was significantly reduced at 10 min following cTBS [F(2, 12) = 7.40, $p < 0.01$] [21] (***d***).

increase in SICI after iTBS. The fact that there does not appear to be a clear relationship between the effects on inhibitory and facilitatory circuits and the effect on MEPs suggests that different circuits are involved in each. This is also supported by a study of cortical volleys before and after cTBS [24].

Cortical volleys were tested before and after cTBS300 in subjects who had cervical epidural electrodes implanted chronically for control of pain [24]. Single-pulse TMS over the primary motor cortex can activate a direct response (D-wave) followed by a number of periodic indirect responses (I-waves). The D-wave is probably produced by stimulating the proximal internodes of the axon of cortical pyramidal cells, while the I-waves are produced by activating excitatory synaptic inputs to the pyramidal cells. The latter is consistent with the fact that the I-waves disappear when the grey matter of the brain is removed [25], suggesting the source of these responses is within the cortex. One possible source is the network of cortical interneurones that synapse on pyramidal neurones. Another source might be the axon collaterals of other pyramidal neurones that run in layers III and V of the cortex. The results demonstrated cTBS300 pronouncedly suppressed the first I-wave (I1-wave), while it affected later I-waves much less. In the subjects in whom the D-wave could be identified, cTBS did not alter the D-wave [24]. This suggests that cTBS does not directly affect the excitability of the corticospinal neurones, but instead specifically affects I1-wave inputs. Together with the concept that I1-wave is produced by a monosynaptic input to corticospinal neurones due to its short latency, we believe that cTBS produces LTD at the excitatory synapse between the I1-wave input and the corticospinal neurone.

The Opposite Effects of Theta Burst Stimulation

It is interesting to find that the pattern of delivery of TBS (continuous vs. intermittent) is crucial in determining the direction of change in synaptic efficiency. A TBS protocol in which the bursts were applied in short trains (2 s; iTBS) induced facilitation, whereas a protocol in which the bursts were applied in a single continuous train (cTBS) induced inhibition. At first sight, the opposing effects of different patterns of TBS are surprising. However, a similar dissociation has been noted in previous work on animal preparations: patterns of iTBS similar to our iTBS paradigm are routinely used to facilitate synaptic connections [20], whereas a small number of studies have used longer trains of a TBS-like paradigm to produce suppression [26, 27]. To investigate the crucial role of the length of bursts and gaps, we tested the effect of a paradigm containing trains and gaps that are both longer than in iTBS but shorter than in cTBS. In this paradigm, which we have called intermediate theta burst stimulation (imTBS), we gave a train lasting 5 s (i.e. 25 bursts), repeated every 15 s for 8 cycles (a total of 600 pulses). As expected, we found imTBS had no effect on MEP [21].

We therefore hypothesise that a mixture of prolonged excitatory and inhibitory effects is induced after conditioning with TBS in our experiments. The overall effect on cortical excitability is determined by the dominant effect. We explored this further by comparing the short-term effects on the amplitude of MEPs after applying just a single train of either the iTBS or the imTBS paradigms (i.e. a train of 10 bursts of TBS or 25 bursts of TBS). A train of 10 bursts (i.e. the individual component of the iTBS pattern) had a purely facilitatory effect on MEPs (fig. 7a), whereas MEPs were initially facilitated after a train of 25 bursts (the component of the imTBS pattern), but then suppressed at 10 s before returning to baseline at 15 s (fig. 7b). [21]. The results support the

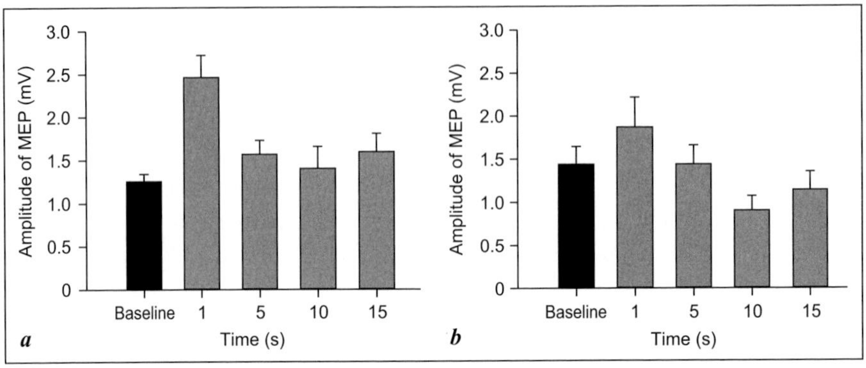

Fig. 7. The effect on MEP size of a short burst of TBS given for either 2 or 5 s. MEP size was measured at baseline and then at 1, 5, 10 and 15 s following the end of stimulation. ***a*** Following a 2-second train of TBS, there was a significant facilitation of the MEP size [$F(4, 16) = 6.99$, $p < 0.005$]. ***b*** In contrast, a 5-second train of TBS produced an initial significant facilitation of the MEP size at 1 s after the end of stimulation ($p < 0.05$) followed by a significant suppression of the MEP size at 10 s ($p < 0.05$) [21].

hypothesis and suggest that in humans TBS produces a mixture of facilitatory and inhibitory effects on synaptic transmission, with facilitation building up faster than inhibition.

There is also indirect evidence in support of this hypothesis from previous animal studies. When Larson et al. [2] first developed the TBS pattern, they actually found that the LTP effect produced by stimulation was considerably smaller when 20 bursts were used compared with 10 bursts. Beierlein et al. [28] have reported an initial facilitation followed by depression during a train of stimulation at frequencies higher than 20 Hz, compatible with the theory that a shorter train of stimulation is excitatory while the longer train is inhibitory.

At a synaptic level, LTP induction appears to be associated with phosphorylation of calcium/calmodulin-dependent protein kinase II, while LTD induction is associated with dephosphorylation of the cyclic-AMP-dependent protein kinase site [29]. A key factor in determining the occurrence and amount of phosphorylation/dephosphorylation is calcium. Calcium can therefore influence the direction of change in synaptic efficiency depending on the concentration and time course over which it is released [30, 31]. In other words, it is not impossible that calcium influx induces concurrent phosphorylation and dephosphorylation that occur in different sites, and that the balance between them is influenced by the pattern of TBS.

Conclusion

We have demonstrated that rTMS given in bursts at high frequency and low intensity is capable of producing consistent and controllable electrophysiological and behavioural changes in the function of the human motor system. These paradigms appear to be safe, and effects are seen after only seconds or a few minutes of rTMS conditioning, which is much quicker than other non-invasive methods of inducing long-term changes in cortical excitability in conscious humans. In particular, we have found that the pattern of delivery of TBS (continuous versus intermittent) is crucial in determining the direction of change in cortical excitability. We have interpreted these changes in excitability and behaviour as being caused by changes in transmission at cortical synapses, and refer to them as 'cortical plasticity'. However, this needs further testing, perhaps with drugs that are known to modify NMDA receptors in the human brain.

The findings have implications for both the use of rTMS in the study of human motor physiology, and the use of rTMS in the treatment of disorders of motor plasticity. Traditional methods of delivering rTMS require lengthy periods of conditioning to produce lasting effects, and the stimulus intensities necessary to do so can be uncomfortable for the subject, and technically difficult due to coil overheating in subjects with high motor thresholds. The effects of such stimulation have been found to have a high interindividual variability, and to be weak, in particular on a behavioural level. The results of studies using traditional methods of rTMS to treat disorders such as Parkinson's disease and dystonia have so far been relatively disappointing. The method of stimulation presented here appears to provide a powerful, controllable and consistent effect on the motor system with very brief periods of conditioning delivered at a low intensity. This TBS-style stimulation might have additional advantages in therapeutic applications both in terms of conditioning time to effect time ratio, the consistency of the effect, and the ease of giving repeated sessions of stimulation.

References

1 Anagnostou E, Sporer B, Steude U, Kempermann U, Buttner U, Botzel K: Contraversive eye deviation during deep brain stimulation of the globus pallidus internus. Neurology 2001;56: 1396–1399.

2 Larson J, Wong D, Lynch G: Patterned stimulation at the theta frequency is optimal for the induction of hippocampal long-term potentiation. Brain Res 1986;368:347–350.

3 Diamond DM, Dunwiddie TV, Rose GM: Characteristics of hippocampal primed burst potentiation in vitro and in the awake rat. J Neurosci 1988;8:4079–4088.

4 Hess G, Aizenman CD, Donoghue JP: Conditions for the induction of long-term potentiation in layer II/III horizontal connections of the rat motor cortex. J Neurophysiol 1996;75:1765–1778.

5 Randic M, Jiang MC, Cerne R: Long-term potentiation and long-term depression of primary afferent neurotransmission in the rat spinal cord. J Neurosci 1993;13:5228–5241.

6 Trepel C, Racine RJ: Long-term potentiation in the neocortex of the adult, freely moving rat. Cereb Cortex 1998;8:719–729.

7 Touge T, Gerschlager W, Brown P, Rothwell JC: Are the after-effects of low-frequency rTMS on motor cortex excitability due to changes in the efficacy of cortical synapses? Clin Neurophysiol 2001;112:2138–2145.

8 Maeda F, Keenan JP, Tormos JM, Topka H, Pascual-Leone A: Interindividual variability of the modulatory effects of repetitive transcranial magnetic stimulation on cortical excitability. Exp Brain Res 2000;133:425–430.

9 Muellbacher W, Ziemann U, Boroojerdi B, Hallett M: Effects of low-frequency transcranial magnetic stimulation on motor excitability and basic motor behavior. Clin Neurophysiol 2000;111: 1002–1007.

10 Schlaghecken F, Munchau A, Bloem BR, Rothwell J, Eimer M: Slow frequency repetitive transcranial magnetic stimulation affects reaction times, but not priming effects, in a masked prime task. Clin Neurophysiol 2003;114:1272–1277.

11 Wassermann EM: Risk and safety of repetitive transcranial magnetic stimulation: report and suggested guidelines from the International Workshop on the Safety of Repetitive Transcranial Magnetic Stimulation, June 5–7, 1996. Electroencephalogr Clin Neurophysiol 1998;108:1–16.

12 Ziemann U, Lonnecker S, Steinhoff BJ, Paulus W: Effects of antiepileptic drugs on motor cortex excitability in humans: a transcranial magnetic stimulation study. Ann Neurol 1996;40: 367–378.

13 Kujirai T, Caramia MD, Rothwell JC, Day BL, Thompson PD, Ferbert A, Wroe S, Asselman P, Marsden CD: Corticocortical inhibition in human motor cortex. *J Physiol* 1993, 471:501–519.

14 Huang YZ, Rothwell JC: The effect of short-duration bursts of high-frequency, low-intensity transcranial magnetic stimulation on the human motor cortex. Clin Neurophysiol 2004;115: 1069–1075.

15 Chen R, Tam A, Butefisch C, Corwell B, Ziemann U, Rothwell JC, Cohen LG: Intracortical inhibition and facilitation in different representations of the human motor cortex. J Neurophysiol 1998;80:2870–2881.

16 Valls-Sole J, Pascual-Leone A, Wassermann EM, Hallett M: Human motor evoked responses to paired transcranial magnetic stimuli. Electroencephalogr Clin Neurophysiol 1992;85:355–364.

17 Ziemann U, Rothwell JC, Ridding MC: Interaction between intracortical inhibition and facilitation in human motor cortex. J Physiol 1996;496(Pt 3):873–881.

18 Sanger TD, Garg RR, Chen R: Interactions between two different inhibitory systems in the human motor cortex. J Physiol 2001;530(Pt 2):307–317.

19 Bestmann S, Siebner HR, Modugno N, Amassian VE, Rothwell JC: Interaction between subthreshold conditioning stimuli in the human motor cortex? A triple-pulse TMS study. Clin Neurophysiol, in press.

20 Capocchi G, Zampolini M, Larson J: Theta burst stimulation is optimal for induction of LTP at both apical and basal dendritic synapses on hippocampal CA1 neurons. Brain Res 1992;591: 332–336.

21 Huang YZ, Edwards MJ, Rounis E, Bhatia KP, Rothwell JC: Theta burst stimulation of the human motor cortex. Neuron 2005;45:201–206.

22 Alagona G, Delvaux V, Gerard P, De Pasqua V, Pennisi G, Delwaide PJ, Nicoletti F, Maertens de Noordhout A: Ipsilateral motor responses to focal transcranial magnetic stimulation in healthy subjects and acute-stroke patients. Stroke 2001;32:1304–1309.

23 Di Lazzaro V, Oliviero A, Profice P, Saturno E, Pilato F, Insola A, Mazzone P, Tonali P, Rothwell JC: Comparison of descending volleys evoked by transcranial magnetic and electric stimulation in conscious humans. Electroencephalogr Clin Neurophysiol 1998;109:397–401.

24 Di Lazzaro V, Pilato F, Saturno E, Oliviero A, Dileone M, Mazzone P, Insola A, Tonali PA, Ranieri F, Huang YZ, et al: Theta-burst repetitive transcranial magnetic stimulation suppresses specific excitatory circuits in the human motor cortex. J Physiol 2005;565(Pt 3):945–950.

25 Patton HD, Amassian VE: Single and multiple-unit analysis of cortical stage of pyramidal tract activation. J Neurophysiol 1954;17:345–363.

26 Heusler P, Cebulla B, Boehmer G, Dinse HR: A repetitive intracortical microstimulation pattern induces long-lasting synaptic depression in brain slices of the rat primary somatosensory cortex. Exp Brain Res 2000;135:300–310.

27 Takita M, Izaki Y, Jay TM, Kaneko H, Suzuki SS: Induction of stable long-term depression in vivo in the hippocampal-prefrontal cortex pathway. Eur J Neurosci 1999;11:4145–4148.
28 Beierlein M, Gibson JR, Connors BW: Two dynamically distinct inhibitory networks in layer 4 of the neocortex. J Neurophysiol 2003;90:2987–3000.
29 Lee HK, Barbarosie M, Kameyama K, Bear MF, Huganir RL: Regulation of distinct AMPA receptor phosphorylation sites during bidirectional synaptic plasticity. Nature 2000;405:955–959.
30 Sheng M, Kim MJ: Postsynaptic signaling and plasticity mechanisms. Science 2002;298: 776–780.
31 Yang SN, Tang YG, Zucker RS: Selective induction of LTP and LTD by postsynaptic $[Ca^{2+}]_i$ elevation. J Neurophysiol 1999;81:781–787.

Prof. John C. Rothwell
Sobell Department of Motor Neuroscience and Movement Disorders
Institute of Neurology, University College London, Queen Square
London WC1N 3BG (UK)
Tel. +44 207 837 3611, ext. 3048, Fax +44 207 278 9836, E-Mail j.rothwell@ion.ucl.ac.uk

Marcolin MA, Padberg F (eds): Transcranial Brain Stimulation for Treatment of Psychiatric Disorders.
Adv Biol Psychiatr. Basel, Karger, 2007, vol 23, pp 204–224

Transcranial Magnetic Stimulation of Deep Brain Regions: Principles and Methods

Yiftach Roth[a], *Frank Padberg*[c], *Abraham Zangen*[b]

[a]Advanced Technology Center, Sheba Medical Center, Tel Hashomer, and [b]The Weizmann Institute of Science, Department of Neurobiology, Rehovot, Israel; [c]Department of Psychiatry and Psychotherapy, Ludwig-Maximilian University Munich, Munich, Germany

Abstract

Repetitive transcranial magnetic stimulation (rTMS) is an established technique for noninvasive brain stimulation and widely used in basic and clinical neurophysiology. Yet, brain stimulation using traditional rTMS systems is limited to superficial, i.e. mainly cortical brain sites laying at the outer cerebral or cerebellar convexity and deeper structures are only modulated by transsynaptic effects primarily stimulated regions exert. Here we report recent developments in extending rTMS to deep brain regions. The Hesed coils (H-coils) are a novel development in rTMS, designed to achieve effective stimulation of deeper neuronal regions without inducing unbearable fields cortically, thus broadly expanding the potential feasibility of TMS for research and treatment of various neuropsychiatric disorders. The construction principles and design of the H-coils and phantom measurements and clinical studies are presented comparing the penetration depth of the H-coils and traditional rTMS coils. Using this approach, transcranial stimulation of subcortical white matter tracts, neurons in the mesial temporal lobe and the ventromedial prefrontal cortex together with the adjacent cingulate gyrus will become available. Moreover, the threshold for neuronal activation depends on the duration of the TMS perturbation through a strength-duration curve. Thus, it may theoretically be possible to exploit the temporal characteristics of the neuronal response, in order to improve dramatically the efficacy and focality of the stimulation of deep brain structures, potentially enabling focused stimulation of deep regions with no activation of cortical brain regions. These considerations will be of particular interest for future treatment options in affective disorders, schizophrenia and drug addiction among others.

Transcranial magnetic stimulation (TMS) is a noninvasive technique used to apply brief magnetic pulses to the brain. The pulses are administered by passing high currents with a stimulator through an electromagnetic coil placed upon the patient's scalp, inducing electric currents in the underlying cortical tissue, thereby producing localized axonal depolarizations. Neuronal stimulation by TMS was first demonstrated in 1985 [1], when a circular coil was placed over a normal subject vertex and evoked action potentials from the abductor digiti minimi. Since then, this technique has become a major research tool in basic and clinical neurophysiology, and has been applied to studying nerve conduction, excitability [2], and functional connectivity in the brain and peripheral nerves. In addition, in recent years, repetitive TMS (rTMS) has become a potentially promising treatment option for various neurobehavioral disorders spanning a wide age range [3–6].

The capacity of TMS to elicit neuronal response has until recently been limited to the cerebral cortex. The coils used for TMS (such as round or figure-of-eight coils) induce stimulation in cortical regions mainly just superficially under the windings of the coil. The intensity of the electric field drops dramatically deeper in the brain as a function of the distance from the coil [7–10]. Therefore, to stimulate deep brain regions, a very high intensity would be needed. Such intensity cannot be reached by standard magnetic stimulators, using the regular figure-of-eight or circular coils. Stimulation of regions at a depth of 3–4 cm, such as for the primary motor area of the leg, may be achieved using coils such as the double-cone coil [11–13], which is a larger figure-of-eight coil with an angle of about 95° between the two wings. However, the intensity needed to stimulate deeper brain regions effectively would stimulate cortical regions and facial nerves over the level that might lead to facial pain, facial and cervical muscle contractions, and may cause epileptic seizures and other undesirable side effects.

The difficulty of efficiently activating deep neuronal structures using TMS emerges from physical properties of the brain, and from physical and physiological aspects of the interaction of a TMS system with the human brain. The purpose of this chapter is to demonstrate how the TMS system, including both the TMS coils and the stimulator, may be optimized for effective stimulation of deeper brain regions. The subsequent section provides neuroanatomical considerations, followed by a section on the basic principles of TMS, a section that describes the construction principles and design of TMS coils for deep brain stimulation, and gives results of clinical studies and phantom measurements obtained with some exemplary coils, and finally a section, in which we outline a method and a TMS system which enable to exploit the temporal characteristics of the neuronal response, in order to improve dramatically the efficiency and focality of stimulation of deep brain structures.

Neuroanatomical Considerations

In the brain, TMS acts on neuronal activity within a three-dimensional neuronal network. Looking at the cortical level, the cytoarchitecture varies between different brain regions, and even the single cerebral lobes, e.g. the frontal lobe, consist of regions with distinct structural differences: e.g. the primate's prefrontal cortex is a homotypical isocortex, clearly laminated, with a well-developed internal granular layer (IV) that differentiates it from the rest of the frontal cortex [14]. This layer becomes thicker and more distinct on approaching the frontal pole, although the cortex as a whole becomes thinner.

Another issue to be considered is the orientation of the magnetic field in relation to the cortical folding. The coil position in relation to the individual gyri and sulci matters for stimulation effects as demonstrated for the primary motor cortex where the orientation of the current flow in relation to the central sulcus changes the amplitude of motor evoked potentials [15]. Moreover, TMS of the motor cortex can evoke D-waves, representing direct stimulation of the corticospinal axon, as well as I-waves that arise from transsynaptic activation of corticospinal neurons [16, 17]. Thus, both corticospinal neurons and interneurons may be stimulated simultaneously. D-waves may be predominantly elicited in corticospinal fibers running horizontally in the primary motor cortex in a direction at right angles to the central sulcus. Accordingly, for intrinsic hand muscles, the motor cortex is excited most readily by coil currents running at right angles to the axis of the precentral gyrus [17]. Presumably, the excitation occurs at the site where the corticospinal fibers bend down into the central sulcus [18]. Therefore, neuronal stimulation will depend on the position of the TMS coil placed tangentially on the skull in relation to the neuronal layer and its main fiber system, i.e. it will probably make a difference whether the target region lays on the outer convexity of a gyrus or the part descending into the sulcus. This assumption may be applicable to both cortical and subcortical regions. To date, however, it is not feasible to target TMS to certain neuronal populations or cortical layers or even to differentially stimulate grey matter and white matter tracts. That means that stimulation effects in the network represent sum or net effects of neuronal and axonal stimulation.

For the motor cortex, a threshold for stimulation effects has been defined, i.e. the resting or active motor threshold which varies interindividually and is also applied to define stimulation intensity at nonmotor sites. Similar thresholds can also be assumed for other cortex regions, e.g. the threshold for eliciting phosphenes over the visual cortex. However, these are not equal to the motor thresholds and not necessarily correlated with them. These threshold measures are specific to neurophysiological phenomena and sum thresholds of component thresholds representing neuronal subpopulations and intracortical, as well as cortico-subcortical networks. As the intensity is increased, a larger volume of the neuronal network is activated above a given threshold and further neuronal populations in the same volume are additionally depolarized. This may be the background for recruitment curves at primary motor sites and intensity-efficacy relationships observed with prefrontal TMS using clinical, neurophysiological or neuroimaging paradigms [19–21].

Similar considerations are important when we turn to deep TMS approaches. However, the situation is even more complex, as the target regions show greater variance in terms of cytoarchitecture compared to neocortical areas and regions or nuclei with fundamentally distinct functions are located in close vicinity to each other. There are particularly interesting deeper brain regions for therapeutic interventions: the anterior cingulate cortex may be a putative target region for the treatment of major depression and schizophrenia, the hippocampus for the treatment of schizophrenia, depressive disorders and dementia, the amygdala for anxiety disorders and depression, the orbital frontal cortex for obsessive-compulsive disorder, the nucleus accumbens/ventral striatum for addiction, obsessive-compulsive disorder and depression, and the basal ganglia for movement disorders. Actually, each specific application may require a different TMS coil design which has to be based on physical calculations and anatomical considerations tested in clinical practice. However, it is important to emphasize the basic principles of specific coil designs which are described in this overview.

Basic Principles of Transcranial Magnetic Stimulation

The Basic TMS Circuit

The TMS circuit consists of a high-voltage power supply that charges a capacitor or a bank of capacitors, which are then rapidly discharged via an electronic switch into the TMS coil to create the briefly changing magnetic field pulse. A typical circuit is shown in figure 1, where low-voltage AC is transformed into high-voltage DC, which charges the capacitor. A crucial component is the thyristor switch, which has to traverse very high current at a very short time of 50–250 μs. The cycle time depends on the capacitance (typically 10–250 μF) and on the coil inductance (typically 10–30 μH). Accepted ranges of peak currents and voltages may be 2,000–10,000 A (typically 5,000 A) and 500–3,000 V (typically 1,500 V), respectively.

The first TMS stimulators produced a monophasic pulse of electric current. Currently, it is accepted to use stimulators with biphasic pulses, for two reasons: (a) a considerable part of the energy returns to the capacitor at the end of the cycle, thus shortening the time for recharging and enabling to save

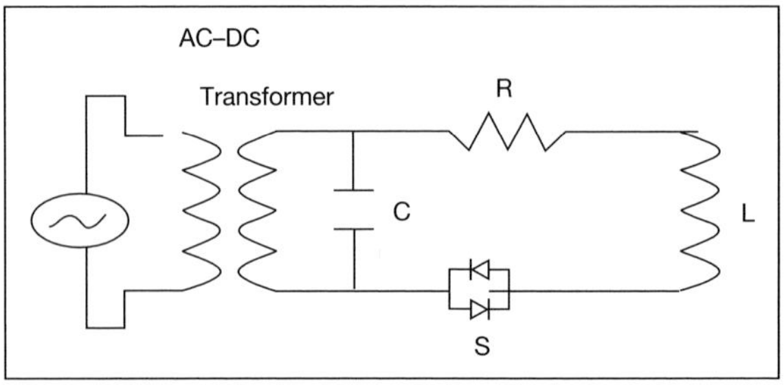

Fig. 1. A schematic TMS circuit, including a DC–AC transformer and amplifier, a capacitor C, high current switch S, resistor R and stimulating coil L.

energy; (b) it was found that the threshold for neuronal activation is generally lower with biphasic compared to monophasic pulses.

During the discharge cycle, the TMS circuit behaves like an RCL circuit, where R, C and L are the total values of the resistance, capacitance and inductance, respectively, in the circuit. The duration τ of one pulse cycle is approximately:

$$\tau = 2\pi\sqrt{(LC)} \qquad (1)$$

The importance of the pulse duration for neuronal activation will be discussed later in this chapter.

Physical and Spatial Factors Affecting Neuronal Activation by TMS

In principle, two related parameters may be relevant for neuronal activation: the electric field strength, and the spatial derivative of the electric field. While the activation of peripheral nerves depends mainly on the derivative of the electric field along the nerve fiber [18], where we deal with neuronal tissue having relatively short axons with bends and branches, such as the brain, it was predicted theoretically [22, 23], and clearly demonstrated experimentally [24–26], that the absolute magnitude of the electric field is the biologically relevant parameter for neuronal stimulation. The electric field is proportional to the rate of change of the current (dI/dt) in the stimulating coil. The brief strong current generates a time-varying magnetic field B. An electric field E_A is generated in every point in space with the direction perpendicular to the magnetic field, and the amplitude proportional to the time rate of change of the vector potential A(r).

Since brain tissue has conducting properties, while the air and skull are almost complete insulators, the vector potential will induce accumulation of electric charge at the brain surface. This charge is another source for an electric field, E_Φ, in addition to E_A. The influence of the electrostatic field E_Φ is in general to oppose the induced field E_A and consequently to reduce the total field E. The amount of surface charge produced and hence the magnitude of E_Φ depends strongly on the coil configuration and orientation. This issue will be elaborated in the following section.

As shown by Heller and Van Hulsteyn [27], the three-dimensional maximum of the electric field intensity will always be located at the brain surface, for any configuration or superposition of TMS coils. It is possible, however, to increase considerably the penetration depth and the percentage of electric field intensity in deep brain regions, relative to the maximal field at the cortex. The next section will outline the construction principles for efficient deep brain stimulation, and will demonstrate several examples of TMS coils designed to accomplish this goal.

Deep Transcranial Magnetic Stimulation Coils

Design Principles

As mentioned above, neuronal stimulation occurs when the electric field magnitude reaches a certain threshold. This threshold, though, depends on the orientation of the induced field. Physiological studies indicate that optimal activation occurs when the field is oriented in the same direction as the nerve fiber [15, 24, 28–33]. Hence, in order to stimulate deep brain regions, it is necessary to use coils in such an orientation that they will produce a significant field in the preferable direction to activate the neuronal structures or axons under consideration.

The construction of deep TMS coils should meet several goals:

(a) high enough electric field intensity in the desired deep brain region that will surpass the threshold for neuronal activation;

(b) high percentage of electric field in the desired deep brain region relative to the maximal intensity in the cortex;

(c) minimal adverse side effects such as pain and activation of facial muscles.

These motivations have led to the development of the Hesed coil (H-coil), a new design of TMS coils, enabling effective stimulation of deep brain regions without inducing an unbearable field in cortical regions [34]. The ability of the H-coil to stimulate deep brain regions was demonstrated using mathematical simulations as well as measurements performed in a phantom brain model [34]. The efficacy of the H-coil in activating distant brain structures was demonstrated clinically in a recent study, where the motor cortex was activated at a distance of 5–6 cm in healthy volunteers, compared to 1.5 cm with a standard figure-of-eight coil [35].

The geometrical features of each specific design are mainly dependent on two goals: (a) the location and size of the deep brain region or regions intended to be activated; (b) the preferred direction or directions of stimulation.

The design of a specific coil is dictated by these goals. Nevertheless, all deep TMS coils have to share the following important features.

(1) *Base complementary to the human head.* The part of the coil close to the head (the base) must be optimally complementary to the human skull at the desired region. In some coils, the base may be flexible and able to receive the shape of an individual patient, and in other coils it may be more robust, i.e. arcuated in a shape that fits the average human skull at the desired region. In this last case, there may be a few similar models designed to fit smaller and larger heads. This feature guarantees that all the wires in the base will be tangential to the head. This configuration maximizes both the intensity and the penetration depth of the electric field induced by the base in the brain.

(2) *Proper orientation of stimulating coil elements.* Coils must be oriented such that they will produce a considerable field in a direction tangential to the surface, which should also be the preferable direction to activate the neuronal structures under consideration.

(3) *Summation of electric impulses.* The induced electric field in the desired deep brain regions is obtained by optimal summation of electric fields, induced by several coil elements with common direction, in different locations around the skull. The principle of summation may be applied in several manners.

(a) *One-point spatial summation.* In this kind of summation, coil elements, leading current in the desired direction, are placed in various locations around the head, in such a configuration to create high electric field intensity in a specific deep brain region, which at the same time is a high percentage of the maximal electric field at the brain cortex.

(b) *Morphological line spatial summation.* The goal of this summation is to induce an electric field at several points along a certain neuronal structure. This line should not be straight and may have a complex bent path. The application of diffusion tensor imaging in MRI for fiber tracking is an evolving field, which may significantly improve the efficacy of TMS treatment. If, for example, we know the path of a certain axonal bundle, a coil shall be designed in a configuration that will produce a significant electric field at several points along the bundle. This configuration may enable the induction of an action potential in this bundle, while minimizing the activation of other brain regions. For example, the TMS coil may be activated in an intensity that will induce a subthreshold electric field at most brain regions, which will not cause an action potential, while the induction of a subthreshold field along the desired path may produce an action potential in this bundle, thus increasing the specificity of the TMS treatment.

(4) *Minimization of nontangential components.* Coil construction is meant to minimize wire elements leading current components which are nontangential to the skull. Electric field intensity in the tissue to be stimulated and the rate of decrease of electric field as a function of the distance from the coil depend on the orientation of the coil elements relative to the tissue surface. It has been shown [8–10, 34] that coil elements which are nontangential to the surface induce accumulation of surface charge, which leads to the cancellation of the perpendicular component of the induced field at all points within the tissue, and usually to the reduction of the electric field in all other directions. At each specific point, the produced electric field is affected by the lengths of the nontangential components, and their distances from this point. Thus, the length of coil elements which are not tangential to the brain tissue surface should be minimized. Furthermore, the nontangential coil elements should be as small as possible and placed as far as possible from the deep region to be activated.

(5) *Remote location of return paths.* The wires leading currents in a direction opposite to the preferred direction (the return paths) should be located far from the base and the desired brain region. This enables a higher absolute electric field in the desired brain region. In some cases, the return paths may be in the air, i.e. far from the head. In other cases, part of the return paths may be adjacent to a different region in the head which is distant from the desired brain region.

(6) *Shielding.* Feature 5 enables the possibility of screening. Since the return paths are far from the main base, it is possible to screen all or part of their field by inserting a shield around them or between them and the base. The shield is comprised of a material with high magnetic permeability, capable of inhibiting or diverting a magnetic field, such as mu-metal, iron or steel core. Alternatively, the shield is comprised of a metal with high conductivity which can cause electric currents or charge accumulation that may oppose the effect produced by the return portions.

Specific deep TMS coils for stimulating different deep brain regions are described below.

Examples of Deep TMS Coils

The biological efficacy of the H-coil was tested [35], using the right abductor pollicis brevis (APB) muscle motor threshold as a measure of a biological effect. The rate of decrease of the electric field as a function of the distance from the coil was measured by gradually increasing the distance of the coil from the skull, and measuring the motor threshold at each distance. A comparison was made to a standard figure-of-eight coil. A sketch of the H-coil version used is shown in figure 2.

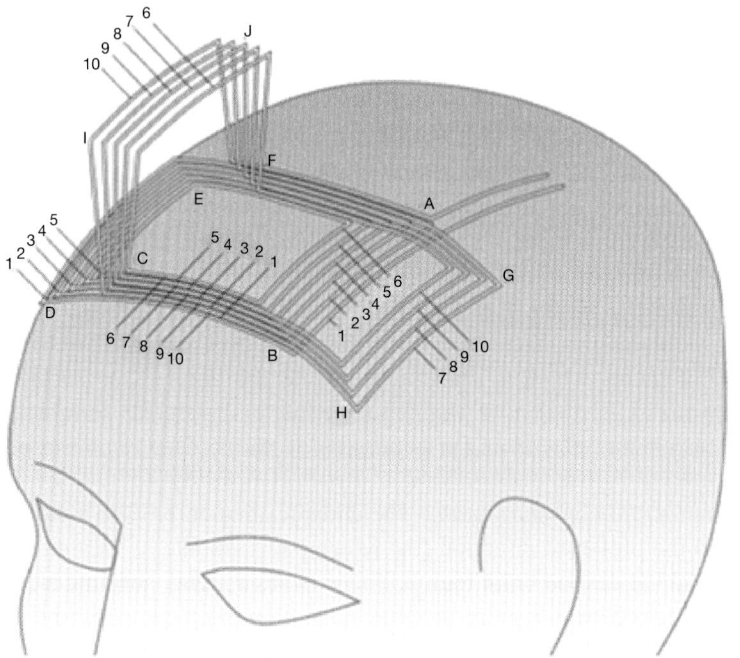

Fig. 2. Sketch of the H-coil version used for activation of the APB, placed on a human head.

The percentage of stimulator output required for APB activation by the H-coil and by a figure-of-eight coil is plotted in figure 3 as a function of the distance from the 'hot spot' on the scalp. It can be seen that the efficacy of the H-coil at large distances from the scalp was significantly greater as compared to the figure-of-eight coil. When using the maximal stimulation power output, the figure-of-eight coil can be effective (reach the stimulation threshold) up to 2 cm away from the coil, while the H-coil can be effective at 5.5 cm away from the coil. Thus, the rate of decay of effectiveness as a function of the distance from the coil is much slower in the H-coil relative to the figure-of-eight coil.

The following example is an H-coil designed for stimulation of deep prefrontal regions [unpubl. data]. Medial prefrontal and orbitofrontal cortices and their connections to deeper brain sites are known to be associated with reward processes and motivation [36–42].

The H-coil version used, termed the H1 coil, was designed for effective activation of cortical and subcortical prefrontal and orbitofrontal neuronal

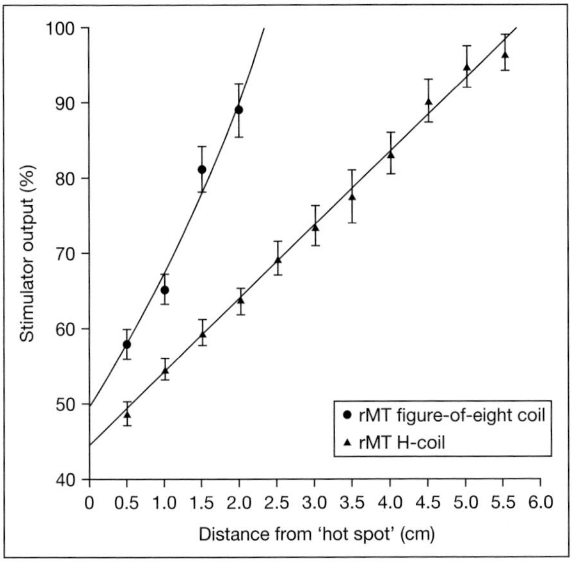

Fig. 3. Intensity needed for APB stimulation at different heights above the scalp. Resting motor threshold (rMT) of the APB was measured at different distances above the 'hot spot' when using either the H-coil or the figure-of-eight coil. The percentage of stimulator power needed to reach the resting motor threshold versus the distance of the coil from the 'hot spot' on the skull is plotted. The points represent means and SDs of 6 healthy volunteers.

structures, with a preference for the left hemisphere. A sketch of the H1 coil version is shown in figure 4.

The electric field distribution produced by the H1 coil was measured in a brain phantom filled with 0.9% weight/volume saline, and compared to a standard Magstim figure-of-eight coil with an internal loop diameter of 7 cm, and a Magstim double-cone coil. The double-cone coil is considered to be able to stimulate deeper brain regions compared to other coils [11–13].

The penetration depth of the coils was tested by measuring the electric field along the up-down line beneath the center of the most effective part of the coil, at 100% output of the Magstim Rapid stimulator. In H1, the most effective part was under strip 8 (lower third of A-I 8 segment in fig. 4), where the probe is oriented in an anterior-posterior direction. In the double-cone coil and the figure-of-eight coil, the most effective part was the junction at the coil center, where the probe is oriented in an anterior-posterior direction. Plots of the total electric field as a function of distance are shown in figure 5.

Figure 6 shows the electric field as a function of distance, relative to the field at a distance of 1 cm, for the three coils.

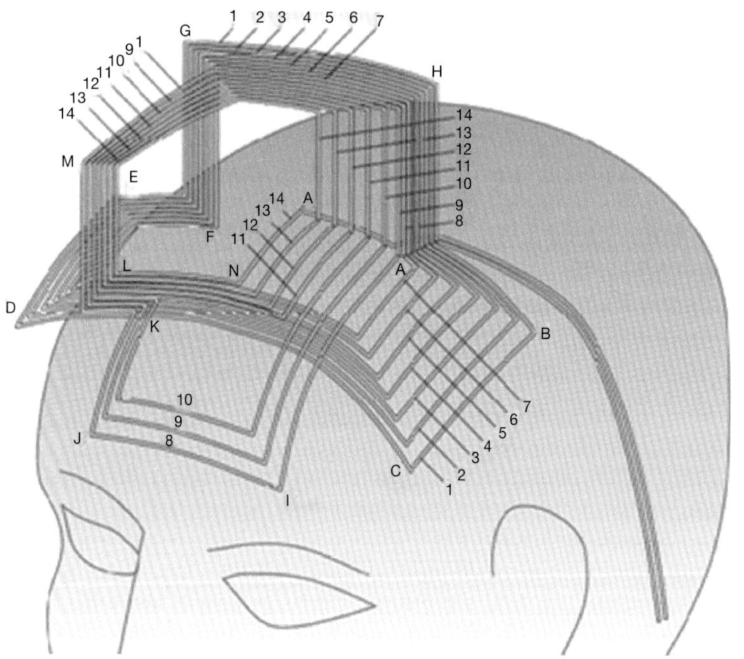

Fig. 4. Sketch of the H1 coil used for effective activation of prefrontal brain regions, placed on a human head.

It can be seen that the total electric field induced by the double-cone coil, and by the figure-of-eight coil, using the maximal output of the stimulator, is markedly greater than the field produced by the H1 coil at a short distances of 1–2 cm. Yet, at distances of above 5 cm, the field of the H1 coil becomes greater, due to its much slower rate of decay. In figure 6, it can be seen that the percentage of depth for the H1 coil is greater than for the two other coils already at a 2-cm distance, and this advantage becomes more prominent with increasing distance. The field produced by the H1 coil at a 6-cm depth is about 63% of the field 1 cm from the coil, while the fields of the double-cone coil and the figure-of-eight coil attenuate to 8–10% at this distance.

In summary, it was demonstrated that the H-coils enable to achieve effective stimulation of deep neuronal regions without inducing an unbearable field in cortical regions. Yet, using H-coils with available TMS stimulators enables effective activation of deep brain regions, but not focal activation. In order to obtain a focused stimulation of deep brain regions, and to considerably enhance the stimulation efficiency, novel TMS systems are required, which account for the temporal properties of neuronal structures. This is the subject of the next section.

5 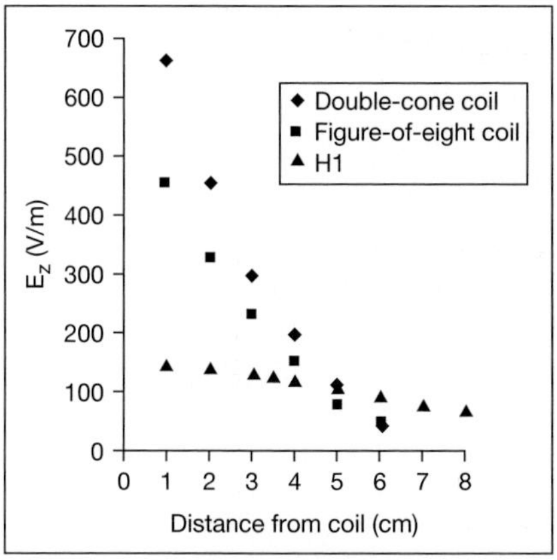

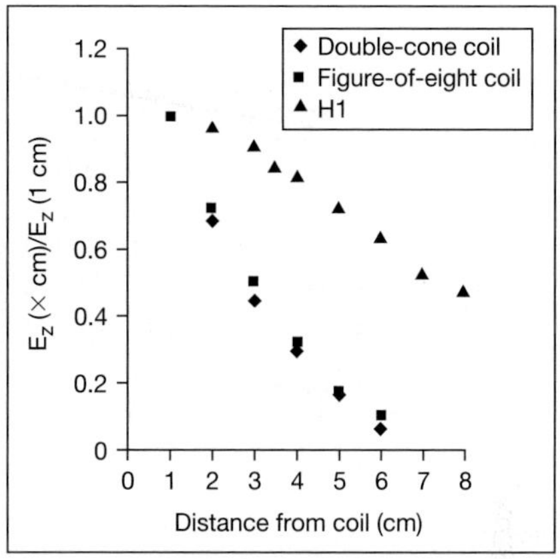 6

Fig. 5. Phanton measurements of the electric field along an anterior-posterior axis, plotted as a function of distance, for the H1 coil, the double-cone coil, and the figure-of-eight coil.

Fig. 6. Electric field relative to the field 1 cm from the coil, as a function of distance, for the H1 coil, the double-cone coil and the figure-of-eight coil, according to the phantom brain measurements.

Novel Deep Transcranial Magnetic Stimulation Systems Based on the Time Summation Principle

Temporal Factors Affecting Neuronal Activation by TMS

In addition to the electric field strength, the neuronal response also strongly depends on the duration of the pulse.

Figure 7 demonstrates the electric field pulse produced by a figure-of-eight coil, as measured by a two-wire probe in a brain phantom filled with saline solution at a physiologic concentration. In rTMS, several such pulses are administered in a train of between 0.2 and 100 Hz, and typically between 1 and 20 Hz.

The longer the pulse duration, the smaller the electric field required to reach neuronal threshold E_{thr}. The dependence of E_{thr} on pulse duration is given by a strength-duration curve [43] of the form:

$$E_{thr} = b(1 + c/\tau) \tag{2}$$

The biological parameters determining neural response are the threshold at infinite duration, termed the rheobase (b, measured in V/m), and the duration at which the threshold is twice the rheobase, termed the chronaxie (c, in μs), which is related to the time constant of the neuronal membrane. The chronaxie and rheobase depend on many biological and experimental factors, such as whether the nerves are myelinated or not (hence peripheral and cortical parameters

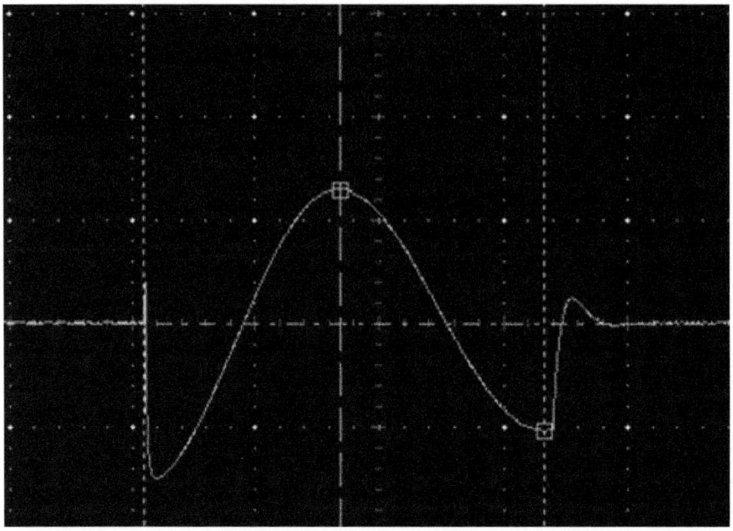

Fig. 7. The induced electric field of a figure-of-eight coil versus time over a TMS pulse cycle. The time scale is 100 μs.

should be different), the pulse shape (i.e. biphasic or monophasic), or train frequency in rTMS, which in general reduces the threshold for stimulation.

In figure 8, a strength-duration curve is shown reflecting the average of 4 subjects, using eight different coils with inductance L of between 6 and 148 μH.

As can be seen from equation 1, the duration of a TMS pulse can be extended in two ways: by increasing the capacitance C, or by increasing the coil inductance L. In regular available stimulators, C is constant. Increasing L is not desired, since it leads to increased power and energy consumption.

Figure 9 shows pulses produced by TMS coils having inductances of 13 and 70 μH. The amplitudes represent the threshold electric field according to points 1 and 2 in the strength-duration curve shown in figure 8. The plots are for resistance and capacitance of $R = 0.1\,\Omega$ and $C = 165\,\mu F$, respectively. It can be seen that when the pulse duration is longer, the required threshold electric field is smaller.

When we want to produce focused activation of deep neuronal structures in the brain, regular TMS stimulators have significant limitations. In available stimulators, the capacitor (or bank of capacitors) is discharged through a single switch to a single coil, hence the current flows simultaneously through all coil elements, and the electric field is produced simultaneously in all brain regions. Thus, the electric field induced in cortical brain regions close to coil elements

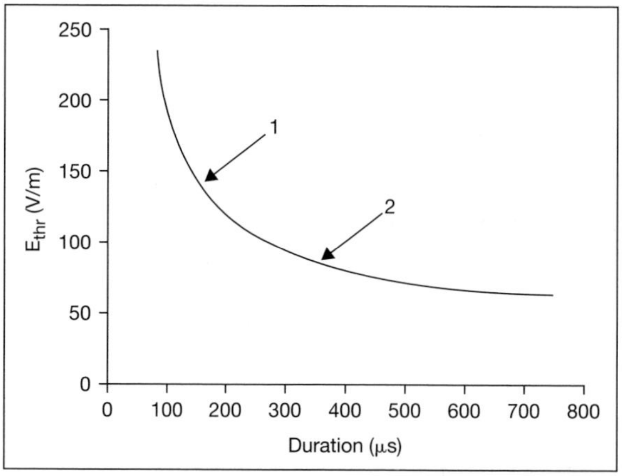

Fig. 8. A strength-duration curve obtained for the hand motor cortex of 4 subjects, using variable coil inductance. Points 1 and 2 represent results obtained with coils having an inductance of 13 and 70 μH, respectively.

will be in general larger than the field induced in deeper brain regions. In the following part, we describe the time summation principle and suited TMS system, which may enable to overcome this difficulty.

Principles of Time Summation Multichannel TMS Systems

The principle of time summation is that various TMS coils may be stimulated consecutively and not simultaneously. As shown in figure 8, the neuronal activation threshold depends on both electric field intensity and the stimulation duration. When we want to stimulate a specific deep brain region, various coils, or alternatively various coil elements connected in parallel, may be scattered around the desired region or path, so that passing a current in each coil will produce a significant field at the desired deep brain region. Each coil may be connected to a separate TMS channel. In such a case, the coils may be activated consecutively, so that at each time period only a certain coil or a group of coils are activated. This way, a significant electric field will be induced in the desired deep brain region at all time periods, while in more cortical regions a significant field will be induced mainly at certain periods, when proximate coils or coil elements are activated. This will enable stimulation of the deep brain structure while minimizing stimulation of other brain regions, and specifically of cortical regions.

The novel TMS systems require several capacitors, which are discharged in different channels through different switches into different TMS coils or different elements of coil connected in parallel. A control unit should control the

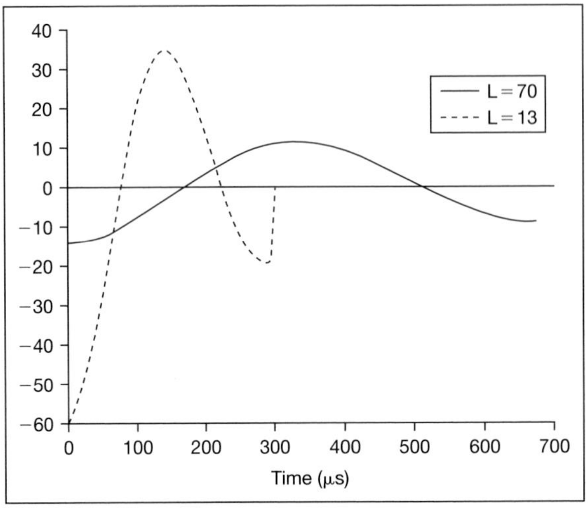

Fig. 9. The electric field pulse produced by two TMS coils with inductances of 13 and 70 μH, as a function of time.

times of charging and discharging of the different capacitors, and the delays between operation times of sequential coils. Various coils or coil elements may be operated sequentially, with delays of between 0 and 1 ms. The relevant time scale for neuronal response is usually on the order of 10–100 μs. In each operation, one TMS cycle is induced through a certain coil or several coils. The number of different coils or coil elements may be different in different applications. In some cases, the delays between consecutive operations of coils will be the same, while in other cases they may be different between different operations and different coils.

A schematic example of a block diagram of a multichannel TMS system that enables to apply the time summation principle is shown in figure 10.

In the example shown in figure 10, there are five channels. The system may include an AC–DC converter, which converts the AC voltage of the electricity mains to a DC voltage. In each channel, there may be a charging circuit, one or more capacitors, and a high current fast switch through which the capacitor/capacitors is/are discharged.

The operator will be able to control the delays between the operation times of the different coils, the number of different channels and coils operated consecutively, the number of times each coil will be activated and the timing of each activation, the polarity of the current in each coil, the frequency of operation (i.e. number of pulses in seconds), the train duration, the number of trains

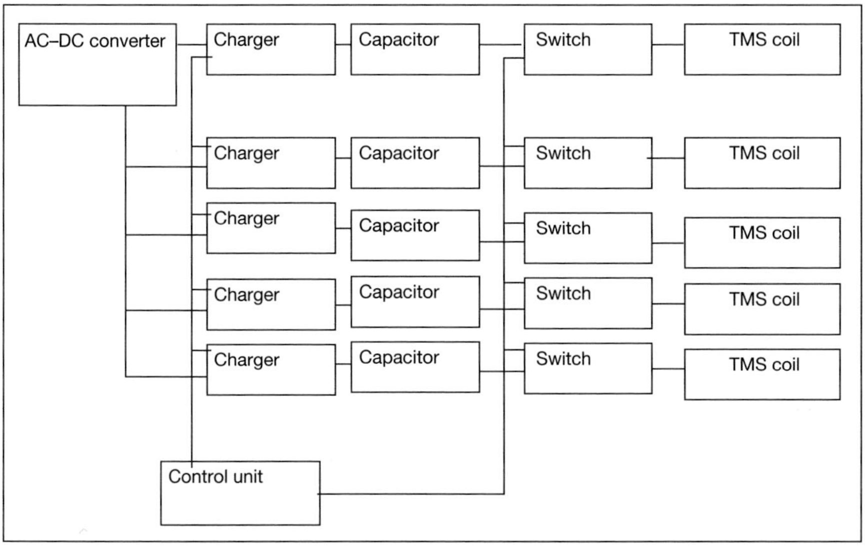

Fig. 10. A schematic diagram of a multichannel TMS system, having 5 channels.

and intertrain intervals, and the power output of operation of each coil. The ability to control the delays between operations of the different coils and the current polarity in each coil enables various kinds of time summation. Several examples are given below.

Examples of Time Summation

Figure 11 shows the electric field pulses induced in a deep brain region and in two cortical regions, where the pulse of the coil close to the second cortical region lags the pulse of the coil close to the first cortical region by a full cycle. In each coil, one pulse cycle is induced, and the switch is disconnected at the end of a cycle when the current is zero. In this and in the following examples, the field intensity in the deep brain region is 50% of the intensity induced in the cortical region close to the equivalent coil (this percentage is realistic with the H-coils), while the field intensity in one of the cortical regions during operation of the coil close to the second cortical region is 5%. Hence in the deep brain region a significant electric field is induced during all the consecutive pulses, while in each of the cortical regions a significant field is induced only during one cycle.

Obviously, the same principles may be applied with more than two coils, and/or with several or all of the coils operated more than once.

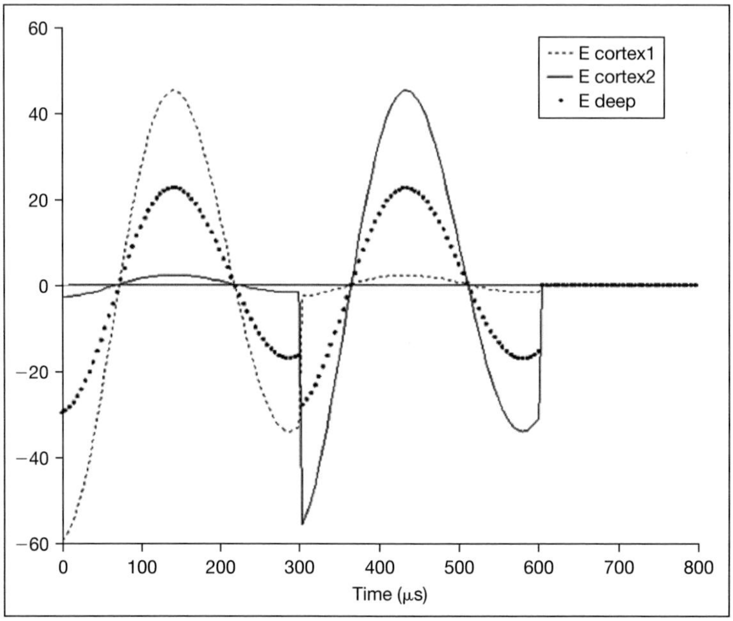

Fig. 11. An example of time summation where the time delay between consecutive pulses is a full cycle. Shown are the electric field pulses induced in cortical regions close to each coil (continuous and dashed curves) and in a deep brain region (dotted curve).

Figure 12 shows the electric field pulses induced in a deep brain region and in three cortical regions, where the delay between two consecutive pulses is half a cycle, and the current polarity in the second pulse is opposite to the polarity in the first and third pulses. In each coil, one pulse cycle is induced, and the switch is disconnected at the end of a cycle when the current is zero. In this example, there is an extension of the duration at which the deep brain region is exposed to a significant field, and in addition there is an increase in intensity after each half cycle. Note that the absolute value of the maximum at the beginning of each pulse is higher than the next maxima due to the decay factor $\alpha = R/2L$, hence at the beginning of the second pulse the relation between the field in the deep brain region and the field in the first cortical region will be higher with higher circuit resistance R, and with lower coil inductance L.

Figure 13 shows the electric field pulses induced in a deep brain region and in three cortical regions, where the current polarity in the second and third pulses is opposite to the polarity in the first pulse. The delay between the first and second pulses is close to 3/4 of a cycle, and the delay between the second and third pulses is about 1/8 of a cycle. In each coil, one pulse cycle is induced,

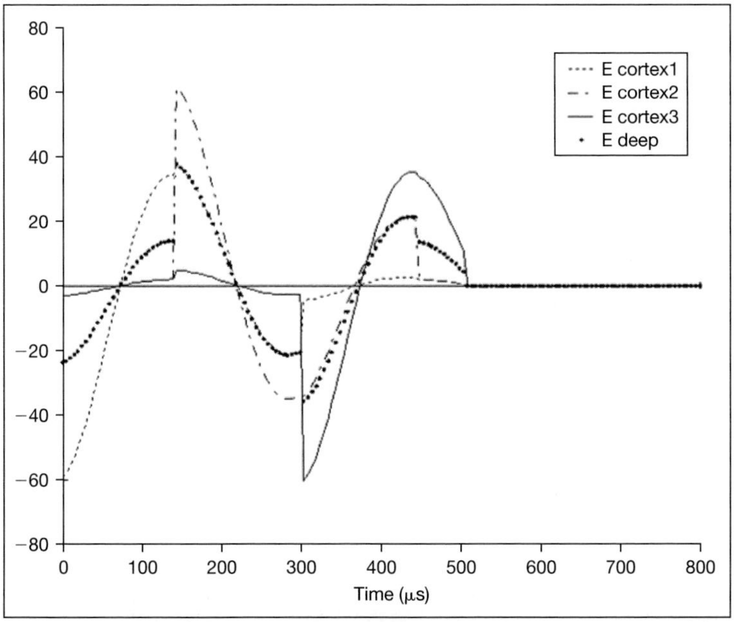

Fig. 12. An example of time summation where the time delay between consecutive pulses is half a cycle, and the current polarity in the second pulse is opposite to the polarity in the first and third pulses. Shown are the electric field pulses induced in cortical regions close to each coil (dashed, dot-dashed and continuous curves) and in a deep brain region (dotted curve).

and the switch is disconnected at the end of a cycle when the current is zero. In this example, there is an extension of the duration of the positive half cycle in the deep brain region, and an increase in intensity. Obviously, the same principles may be applied with more than three coils, and/or with several or all of the coils operated more than once. In different applications, more than one pulse may be induced in part or all of the coils. This way, the time duration at which the deep brain region experiences a significant induced field may be extended. Thus, the stimulator power output required to activate neuronal structures in this deep brain region may be lowered, and the ability to activate the deep brain region without activating cortical regions – or with minimally activating cortical regions – may be improved.

The efficiency and focality of stimulation of deep brain regions using the time summation principle with a multichannel TMS system depend on the penetration depth of the electric field induced by the TMS coils of the various channels. Where we have better penetration depth, it is easier to obtain neuronal

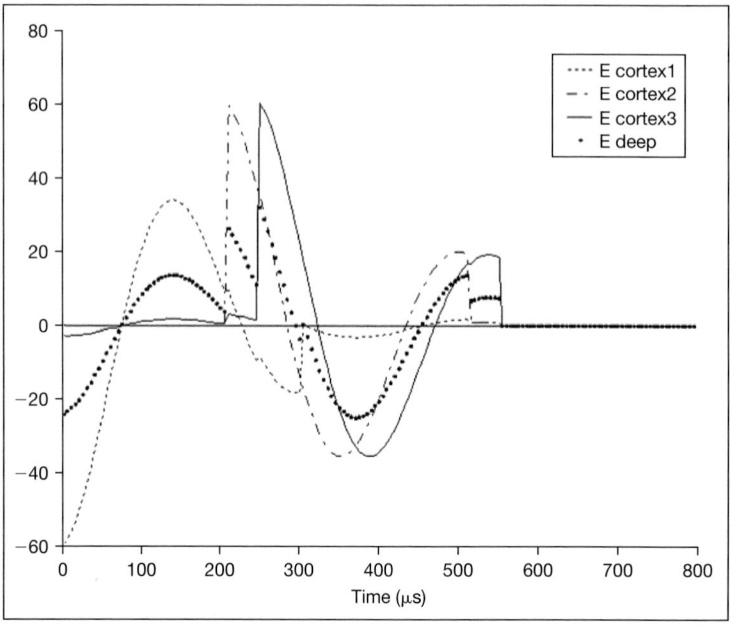

Fig. 13. An example of time summation where the current polarity in the second and third pulses is opposite to the polarity in the first pulses, and there is an extension of the duration of the positive half cycle in the deep brain region, and an increase in the intensity. Shown are the electric field pulses induced in cortical regions close to each coil (dashed, dot-dashed and continuous curves) and in a deep brain region (dotted curve).

stimulation in the desired deep brain region without activating superficial regions. The H-coils are optimized to achieve both maximal absolute field strength at depth, and a high percentage of field relative to the cortex. Hence the usage of coils designed according to the construction principles of the H-coils, as the stimulating coils of the various channels, is predicted to be advantageous in terms of efficiency, focality, flexibility, and energy and power consumption.

References

1 Barker AT, Jalinous R, Freeston IL: Non-invasive magnetic stimulation of the human motor cortex. Lancet 1985;i:1106–1107.
2 Ziemann U: TMS induced plasticity in human cortex. Rev Neurosci 2004;15:253–266.
3 Kirkcaldie MT, Pridmore SA, Pascual-Leone A: Transcranial magnetic stimulation as therapy for depression and other disorders. Aust NZ J Psychiatry 1997;31:264–272.

4 Wassermann EM, Lisanby SH: Therapeutic application of repetitive transcranial magnetic stimulation: a review. Clin Neurophysiol 2001;112:1367–1377.
5 Lin KL, Pascual-Leone A: Transcranial magnetic stimulation and its applications in children. Chang Gung Med J 2002;25:424–436.
6 Fregni F, Pascual-Leone A: Transcranial magnetic stimulation for the treatment of depression in neurologic disorders. Curr Psychiatry Rep 2005;7:381–390.
7 Maccabee PJ, Eberle L, Amassian VE, Cracco RQ, Rudell A, Jayachandra M: Spatial distribution of the electric field induced in volume by round and figure '8' magnetic coils: relevance to activation of sensory nerve fibers. Electroencephalogr Clin Neurophysiol 1990;76:131–141.
8 Tofts PS: The distribution of induced currents in magnetic stimulation of the brain. Phys Med Biol 1990;35:1119–1128.
9 Tofts PS, Branston NM: The measurement of electric field, and the influence of surface charge, in magnetic stimulation. Electroencephalogr Clin Neurophysiol 1991;81:238–239.
10 Eaton H: Electric field induced in a spherical volume conductor from arbitrary coils: application to magnetic stimulation and MEG. Med Biol Eng Comput 1992;30:433–440.
11 Stokic DS, McKay WB, Scott L, Sherwood AM, Dimitrijevic MR: Intracortical inhibition of lower limb motor-evoked potentials after paired transcranial magnetic stimulation. Exp Brain Res 1997;117:437–443.
12 Terao Y, Ugawa Y, Sakai K, Uesaka Y, Kanazawa I: Transcranial magnetic stimulation of the leg area of the motor cortex in humans. Acta Neurol Scand 1994;89:378–383.
13 Terao Y, Ugawa Y, Hanajima R, Machii K, Furubayashi T, Mochizuki H, Enomoto H, Shiio Y, Uesugi H, Iwata NK, Kanazawa I: Predominant activation of I1-waves from the leg motor area by transcranial magnetic stimulation. Brain Res 2000;859:137–146.
14 Fuster JM: The Prefrontal Cortex, ed 3. Philadelphia, Lippincott-Raven, 1997.
15 Brasil-Neto JP, Cohen LG, Panizza M, Nilsson J, Roth BJ, Hallett M: Optimal focal transcranial magnetic activation of the human motor cortex: effects of coil orientation, shape of the induced current pulse, and stimulus intensity. J Clin Neurophysiol 1992;9:132–136.
16 Rothwell JC, Thompson PD, Day BL, Boyd S, Marsden CD: Stimulation of the human motor cortex through the scalp. Exp Physiol 1991;76:159–200.
17 Terao Y, Ugawa Y: Basic mechanisms of TMS. J Clin Neurophysiol 2002;19:322–343.
18 Maccabee PJ, Amassian VE, Eberle VE, Cracco RQ: Magnetic coil stimulation of straight and bent amphibian and mammalian peripheral nerve in vitro: locus of excitation. J Physiol 1993;460: 201–219.
19 Nahas Z, Lomarev M, Roberts DR, Shastri A, Lorberbaum JP, Teneback C, McConnell K, Vincent DJ, Li X, George MS, Bohning DE: Unilateral left prefrontal transcranial magnetic stimulation (TMS) produces intensity-dependent bilateral effects as measured by interleaved BOLD fMRI. Biol Psychiatry 2001;50:712–720.
20 Padberg F, Zwanzger P, Keck ME, Kathmann N, Mikhaiel P, Ella R, Rupprecht P, Thoma H, Hampel H, Toschi N, Möller HJ: Repetitive transcranial magnetic stimulation (rTMS) in major depression: relation between efficacy and stimulation intensity. Neuropsychopharmacology 2002;27:638–645.
21 Kähkonen S, Komssi S, Wilenius J, Ilmoniemi RJ: Prefrontal transcranial stimulation produces intensity-dependent EEG responses in humans. Neuroimage 2005;24:955–960.
22 Amassian VE, Eberle L, Maccabee PJ, Cracco RQ: Modeling magnetic coil excitation of human cerebral cortex with a peripheral nerve immersed in a brain-shaped volume conductor: the significance of fiber bending in excitation. Electroencephalogr Clin Neurophysiol 1992;85:291–301.
23 Ilmoniemi RJ, Ruhonen J, Karhu J: Transcranial magnetic stimulation – A new tool for functional imaging of the brain. Crit Rev Biomed Eng 1999;27:241–284.
24 Kammer T, Beck S, Thielscher A, Laubis-Herrmann U, Topka H: Motor thresholds in humans. A transcranial magnetic stimulation study comparing different pulse waveforms, current directions and stimulator types. Clin Neurophysiol 2001;112:250–258.
25 Stewart LM, Walsh V, Rothwell JC: Motor and phosphene thresholds: a transcranial magnetic stimulation correlation study. Neuropsychologia 2001;39:415–419.
26 Thielscher A, Kammer T: Linking physics with physiology in TMS: a spherical field model to determine the cortical stimulation site in TMS. Neuroimage 2002;17:1117–1130.

27 Heller L, van Hulsteyn DB: Brain stimulation using electromagnetic sources: theoretical aspects. Biophys J 1992;63:129–138.

28 Durand D, Ferguson AS, Dalbasti T: Induced electric fields by magnetic stimulation in non-homogeneous conducting media. IEEE Eng Med Biol Soc 11th Annu Int Conf, Seattle, 1989, vol 6, pp 1252–1253.

29 Roth BJ, Basser PJ: A model of the stimulation of a nerve fiber by electromagnetic radiation. IEEE Trans Biomed Eng 1990;37:588–597.

30 Basser PJ, Roth BJ: Stimulation of a myelinated nerve axon by electromagnetic induction. Med Biol Eng Comput 1991;29:261–268.

31 Mills KR, Boniface SJ, Schubert M: Magnetic brain stimulation with a double coil: the importance of coil orientation. Electroencephalogr Clin Neurophysiol 1992;85:17–21.

32 Pascual-Leone A, Cohen LG, Brasil-Neto JP, Hallett M: Non-invasive differentiation of motor cortical representation of hand muscles by mapping of optimal current directions. Electroencephalogr Clin Neurophysiol 1994;93:42–48.

33 Niehaus L, Meyer BU, Weyh T: Influence of pulse configuration and direction of coil current on excitatory effects of magnetic motor cortex and nerve stimulation. Clin Neurophysiol 2000;111:75–80.

34 Roth Y, Zangen A, Hallett M: A coil design for transcranial magnetic stimulation of deep brain regions. J Clin Neurophysiol 2002;19:361–370.

35 Zangen A, Roth Y, Voller B, Hallett M: Transcranial magnetic stimulation of deep brain regions: evidence for efficacy of the H-coil. Clin Neurophysiol 2005;116:775–779.

36 Breiter HC, Rosen BR: Functional magnetic resonance imaging of brain reward circuitry in the human. Ann NY Acad Sci 1999;877:523–547.

37 Jentsch JD, Taylor JR: Impulsivity resulting from frontostriatal dysfunction in drug abuse: implications for the control of behavior by reward-related behaviors. Psychopharmacology 1999;146: 373–390.

38 Kalivas PW, Nakamura M: Neural systems for behavioral activation and reward. Curr Opin Neurobiol 1999;9:223–227.

39 Tremblay L, Schultz W: Relative reward preference in primate orbitofrontal cortex. Nature 1999;22:704–708.

40 Parkinson JA, Cardinal RN, Everitt BJ: Limbic cortical-ventral striatal systems underlying appetitive conditioning. Prog Brain Res 2000;126:263–285.

41 Volkow ND, Fowler JS: Addiction, a disease of compulsion and drive: involvement of the orbitofrontal cortex. Cereb Cortex 2000;10:318–325.

42 Kalivas PW, Volkow ND: The neural basis of addiction: a pathology of motivation and choice. Am J Psychiatry 2005;162:1403–1413.

43 Bourland JD, Nyenhuis JA, Noe WA, Schaefer JD, Foster KS, Geddes LA: Motor and sensory strength-duration curves for MRI gradient fields. Proc Int Soc Magn Reson Med 4th Sci Meet Exhibit, New York, 1996, p 1724.

Abraham Zangen, PhD
The Weizmann Institute of Science, Department of Neurobiology
Rehovot, 76100 (Israel)
Tel. +972 8 934 4415, Fax +972 8 934 4131, E-Mail a.zangen@weizmann.ac.il

Author Index

Subject Index